Current Clinical Practice

Series Editor
Neil S. Skolnik, MD

For further volumes:
http://www.springer.com/series/7633

Matthew J. Sorrentino
Editor

Hyperlipidemia in Primary Care

A Practical Guide to Risk Reduction

Foreword by Neil S. Skolnik

Humana Press

Editor
Matthew J. Sorrentino
Department of Medicine
Section of Cardiology
University of Chicago Pritzker School of Medicine
Chicago, IL 60637, USA
msorrent@medicine.bsd.uchicago.edu

ISBN 978-1-60327-501-9 e-ISBN 978-1-60327-502-6
DOI 10.1007/978-1-60327-502-6
Springer New York Dordrecht Heidelberg London

Library of Congress Control Number: 2011932354

Printed on acid-free paper

Humana Press is part of Springer Science+Business Media (www.springer.com)

Foreword

Cardiac disease is the number one cause of mortality in the USA. It is also the number one cause of preventable deaths, with the largest opportunity for improvement in health to be had through the careful control of cardiac risk factors. These risk factors are generally amenable to improvement both through lifestyle interventions and through pharmacologic intervention. Both approaches are important, and the challenge for the primary care physician is to decide which patient warrants which form of therapy at what time, and once a given therapy is decided upon, how to help patients comply with recommendations.

In developing an accessible, readable book, *Hyperlipidemia in Primary Care: A Practical Guide to Risk Reduction,* Dr. Sorrentino helps us in our job as primary care physicians in tackling hyperlipidemia, a major cardiac risk factor which primary care physicians address many times every day in the office. In fact, based on the National Ambulatory Medical Care Survey and the National Hospital Ambulatory Medical Care Survey, there were over 100 million visits for hyperlipidemia to primary care clinicians in 2008 [1].

Appropriate treatment of high cholesterol should be viewed as one of the most important medical achievements of the last 40 years. According to data from the CDC, in 1960–1962, 33% of the population in the USA had high total cholesterol values (defined as total cholesterol over 240 mg/dl); by 2003–2006 only 16% of the population had high total cholesterol [2]. This improvement in cholesterol levels, which has contributed to the decrease in age-adjusted rates of coronary heart disease in the USA, has occurred in the context of an obesity epidemic where the number of individuals in the USA who are obese has more than doubled over the last 25 years.

Our need for knowledge to guide our decisions in cardiac risk factor management and hyperlipidemia is large and important. We owe Dr. Sorrentino thanks for the development and publication of this accessible book that should provide a ready source of knowledge and help all of us who care for patients with elevated cardiac risk utilize appropriate risk-based decisions regarding the treatment of elevated cholesterol levels to get the right treatment to the right person at the right time.

Abington, PA, USA Neil S. Skolnik, MD

1. Visits to Primary Care Delivery Sites: United States, 2008. http://www.cdc.gov/nchs/data/databriefs/db47.htm. Accessed 27 October 2010.
2. Health, United States, 2009. http://www.cdc.gov/nchs/data/hus/hus09.pdf. Accessed 27 October 2010.

Preface

Cardiovascular disease is the number one cause of death for men and women in this country, surpassing the deaths due to all cancers combined. Better awareness of heart disease risk factors and improved treatment modalities has produced great progress in reducing the number of deaths due to myocardial infarction and stroke over the past few decades. Approximately, half of the decline in US deaths from coronary artery disease can be attributable to reductions in major cardiovascular disease (CVD) risk factors.

Unfortunately, about half of all first coronary events occur in individuals who have no cardiac symptoms and no previously diagnosed heart disease. The primary care physician, therefore, has an important role in identifying at-risk individuals and beginning preventive modalities.

The first step in reducing cardiovascular risk is to determine an individual's CVD risk category. Preventive treatment algorithms are based on the patient's category of risk. The first goal of this book is to review methods of assessing risk in our patients, understanding that there are limitations in how well we will be able to categorize a patient. The Framingham risk algorithm is commonly used to assess CVD risk. Despite some concerns about limitations of this algorithm, the Framingham risk score has proven to be remarkably predictive of future CVD risk. There are a number of approaches that can go beyond the Framingham risk score as a prediction tool including assessment of family history, the presence of metabolic syndrome, the measurement of inflammatory factors, and the use of noninvasive imaging to detect subclinical atherosclerosis. Subsequent chapters in this book look critically at these approaches and help you to determine how to use them in clinical practice.

The second goal of this book is to review the evolving world of lipidology and how to apply many of the newer lipid tests to our patients in daily practice. When assessing any new test, two very simple questions need to be asked about the test as it applies to practice. The first question to ask is will the test change any treatment recommendation for my patient. Second, will this treatment change lead to an improvement in the outcome of my patient. If we keep these simple questions in mind, we can devise a practical approach to the myriad of new tests that are now offered to further subdivide lipid particles. This book attempts to put these tests into proper perspective and offers a rational approach to using them in practice.

Finally, treatment decisions will need to be made for individuals who are at increased CVD risk. As treatment has expanded to more risk groups, a number of different guidelines have been published with recommended lipid goals. This is an evolving area of research and newer guidelines are expected that will likely expand the pool of high-risk patients. A number of these patient risk groups, such as patients with chronic kidney disease and HIV disease, are highlighted in this book.

Our goal in organizing and writing this book is to offer a reasonable approach to risk assessment and treatment of individuals at increased cardiovascular risk. Evidence-based medicine is used whenever data are available. At times, however, a clinical trial may not give us the full confidence that evidence applies to an individual patient in our office. We must then extrapolate what we know about the development of atherosclerotic disease and the lipid hypothesis to determine the best treatment. The goal of this book is to give the background needed to make scientifically based decisions to ultimately help our patients reduce the impact of cardiovascular disease.

I would like to thank all the contributors who took the time and effort to make this book a reality. The care put into the chapters by the authors has made this a better book. We hope that this book will prove useful in your daily crusade to reduce the impact of heart disease.

Chicago, IL, USA Matthew J. Sorrentino, MD

Contents

Contributors

Bashar Almadani, MD, MPH Division of Cardiology, Feinberg School of Medicine, Northwestern Memorial Hospital, Chicago, IL 60611, USA

Sonal Chandra, MD Department of Medicine, Section of Cardiology, University of Chicago Pritzker School of Medicine, Chicago, IL 60637, USA

Michael H. Davidson, MD Department of Medicine, Section of Cardiology, University of Chicago Pritzker School of Medicine, Chicago, IL 60637, USA

Ewa Dembowski, MD Central DuPage Hospital, Winfield, IL, USA

Rajesh Gupta, MD Division of Cardiology, Feinberg School of Medicine, Northwestern Memorial Hospital, Chicago, IL 60611, USA

Tochi Okwuosa, MD Division of Cardiology, Wayne State University School of Medicine, Detroit, MI 48201, USA

Tamar S. Polonsky, MD Department of Medicine, Section of Cardiology, University of Chicago, Chicago, IL 60637, USA

Robert S. Rosenson, MD, FACP, FACC, FAHA Mount Sinai School of Medicine, New York, NY 10029-6324, USA

Matthew J. Sorrentino, MD Department of Medicine, Section of Cardiology, University of Chicago Pritzker School of Medicine, Chicago, IL 60637, USA

Neil Stone, MD, MACP, FACC, FAHA Division of Cardiology, Feinberg School of Medicine, Northwestern Memorial Hospital, Chicago, IL 60611, USA

R. Parker Ward, MD Department of Medicine, Section of Cardiology, University of Chicago Pritzker School of Medicine, Chicago, IL 60637, USA

Chapter 1
Cardiovascular Risk Assessment

Matthew J. Sorrentino

Keywords Framingham risk score • Reynolds risk score • High-sensitivity C-reactive protein • Family history

Cardiovascular disease remains the number one cause of death for men and women in this country. Despite this fact, great progress has been made over the past few decades in reducing the number of deaths due to myocardial infarction and stroke. Data from the National Center for Health Statistics from 1970 through 2002 have shown a decline in age-adjusted death rates with the largest percentage decreases in death rates from strokes (63%) and heart disease (52%) [1]. Approximately half of the decline in US deaths from coronary artery disease can be attributable to reductions in major cardiovascular disease (CVD) risk factors including reductions in total cholesterol (24%), systolic blood pressure (20%), smoking (12%), and physical inactivity (5%) [2]. Unfortunately, these reductions were partially offset by the increase in obesity and diabetes which accounted for an increased number of deaths (8% and 10%, respectively) due to heart disease.

Approximately half of first coronary events occur in patients who have no cardiac symptoms and no previously diagnosed heart disease. The primary prevention of cardiac disease, therefore, needs to identify at risk individuals. The first step prior to initiating risk reduction therapy is to determine an individual's CVD risk category. Treatment algorithms are based on what category of risk a patient is placed. In general, risk is assessed by counting the number of cardiovascular risk factors an individual may have. Risk is highly dependent on age since the prevalence of heart

M.J. Sorrentino (✉)
Department of Medicine, Section of Cardiology,
University of Chicago Pritzker School of Medicine, Chicago, IL 60637, USA
e-mail: msorrent@medicine.bsd.uchicago.edu

M.J. Sorrentino (ed.), *Hyperlipidemia in Primary Care: A Practical Guide to Risk Reduction*, Current Clinical Practice, DOI 10.1007/978-1-60327-502-6_1,

disease increases with age. Factors that have been shown to be independently associated with heart disease by logistic regression analysis of large epidemiological studies carry the largest weight in determining future risk.

Framingham Risk Calculator

Framingham, Massachusetts is a town near Boston that was chosen by the National Institutes of Health in the 1940s as a study site for the assessment of cardiovascular disease. The initial cohort consisted of over 5,000 men and women aged 30–62 years free of coronary heart disease at baseline. The population was nearly all Caucasian. Participants were seen every other year for an extensive history, physical examination, and laboratory evaluation. The Framingham Offspring Study evaluated the children and their spouses of the original cohort in a similar study beginning in 1970. These data were used to develop a coronary prediction model using pooled information from the original and offspring cohorts followed for 12 years establishing independent and biologically important CVD risk factors [3]. The National Cholesterol Education Program (NCEP) adapted the Framingham scoring system to calculate 10-year risk for persons with multiple risk factors [4]. Risk calculators are available at http://www.nhlbi.nih.gov/guidelines/cholesterol (see Tables 1.1 and 1.2 for risk calculators for coronary heart disease risk for men and women).

Table 1.1 Estimate of 10-year risk for men

Framingham point scores by age group

Age	Points
20–34	–9
35–39	–4
40–44	0
45–49	3
50–54	6
55–59	8
60–64	10
65–69	11
70–74	12
75–79	13

Framingham point scores by age group and total cholesterol

Total cholesterol	Age 20–39	Age 40–49	Age 50–59	Age 60–69	Age 70–79
<160	0	0	0	0	0
160–199	4	3	2	1	0
200–239	7	5	3	1	0
240–279	9	6	4	2	1
280+	11	8	5	3	1

(continued)

Table 1.1 (continued)

Framingham point scores by age and smoking status

	Age 20–39	Age 40–49	Age 50–59	Age 60–69	Age 70–79
Nonsmoker	0	0	0	0	0
Smoker	8	5	3	1	1

Framingham point scores by HDL level

HDL	Points
60+	−1
50–59	0
40–49	1
<40	2

Framingham point scores by systolic blood pressure and treatment status

Systolic BP	If untreated	If treated
<120	0	0
120–129	0	1
130–139	1	2
140–159	1	2
160+	2	3

10-Year risk by total Framingham point scores

Point total	10-Year risk (%)
<0	<1
0	1
1	1
2	1
3	1
4	1
5	2
6	2
7	3
8	4
9	5
10	6
11	8
12	10
13	12
14	16
15	20
16	25
17 or more	≥30

Table 1.2 Estimates of 10-year risk for women

Framingham point scores by age group

Age	Points
20–34	−7
35–39	−3
40–44	0
45–49	3
50–54	6
55–59	8
60–64	10
65–69	12
70–74	14
75–79	16

Framingham point scores by age group and total cholesterol

Total cholesterol	Age 20–39	Age 40–49	Age 50–59	Age 60–69	Age 70–79
<160	0	0	0	0	0
160–199	4	3	2	1	1
200–239	8	6	4	2	1
240–279	11	8	5	3	2
280+	13	10	7	4	2

Framingham point scores by age and smoking status

	Age 20–39	Age 40–49	Age 50–59	Age 60–69	Age 70–79
Nonsmoker	0	0	0	0	0
Smoker	9	7	4	2	1

Framingham point scores by HDL level

HDL	Points
60+	−1
50–59	0
40–49	1
<40	2

Framingham point scores by systolic blood pressure and treatment status

Systolic BP	If untreated	If treated
<120	0	0
120–129	1	3
130–139	2	4
140–159	3	5
160+	4	6

(continued)

Table 1.2 (continued)

10-Year risk by total Framingham point scores	
Point total	10-Year risk (%)
<9	<1
9	1
10	1
11	1
12	1
13	2
14	2
15	3
16	4
17	5
18	6
19	8
20	11
21	14
22	17
23	22
24	27
25 or more	≥30

Table 1.3 Traditional CVD risk factors

1. Advancing age
2. Elevated total and LDL cholesterol
3. Low HDL cholesterol
4. Elevated blood pressure
5. Cigarette smoking
6. Diabetes mellitus

A patient's risk status is determined by evaluating for the presence of clinical atherosclerotic disease and for major cardiovascular risk factors. Major independent risk factors as determined by the Framingham Heart Study include advancing age, elevated total and low-density lipoprotein (LDL) cholesterol, low high-density lipoprotein (HDL) cholesterol, elevated blood pressure, cigarette smoking, and diabetes mellitus (Table 1.3). Individuals can be classified into three risk categories for a cardiac event:

- Low risk (<10% 10-year risk of a coronary event)
- Moderate risk (10–20% 10-year risk)
- High risk (>20% 10-year risk)

When only 0–1 risk factors are present, calculating a Framingham risk score is usually not necessary and patients are generally considered low risk. The high-risk category includes patients with established coronary heart disease (CHD) as well as non-CHD patients who carry the same risk for major coronary events as CHD patients. This includes patients with diabetes mellitus and patients with other clinical forms of atherosclerosis (referred to as CHD-risk equivalent disease) such as symptomatic carotid artery disease, an abdominal aortic aneurysm, or peripheral arterial disease. Moderate-risk patients have a 10–20% 10-year CHD risk. Patients who do not have clinical CHD or diabetes but have two or more CVD risk factors can be assessed by Framingham scoring. If the score calculates at >20% 10-year risk, they would be considered to be in the high-risk category.

There are a number of limitations that need to be considered when using the Framingham risk score assessment. The Framingham score is derived from measurements that were obtained some years ago and may not reflect the impact of these risk factors at the present time. The Framingham population was mostly Caucasian and the risk factors may not have the same significance for different ethnic groups. Finally, the Framingham score only uses the risk factors that were independent factors after multivariate analysis and therefore may not include factors that may have a significant impact on risk or were not fully measured in the earlier cohorts. Factors such as those associated with the metabolic syndrome, inflammatory factors such as C-reactive protein (CRP), and family history are not considered in the Framingham score.

The Framingham score is highly dependent on age because the prevalence of heart disease increases with age. The Framingham score calculates a short term (10-year) risk that will change as an individual ages. Recently, there has been increasing emphasis placed on determining the absolute lifetime risk of developing CHD. Longer-term risk assessment is particularly relevant for younger individuals who will likely have a low 10-year risk score by the Framingham calculator but may have a long-term exposure to a risk factor that may lead to a high absolute life time risk for developing CHD. Framingham investigators have reported lifetime risk of CHD for total cholesterol levels. For example, at an age of 40 years, the lifetime risk for CHD through age 80 for men with total cholesterol levels <200 mg/dL, 200–239 mg/dL, and 240 mg/dL or greater were 31%, 43%, and 57%, respectively [5].

A family history of cardiac death or premature atherosclerosis is not included in the Framingham risk calculator. The Framingham study, however, has observed that CHD tends to cluster within families. Parental history of CHD death was found to be an independent risk factor for CHD but concerns were raised about the validation of the reported events [6]. Because of the long follow-up of the Framingham data base, it is now possible to have enough validated events to determine if family history is an independent risk factor for CHD. Premature family history was defined as a validated parental event before age 55 in a father or age 65 in a mother [7]. After adjustment for other risk factors, premature CVD in a least one parent was associated with a significant twofold CVD risk for middle-aged men and a 70% increased risk for women. In addition, validated sibling CVD events were found to significantly increase the risk of future CVD events above and beyond both traditional risk factors and parental CVD history [8]. Prospective studies have shown that the Framingham calculated 10-year risk markedly underestimates the observed incidence of CHD events in initially healthy young brothers of patients with documented CHD [9].

The knowledge of an individual's family history may not make a major impact on risk assessment of a high- or low-risk individual. Knowledge of the family history in these categories would not likely change treatment strategies. For patients in the moderate-risk group, however, the additional information provided by a positive family history may change the probability of developing a CVD event enough to consider change in risk reduction therapy. In addition, a positive family history can alert the physician to the possibility of a genetic abnormality that may confer an increased cardiovascular risk.

The Framingham risk calculation may not give an accurate risk assessment of populations different from the largely Caucasian Framingham cohort. The Reduction of Atherothrombosis for Continued Health (REACH) Registry is a large international data base that collected data on risk factors in nearly 68,000 individuals and showed that the classic cardiovascular risk factors are remarkably consistent throughout the world [10]. Some variability among risk factors, however, has been noted. For example, hypertension was found to be a more powerful predictor of CHD events in black than in white patients in the Atherosclerosis Risk in Communities (ARIC) study [11]. Overall, however, the incidence rates of CHD were similar in black and white persons. The Framingham risk calculator was evaluated using data bases in other populations including other groups of whites, blacks, Asian Americans, Hispanics, and Native Americans [12]. The Framingham score was found to function well among whites and blacks. CHD risk was overestimated in Japanese American men, Hispanic men, and Native American women. This overestimation was easily corrected by a process of recalibration.

The Framingham risk score may not be as helpful in determining CHD risk in women as in men in part due to the lower prevalence of heart disease in women below the age of 65 years. It has been estimated that up to 20% of coronary events in women occur in the absence of traditional Framingham risk factors [13]. A study of women under the age of 65 years with a first myocardial infarction and no known previous heart disease found that the Framingham risk score would have classified only 18% of the women into a risk group recommending the initiation of pharmacotherapy [14]. None of the women in this cohort had a calculated risk of >20% and the majority of the women had a 10-year risk that classified them in the low-risk category.

Reynolds Risk Score

The concern about the utility of the Framingham risk score in younger women led investigators to develop new cardiovascular risk algorithms based on a large panel of traditional and novel risk factors. Using the data base from the large Women's Health Study of nearly 25,000 women, the best model used the traditional Framingham risk factors plus family history of heart disease and high-sensitivity C-reactive protein (hs-CRP) [15]. The best model is referred to as the Reynolds risk score (the name is taken from the Donald W. Reynolds Foundation which helped to support the research). Using the Reynolds score, 40–50% of women at moderate Framingham risk were reclassified into the high- or low-risk categories. The variables used in

Table 1.4 Reynolds risk score from reynoldsriskscore.org to calculate 10-year cardiovascular disease risk

Gender	☐ Male ☐ Female
Age	☐ Years (Maximum age must be 80)
Do you currently smoke?	☐ Yes ☐ No
Systolic Blood Pressure (SBP)	☐ mm/Hg
Total Cholesterol	☐ mg/DL (or) ☐ mmol/L
HDL or "Good" Cholesterol	☐ mg/DL (or) ☐ mmol/L
High Sensitivity C-Reactive Protein (hsCRP)	☐ mg/L
Did your Mother or Father have a heart attack before age 60 ?	☐ Yes ☐ No

calculating the Reynolds risk are age, systolic blood pressure, hemoglobin A_{1c} if diabetic, current smoking, total and HDL cholesterol, hs-CRP, and parental history of myocardial infarction before the age of 60 years. The Reynolds risk score has since been validated for men. The Reynolds risk score can be found at www.reynoldsriskscore.org and is reproduced in Table 1.4.

The addition of hs-CRP to risk prediction models has generated controversy regarding its ability to improve risk prediction above and beyond traditional risk factors. An analysis of a cohort from the Framingham study evaluated the prognostic information of adding an elevated hs-CRP to the traditional risk models [16]. No additional predictive value of hs-CRP measurements in estimating the risk of new cardiovascular events was found in this group. The ability to discriminate CVD cases was evaluated by calculation of the C statistic which measures the discrimination of cases vs. noncases. The C statistic for major CHD events using traditional risk factors was 0.80 meaning that for any two individuals we have a 80% chance of correctly predicting the individual who will develop a CHD event vs. the individual who will not. The addition of hs-CRP did not change the C statistic.

This illustrates that the use of traditional risk factor analysis as in the Framingham risk score is fairly robust in CVD risk estimation. Any new test being evaluated for risk determination should be evaluated against an assessment of traditional risk factors. Since the traditional factors yield a risk prediction of about 80%, any new test would have to have a very high predictive value to significantly change our ability to predict risk. To determine the utility of a new test, receiver operator characteristic (ROC) curves, a plot of the true-positive rate vs. the false-positive rate over the entire range of possible cutoff values, and calculation of the C statistic are performed. The area under the ROC curve (C statistic) indicates the probability of being able to discriminate randomly selected affected and unaffected persons based on their scores [17]. The closer the score is to 1.0 (100%), the better the test. An area of 0.5 indicates a worthless test or one that is no better than chance.

Investigators from other study groups have evaluated emerging risk factors to assess their usefulness in CHD prediction models. Nineteen novel risk markers including hs-CRP were studied in the ARIC study [18]. The traditional risk factor model predicted incident CHD well with a C statistic of about 0.8. The CRP level did not add significantly to the area under the curve (AUC) with an increase of only 0.003 and neither did the other risk factors studied. Investigators using the Framingham Offspring Study evaluated ten biomarkers and found only modest improvement in risk prediction when a model of traditional risk factors was compared to a model of risk factors plus all ten of the biomarkers (C statistic 0.76 vs. 0.77) [19]. A similar analysis of a large cohort from Sweden analyzing multiple biomarkers including CRP found that the addition of individual biomarkers did not increase the C statistic appreciably [20].

Why do these emerging risk factors fail to improve our ability to predict CVD risk? A new biomarker has to be compared to multiple proven predictive and causal risk factors such as cholesterol, blood pressure, and diabetes. Comparing the strength of a new individual factor can be statistically difficult and many of these factors may track the causal factors already identified.

This does not mean that new and emerging factors may not be important. It is possible that newer factors may improve our risk prediction based on traditional models. For individuals placed in either the high- or low-risk categories, it is unlikely that newer risk factors will substantially change risk prediction or therapeutic decisions. Newer biomarkers may have some utility in the moderate-risk group especially if studies can show that a substantial number of individuals can be reclassified into a higher or lower risk group. This may then lead to a change in therapy. Studies will need to be done to prove that this change in risk category generated by the new biomarker leading to a change in therapy will translate into a change in outcomes. This same analysis will need to apply to noninvasive imaging for subclincal atherosclerosis with such modalities as coronary artery calcium scoring, carotid intima media thickness, and the ankle brachial index.

How to Perform CVD Risk Assessment

The primary prevention of CVD begins with the assessment of cardiac risk factors. Patients can be classified into low-, moderate-, and high-risk groups. A simplified approach to risk assessment is outlined in Table 1.5. First, determine if the patient is in high risk. Does the patient have clinical coronary heart disease, e.g., history of a previous myocardial infarction or coronary intervention? If so they are high risk.

Table 1.5 How to perform CVD risk assessment

1. Does patient have established atherosclerotic CVD (CHD, carotid, aortic, and peripheral arterial disease) or diabetes mellitus?
   - If *yes*: high risk
   - If *no*: go to question #2
2. What is patient's number of traditional risk factors?
   - If 0–1: low risk
   - If ≥2: go to question #3
3. Calculate the Framingham risk score
   - If <10%: low risk
   - If 10–20%: moderate risk
   - If >20%: high risk

Does the patient have CHD risk equivalent disease? This would include diabetes mellitus, symptomatic carotid artery disease, aortic aneurysm, and peripheral arterial disease. If present, these individuals would be classified as high risk. It is possible that additional categories of patients, such as chronic kidney disease and patients with a history of a cerebrovascular event, will be included in the high-risk category in the future.

If a patient does not have CHD or fit a CHD risk equivalent category, the next step is to count the number of traditional risk factors (Table 1.3). If an individual has 0–1 risk factors, they would be considered low risk and it is usually not necessary to calculate a Framingham risk score. If an individual has two or more traditional risk factors, then it is recommended to calculate the Framingham risk score (Tables 1.1 and 1.2). If the risk calculation is >20%, the patient is high risk, 10–20% moderate risk, and <10% low risk.

If the patient is in the moderate-risk group, there may be a number of treatment options and goals available. In addition, there may be concern that an individual's risk score may not fully predict future risk. This may be important in younger women, individuals with a prominent family history of heart disease, or in individuals in different ethnic groups. In these individuals, it may be appropriate to consider measuring additional novel risk factors or using alternative risk scoring systems such as the Reynolds risk score. We would recommend obtaining further risk assessment only if the results would likely lead to a change in treatment. Since a change in treatment or a reclassification of risk is unlikely to occur in the low- and high-risk categories, further risk assessment testing is not likely to be helpful in these two groups.

References

1. Jemal A, Ward E, Hao Y, Thun M. Trends in the leading causes of death in the United States, 1970–2002. JAMA. 2005;294(10):1255–9.
2. Ford ES, Ajani UA, Croft JB, et al. Explaining the decrease in U.S. deaths from coronary disease, 1980–2000. N Engl J Med. 2007;356(23):2388–98.

3. Wilson PW, D'Agostino RB, Levy D, Belanger AM, Silbershatz H, Kannel WB. Prediction of coronary heart disease using risk factor categories. Circulation. 1998;97(18):1837–47.
4. Expert Panel on Detection, Evaluation, and Treatment of High Blood Cholesterol in Adults. Executive Summary of The Third Report of The National Cholesterol Education Program (NCEP) Expert Panel on Detection, Evaluation, And Treatment of High Blood Cholesterol In Adults (Adult Treatment Panel III). JAMA. 2001;285(19):2486–97.
5. Lloyd-Jones DM, Wilson PW, Larson MG, et al. Lifetime risk of coronary heart disease by cholesterol levels at selected ages. Arch Intern Med. 2003;163(16):1966–72.
6. Myers RH, Kiely DK, Cupples LA, Kannel WB. Parental history is an independent risk factor for coronary artery disease: the Framingham Study. Am Heart J. 1990;120(4):963–9.
7. Lloyd-Jones DM, Nam BH, D'Agostino Sr RB, et al. Parental cardiovascular disease as a risk factor for cardiovascular disease in middle-aged adults: a prospective study of parents and offspring. JAMA. 2004;291(18):2204–11.
8. Murabito JM, Pencina MJ, Nam BH, et al. Sibling cardiovascular disease as a risk factor for cardiovascular disease in middle-aged adults. JAMA. 2005;294(24):3117–23.
9. Vaidya D, Yanek LR, Moy TF, Pearson TA, Becker LC, Becker DM. Incidence of coronary artery disease in siblings of patients with premature coronary artery disease: 10 years of follow up. Am J Cardiol. 2007;100(9):1410–5.
10. Bhatt DL, Steg PG, Ohman EM, et al. International prevalence, recognition, and treatment of cardiovascular risk factors in outpatients with atherothrombosis. JAMA. 2006;295(2):180–9.
11. Jones DW, Chambless LE, Folsom AR, et al. Risk factors for coronary heart disease in African Americans: the atherosclerosis risk in communities study, 1987–1997. Arch Intern Med. 2002;162(22):2565–71.
12. D'Agostino Sr RB, Grundy S, Sullivan LM, Wilson P. Validation of the Framingham coronary heart disease prediction scores: results of a multiple ethnic groups investigation. JAMA. 2001;286(2):180–7.
13. Khot UN, Khot MB, Bajzer CT, et al. Prevalence of conventional risk factors in patients with coronary heart disease. JAMA. 2003;290(7):898–904.
14. Akosah KO, Schaper A, Cogbill C, Schoenfeld P. Preventing myocardial infarction in the young adult in the first place: how do the National Cholesterol Education Panel III guidelines perform? J Am Coll Cardiol. 2003;41(9):1475–9.
15. Ridker PM, Buring JE, Rifai N, Cook NR. Development and validation of improved algorithms for the assessment of global cardiovascular risk in women: the Reynolds Risk Score. JAMA. 2007;297(6):611–9.
16. Wilson PW, Nam BH, Pencina M, D'Agostino Sr RB, Benjamin EJ, O'Donnell CJ. C-reactive protein and risk of cardiovascular disease in men and women from the Framingham Heart Study. Arch Intern Med. 2005;165(21):2473–8.
17. Greenland P, O'Malley PG. When is a new prediction marker useful? A consideration of lipoprotein-associated phospholipase A2 and C-reactive protein for stroke risk. Arch Intern Med. 2005;165(21):2454–6.
18. Folsom AR, Chambless LE, Ballantyne CM, et al. An assessment of incremental coronary risk prediction using C-reactive protein and other novel risk markers: the atherosclerosis risk in communities study. Arch Intern Med. 2006;166(13):1368–73.
19. Wang TJ, Gona P, Larson MG, et al. Multiple biomarkers for the prediction of first major cardiovascular events and death. N Engl J Med. 2006;355(25):2631–9.
20. Melander O, Newton-Cheh C, Almgren P, et al. Novel and conventional biomarkers for prediction of incident cardiovascular events in the community. JAMA. 2009;302(1):49–57.

Chapter 2
The Metabolic Syndrome

Matthew J. Sorrentino

Keywords Waist circumference • Abdominal obesity • Impaired fasting glucose • HDL-cholesterol • Triglycerides

Metabolic syndrome is the designation given to a clustering of interrelated metabolic factors that increase the future risk of the development of diabetes mellitus and cardiovascular disease. Intraabdominal or visceral obesity appears to be the underlying component of the syndrome that leads to the development of an atherogenic dyslipidemia, endothelial dysfunction and hypertension, insulin resistance, a prothrombotic, and a proinflammatory state. The risk attributed to the metabolic syndrome is likely due to the sum of its individual components. As such, the designation of the metabolic syndrome is an easy and convenient way of characterizing individuals who may be at increased risk for developing diabetes and cardiovascular disease.

Definition of the Metabolic Syndrome

The National Cholesterol Educational Program (NCEP) Adult Treatment Panel III (ATP III) recognized the metabolic syndrome as a secondary target of risk-reduction therapy in the guidelines published in 2001 [1]. The ATP III suggested that a diagnosis of the metabolic syndrome can be made when three or more of five designated risk factors are present (Table 2.1). The American Diabetes Association (ADA) subsequently redefined impaired fasting glucose (IFG) as a fasting glucose from 100 to

M.J. Sorrentino (✉)
Department of Medicine, Section of Cardiology,
University of Chicago Pritzker School of Medicine, Chicago, IL 60637, USA
e-mail: msorrent@medicine.bsd.uchicago.edu

M.J. Sorrentino (ed.), *Hyperlipidemia in Primary Care: A Practical Guide to Risk Reduction*, Current Clinical Practice, DOI 10.1007/978-1-60327-502-6_2,

Table 2.1 Clinical factors that define the metabolic syndrome [1]

1. Abdominal obesity (waist circumference)	
a. Men	>102 cm (>40 in.)
b. Women	>88 cm (>35 in.)
2. Triglycerides	≥150 mg/dl
3. High-density lipoprotein cholesterol (HDL)	
a. Men	<40 mg/dl
b. Women	<50 mg/dl
4. Blood pressure	≥130/≥85 mmHg
5. Fasting glucose	≥110 mg/dl[a]

Any three of the five risk factors designate the metabolic syndrome
[a] American Diabetes Association [2] definition of impaired fasting glucose: fasting glucose 100 mg/dl or greater, accepted as criteria for metabolic syndrome

125 mg/dl [2] and an elevated fasting glucose of ≥100 mg/dl is now an accepted criteria for the metabolic syndrome [3].

The International Diabetes Federation (IDF) produced a new set of criteria for a worldwide definition of the metabolic syndrome recognizing that the obesity epidemic is one of the main drivers of the high prevalence of this syndrome [4]. The IDF definition differs from the ATP III definition in that it requires the presence of central obesity for the diagnosis of the metabolic syndrome because it is highly correlated with insulin resistance. The IDF recommended waist circumference measurements of central obesity with gender and ethnic-group specific cut-points. The additional components of the IDF definition are otherwise the same as the ATP III definition.

Components of the Metabolic Syndrome

Abdominal Obesity

In 1998, the National Heart, Lung, and Blood Institute of the National Institutes of Health (NIH) released a clinical guideline on the identification, evaluation, and treatment of overweight and obese adults and proposed a classification of six body mass index (BMI) categories and two waist circumference categories (normal or high) (Table 2.2) [5]. The waist circumference cutoffs were taken from a study of over 2,000 individuals in North Glasgow that corresponded to a BMI of 30 or above at the point in which symptoms of breathlessness, arthritis, and increased health risk occurred [6]. The NCEP adopted these cutoffs for the definition of metabolic syndrome.

Visceral or intraabdominal adiposity is more metabolically active than subcutaneous fat accumulation. In addition, visceral adiposity correlates with markers of

Table 2.2 Body mass index (BMI) and waist circumference categories – disease risk for type II diabetes, hypertension, and cardiovascular disease (adapted from [5])

	BMI (kg/m^2)	Disease risk relative to normal weight and waist circumference Men ≤ 102 cm Women ≤ 88 cm	Men > 102 cm Women > 88 cm
Underweight	<18.5		
Normal	18.5–24.9		Increased
Overweight	25.0–29.9	Increased	High
Obesity, class I	30.0–34.9	High	Very high
Class II	35.0–39.9	Very high	Very high
Class III (extreme obesity)	≥40	Extremely high	Extremely high

dyslipidemia, hypertension, insulin resistance, and inflammation. Waist circumference correlates better than BMI or waist-to-hip ratio (WHR) to the quantity of adipose tissue in the abdominal cavity as measured by CT scanning [7]. In the Nurses Health Study, a higher waist circumference was independently associated with an increased risk of coronary heart disease (CHD) [8]. A waist circumference of 30 cm was associated with more than a twofold higher coronary risk and a waist circumference of 38 cm was associated with a greater than threefold risk. Nearly 15,000 subjects in the Third National Health and Nutrition Examination Survey (NHANES) were evaluated to determine if the NIH waist circumference cutoffs helped to identify individuals at increased health risk [9]. Within the three BMI categories of normal weight, overweight, and class I obese, individuals with high waist circumference values (men > 102 cm, women > 88 cm) were increasingly likely to have hypertension, diabetes, dyslipidemia, and the metabolic syndrome. Thus, it appears that the waist circumference cutoffs chosen for the American population are a reasonable measurement to help determine risk. Non-US populations, however, may be at increased risk at different levels of visceral obesity. The International Diabetes Federation recommends ethnic-group specific waist circumference thresholds because of emerging information on the variable relationship between waist circumference and metabolic abnormalities and has acknowledged that more research is needed to determine the optimal cutoffs [4].

High-Density Lipoprotein Cholesterol

A low high-density lipoprotein cholesterol (HDL-C) is a well-known independent predictor of CHD especially in women. The criteria for the metabolic syndrome uses a lower than average HDL-C as one of the major components of the syndrome. The HDL-C cutoff chosen is a value below the 50th percentile for HDL-C for the American population. Women tend to have higher HDL-C than men so the HDL threshold is higher for women. The National Health and Nutrition Surveys have tracked the trends in lipid levels for the USA over the last four decades. From the 1999–2002 survey, the average HDL-C for men ≥20 years of age in this country was 45.9 mg/dl and the average HDL-C for women was 56.2 mg/dl [10]. From 1988 to the present, there has been a steady decline in total and low-density lipoprotein cholesterol (LDL-C) but substantially no change in the average HDL-C levels. The HDL-C criteria used for the metabolic syndrome are an HDL-C < 40 mg/dl for men and an HDL-C < 50 mg/dl for women.

Triglycerides

The NCEP ATPIII redefined fasting serum triglycerides and classified triglycerides values less than 150 mg/dl as normal (Table 2.3). Elevated serum triglycerides are a common lipid abnormality in the metabolic syndrome. A high triglyceride value is associated with smaller and denser LDL particles that are thought to be more atherogenic. Triglyceride levels and the ratio of triglycerides to HDL have correlated well with the presence of insulin resistance. A triglyceride/HDL ratio of 3.5 or greater predicts insulin resistance as well as the criteria for metabolic syndrome [11].

There is emerging evidence that nonfasting serum triglyceride levels are associated with an increased risk of atherosclerosis. Two recent large cohort studies found that nonfasting triglycerides were a significant risk factor for CHD and death in men and women and were a more robust indicator of risk than fasting levels [12, 13]. These data suggested that a postprandial triglyceride tolerance test can be developed with measurement of triglyceride values 2–4 h after a standard meal. A postprandial cutoff value for triglycerides has not been established although in the Danish study there appeared to be a jump in risk in individuals with a postprandial triglyceride value greater than 5 mmol/L (442.5 mg/dl) [13]. Finally, there is now evidence to suggest that patients with insulin resistance accumulate triglycerides in myocardial cells and that this is associated with diastolic abnormalities and may be an early marker for cardiac dysfunction [14].

Elevated Blood Pressure

The NCEP ATP III definition of metabolic syndrome uses a blood pressure of 130/85 or greater as one of the criteria for the syndrome. Although this cutoff is somewhat arbitrary, there is a clear increased prevalence of cardiovascular events

Table 2.3 Classification of serum triglycerides (from [1])

Normal triglycerides	<150 mg/dl
Borderline high triglycerides	150–199 mg/dl
High triglycerides	200–499 mg/dl
Very high triglycerides	≥500 mg/dl

associated with increasing blood pressure that is continuous and independent of other risk factors. For individuals aged 40–70 years, each incremental increase in 20 mmHg systolic or 10 mmHg diastolic blood pressure doubles cardiovascular risk across the entire blood pressure range beginning at 115/75 mmHg [15].

Hypertension is the most common chronic health condition associated with obesity. Insulin resistance has long been linked to essential hypertension [16] and studies suggest that the presence of hyperinsulinemia predicts the development of hypertension [17]. Visceral adiposity may contribute to the development of hypertension by releasing free fatty acids and inflammatory mediators into the circulation and change levels of adipocytokines that can lead to endothelial dysfunction. Individuals with high triglycerides and a low HDL-C and increased blood pressure are at significantly higher cardiovascular risk than those with normal pressure [18].

Impaired Fasting Glucose

The American Diabetes Association (ADA) has defined IFG as fasting plasma glucose levels of 100–125 mg/dl [2]. Patients with IFG are referred to as having "prediabetes" since they have a high risk of developing diabetes. IFG is also a risk factor for cardiovascular disease. Since this definition of IFG was proposed after the NCEP ATPIII definition of metabolic syndrome was formulated, the cutoff for fasting glucose is different in the two definitions. The current ADA definition is generally accepted as the cutoff for the metabolic syndrome designation as well.

Impaired glucose tolerance (IGT) can also be used to identify individuals with insulin resistance. IGT patients are defined as individuals who have 2-h values in the oral glucose tolerance test of ≥140 mg/dl but less than 200 mg/dl [17]. Many patients with IGT will have normal fasting glucose values and normal glycated hemoglobin levels.

A patient's lipoprotein level may also predict insulin resistance. The triglyceride/HDL ratio has been shown to predict cardiovascular events and is associated with small, dense LDL particles. A triglyceride/HDL ratio of 3.5 or higher can identify insulin resistant individuals with a sensitivity and specificity similar to the metabolic syndrome criteria [11]. Of note, this ratio did not correlate with insulin resistance in an African American population [19]. Patients with a high triglyceride/HDL ratio and normal fasting plasma glucose values may be a group to consider further evaluation with an oral glucose tolerance test.

Prothrombotic State

Patients identified with the metabolic syndrome exhibit a pattern of coagulation factors that are prothrombotic. Fibrinolysis is induced by plasmin which is formed from plasminogen by tissue plasminogen activators and neutralized by plasminogen activator inhibitor-1 (PAI-1). Increased concentrations of insulin and proinsulin in the plasma can increase plasma PAI-1 levels and is associated with decreased fibrinolytic activity in the blood [20]. The metabolic syndrome and insulin resistance has also been associated with increased coagulation factors VII–IX, von Willebrand factor, and blood viscosity [21]. The combination of all these findings may increase the potential for increased cardiovascular events.

Proinflammatory State

Visceral adiposity is highly metabolically active and produces a large number of inflammatory molecules either from the adipocytes or associated macrophages. Tumor necrosis factor-alpha (TNF-α) and Interleukin-6 are two inflammatory molecules that are increased in patients with central obesity and metabolic syndrome. These factors circulate to the liver and stimulate the production of C-reactive protein (CRP). CRP levels are directly associated with the number of metabolic syndrome factors [22]. Inflammation is thought to play a significant role in the progression of coronary atherosclerosis and plaque rupture and may be a marker for individuals at increased CVD risk.

Other Metabolic Abnormalities

The metabolic syndrome is a clustering of multiple factors that together increase the risk of developing diabetes or cardiovascular disease. Because it is not known if there is an underlying factor that ties all of these risk markers together, the syndrome was first labeled as syndrome x, where x is the unknown. It is likely that visceral obesity may be the underlying source of many of the metabolic parameters described in this syndrome. Table 2.4 lists many of the metabolic abnormalities that are thought to cluster in individuals with the metabolic syndrome.

How to Diagnose the Metabolic Syndrome

The metabolic syndrome is diagnosed when a patient has three or more of the components of the metabolic syndrome as defined by the NCEP panel. Of note, a patient would be considered to have a component of the metabolic syndrome even if one of the factors is treated and normalized. The definition of metabolic syndrome includes a fasting glucose of ≥110 mg/dl (or we can use the newer ADA definition of a fasting glucose ≥100 mg/dl). This definition includes patients with a fasting glucose

Table 2.4 Clustering of factors associated with the metabolic syndrome

1. Prothrombotic factors
   a. Coagulation factors VII–IX
   b. von Willebrand factor
   c. Fibrinogen
   d. Plasminogen activator inhibitor-1 (PAI-1)
   e. Increased blood viscosity
2. Inflammatory factors
   a. Hs-CRP
   b. Interleukins
   c. High WBC
   d. Tumor necrosis factor-alpha (TNF-α)
3. Renal factors
   a. Microalbuminuria
   b. Hyperuricemia
4. Adipocytokines
   a. High leptin levels with leptin resistance
   b. Decreased adiponectin levels
5. Lipoproteins
   a. Increased VLDL – Triglycerides
   b. Low HDL-C
   c. Increased small, dense LDL and oxidized LDL
   d. Increased free fatty acids
6. Endothelial dysfunction
   a. Decreased endothelial-dependent relaxation
   b. Increased adhesion molecules
   c. Raised blood pressure
7. Insulin resistance
   a. Hyperinsulinemia
   b. Hyperglycemia

level in the diabetic range and diabetic patients can be designated as having metabolic syndrome in addition to diabetes. Metabolic syndrome can then identify a diabetic patient with additional multiple cardiovascular risk factors and therefore at higher cardiovascular risk.

Plasma lipid levels should be measured after a 9–12 h fast. This will eliminate chylomicrons from the circulation and give a fasting triglyceride value that can be used to calculate an LDL-C level. For some patients, a nonfasting triglyceride value may give additional prognostic information especially if it is greater than 400 mg/dl. Waist circumference is recommended as a measurement of visceral adiposity and correlates with the risk factors of metabolic syndrome better than BMI. Waist circumference can be measured by locating the top of the right iliac crest and placing a tape measure in the horizontal plane around the abdomen making the measurement at end expiration.

How to Use Metabolic Syndrome in Risk Assessment

The standard method for calculating an individual's cardiovascular risk is to count traditional independent risk factors and use an algorithm based on large epidemiological studies such as the Framingham study. This analysis can predict a 10-year cardiovascular risk with an accuracy of approximately 75% [23]. Many individuals with two or more risk factors will fall into the intermediate risk group defined as a yearly cardiovascular risk between 1 and 2%. The presence of metabolic syndrome can modify this risk prediction by adding additional risk factors to the total number of factors. This may have treatment implications when considering treatment goals. As a general rule, the more risk factors that are present, the higher the possibility of a cardiovascular event suggesting a more aggressive risk factor modification treatment approach.

Prevalence of the Metabolic Syndrome

Data from the Third National Health and Nutrition Survey (NHANES) gathered between 1988 and 1994 were used to determine the prevalence of the metabolic syndrome in ambulatory Americans using the ATPIII definition of metabolic syndrome [24]. The prevalence of the metabolic syndrome is about 22% for the US population. For participants aged 60–69 years of age, the prevalence is 43%. Mexican Americans have the highest prevalence of metabolic syndrome at nearly 32%. Men and women have a similar prevalence except among African Americans where women have a 57% higher prevalence than men. Using 2000 census data, it is estimated that about 47 million Americans have the metabolic syndrome. In addition to the high prevalence in Mexican Americans, American Indians have a very high prevalence of metabolic syndrome as well. The Strong Heart Study showed a 35% prevalence of metabolic syndrome in American Indians aged 45–74 years [25].

Worldwide prevalence of metabolic syndrome approaches the prevalence in the USA especially as countries adopt a Western style diet. A study based on 11 prospective European cohorts of men and women aged 30–89 years without diabetes using a World Health Organization (WHO) definition of metabolic syndrome found a 14–15% prevalence of the condition [26]. In developing countries, the prevalence of metabolic syndrome is also approaching Western numbers. A study from eastern China using NCEP criteria and ethnic-group specific waist circumference found a 12.7% prevalence of metabolic syndrome in urban males and a 10.1% prevalence in urban females [27].

The prevalence of the metabolic syndrome will likely continue to increase as the average weight of populations increase. From NHANES data, the age-adjusted prevalence of obesity in this country was 30.5% in 1999–2000 compared with 22.9% in 1988–1994 [28]. Even more alarming is the increasing prevalence of class 3 obesity (BMI≥40). In 2000, 2.2% of adults in this country have class 3 obesity with the highest prevalence among African American women at 6.0% [29]. Epidemiological data have shown a decreased mortality from CHD with approximately half of this decline attributable to reductions in major risk factors [30]. These reductions have been partially offset by increases in BMI and the increased prevalence of diabetes which is estimated to account for an increased number of deaths (8% and 10%, respectively).

The consumption of a Western style diet may have a significant role in the obesity epidemic and promote the incidence of metabolic syndrome. Dietary intake was assessed in the Atherosclerosis Risk in Communities (ARIC) study comparing a Western and prudent diet [31]. A Western diet pattern was associated with incident metabolic syndrome with meat, fried foods, and diet soda adversely associated with metabolic syndrome and dairy consumption found to be beneficial. The Framingham Heart Study has also found that the intake of at least one regular or diet soft drink per day is associated with a >50% higher incidence of the metabolic syndrome [32]. Although it seems counterintuitive that diet drinks may lead to weight gain, individuals who consume these products may have a greater preference for the intake of sweets and fats in the diet and are more likely to have a sedentary lifestyle. To address the emerging obesity epidemic in this country, the American Heart Association has recommended reductions in added sugar intake to no more than 100–150 kcal/day for most Americans [33].

Metabolic Syndrome and Diabetes

The metabolic syndrome can be thought of as a prediabetic state and can predict the incidence of type 2 diabetes mellitus. A study in Finnish middle-aged men indicated that individuals with the metabolic syndrome by either the WHO or NCEP definition were seven times more likely to develop diabetes during a 4-year follow-up than age-matched controls without metabolic syndrome [34]. Middle-aged individuals of different ethnicities in the Insulin Resistance Atherosclerosis Study with metabolic syndrome had a 3.4–5.4 increased risk of developing diabetes [35]. From the Framingham Offspring cohort, the odds of developing diabetes were 6.92-fold over an 8-year period similar for men and women [36]. Metabolic syndrome accounted for about 50% of the new cases of type 2 diabetes. From this study group, a simple clinical model was developed that was able to identify subjects with an elevated risk for diabetes [37]. The variables that predict type 2 diabetes include a parental history of diabetes, obesity, hypertension, low HDL-C, elevated triglycerides, and IFG. In other words, the metabolic syndrome parameters effectively predict the development of diabetes mellitus.

Metabolic syndrome can be thought of as an earlier stage in the development of insulin resistance and diabetes mellitus in many individuals. Classification of individuals with this syndrome may allow identification of those destined to become diabetic at a time 10–15 years earlier than frank hyperglycemia. Since diabetes is a known CHD risk equivalent, the presence of metabolic syndrome may give time to

Table 2.5 Diagnosis of diabetes mellitus (from [2])

Diabetes mellitus can be diagnosed when any of the following are present:
1. Symptoms of diabetes with a casual plasma glucose ≥ 200 mg/dl (symptoms include polyuria, polydipsia, and unexplained weight loss)
2. Fasting plasma glucose ≥ 126 mg/dl
3. 2-h Postload glucose ≥ 200 mg/dl during a 75 g oral glucose tolerance test

The results from each method are confirmed on a different day unless definite symptoms of hyperglycemia are present

begin risk-reduction therapy that may both prevent the development of diabetes and reduce cardiovascular risk.

The diagnosis of diabetes is delayed or unrecognized in many patients. The designation of metabolic syndrome may allow earlier diagnosis and treatment of diabetes. An oral glucose tolerance test can be considered in patients with metabolic syndrome who do not reach criteria for diabetes with a fasting sugar. The criteria for the diagnosis of diabetes as outlined by the American Diabetes Associations are presented in Table 2.5.

Metabolic Syndrome and Cardiovascular Risk

Studies have consistently shown that the metabolic syndrome is associated with an increased incidence of cardiovascular disease including an increased risk for myocardial infarction and stroke as well as increased cardiovascular and all-cause death. The NCEP ATPIII metabolic syndrome criteria was applied to the NHANES III data base of over 10,000 subjects and showed that the metabolic syndrome was significantly related in a multivariate analysis to myocardial infarction [odds ratio (OR) 2.01] and stroke (OR 2.16) [38]. This association was similar for men and women. Non-Hispanic black subjects had significantly higher odds ratios compared with non-Hispanic white subjects particularly for stroke.

Other epidemiological surveys have shown similar results. In the Framingham Offspring Study of over 3,000 middle-aged adults, the metabolic syndrome age-adjusted relative risk of cardiovascular disease was 2.88 [36]. European surveys, usually using the WHO definition of metabolic syndrome, concur with these risk assessments. In the Kuopio Ischaemic Heart Disease Risk Factor Study, middle-aged men with metabolic syndrome by NCEP criteria were 2.9 times and by WHO criteria 4.2 times more likely to die of CHD after adjustment for conventional cardiovascular risk factors than those who did not fit criteria for the syndrome [39]. A report based on 11 prospective European cohort studies using a modified WHO definition of the metabolic syndrome found an increased cardiovascular mortality of 2.26 in men and 2.78 in women after adjustment for age, blood cholesterol levels, and smoking [26].

The different definitions of the metabolic syndrome and different populations (lower- and higher-risk groups) have led to some variability in the relative risk of having the metabolic syndrome. A large meta-analysis of 37 studies with 43 cohorts and over 170,000 individuals showed that the metabolic syndrome had a relative risk of cardiovascular events and death of 1.78 [40]. This association was stronger in women (RR 2.63 vs. 1.98, $p=0.09$) and if the analysis used the WHO definition of metabolic syndrome. The association remained significant after adjusting for traditional risk factors (RR 1.54, 95% CI 1.32–1.79).

How does the metabolic syndrome compare with traditional risk factor analysis in predicting cardiovascular events? A prospective study of over 5,000 middle-aged men in Britain with no history of cardiovascular disease or diabetes was observed for 20 years [41]. Using the NCEP definition of metabolic syndrome, men fitting the criteria of the syndrome at baseline had a significantly higher relative risk of developing CHD (RR 1.64), stroke (RR 1.62), and diabetes (RR 3.57). The probability of having a CHD event over 20 years increased from 7.1% for individuals with no metabolic syndrome abnormalities to 20.2% in those with three of the criteria to 24.5% in those with four or five of the abnormalities. The Framingham risk score, however, was a better predictor of CHD than the number of metabolic abnormalities. In a multivariate model, metabolic syndrome provided no additional predictive value for CHD when the Framingham risk score was included in the model but it did remain strongly associated with diabetes.

This type of analysis suggests that the designation of the metabolic syndrome does not appear to confer greater CHD risk than the sum of its individual parts. A number of additional studies have also concluded that once the individual components of the metabolic syndrome are accounted for, the predictive power of the syndrome as a discrete entity disappears [42]. In other words, no additional information regarding risk is added when considering the combination of the components of the metabolic syndrome than considering the risk factors individually in a typical Framingham-type model. This has led some groups, such as the American Diabetes Association, to question the utility of using the metabolic syndrome as a risk predictor.

Designating a patient with the metabolic syndrome, however, is a convenient way of recognizing a patient who has a clustering of cardiometabolic risk factors and is at an increased risk of developing diabetes. This designation can alert both physicians and patients that an individual is at an intermediate risk level and can focus therapy goals to reduce risk. In addition, the designation of metabolic syndrome highlights factors that are not included in the traditional Framingham risk assessment tool such as visceral obesity, elevated triglycerides, and IFG. By identifying these factors, a focused treatment plan can be formulated that addresses these components. Although there are no studies that have determined if patient motivation is improved if they are diagnosed with the metabolic syndrome, increased awareness of multiple risk factors should at least alert a physician to considering a more aggressive multifactorial treatment approach for risk reduction.

The metabolic syndrome may also predict a population that is at increased risk for other diseases as well. A prospective study in Japan of over 28,000 participants showed that the metabolic syndrome was associated with an increased risk of atrial fibrillation [43]. Microalbuminuria has been associated with the metabolic syndrome suggesting that clinically important renal dysfunction may be an important risk for patients with the syndrome especially those individuals with increased blood pressure and IFG [44]. Elderly patients with the metabolic syndrome were more likely to have cognitive impairment than those without [45]. This emerging data support the contention that the metabolic syndrome can easily identify a higher-risk cohort that should be considered for more aggressive risk management.

Management of the Metabolic Syndrome

Lifestyle Modification

The NCEP ATPIII recognized the metabolic syndrome as a secondary target for risk reduction after addressing LDL-C. The NCEP recommended that first line therapy for all of the risk factors associated with the metabolic syndrome is weight reduction and increased exercise [1]. The NCEP pointed out that weight reduction and exercise can help further lower the LDL-C as well as improve all the lipid and nonlipid components of the syndrome. The American Heart Association/National Heart, Lung, and Blood Institute published a scientific statement that recommended a general outline of the therapeutic targets and goals of a lifestyle treatment program for the long-term prevention of both CVD and diabetes for patients with the metabolic syndrome [3]. These recommendations are summarized in Table 2.6.

Abdominal obesity is a major underlying cause of many of the metabolic abnormalities of the metabolic syndrome so it should be a primary target of therapy. Individuals with the metabolic syndrome should try to reduce body weight by 7–10% in the first year of treatment. Ideally, strategies should be adopted to ultimately achieve a body weight in the normal BMI category. Calorie reduction is an essential component of any weight loss plan if any significant progress is to be achieved. Restricting high caloric products (fatty foods) and avoiding highly processed foods may help further reduce weight. Whole foods should be consumed in preference to refined products. Foods that have high fructose content may contribute to a prediabetic state by contributing to tissue insulin insensitivity [46]. Patients should be counseled to reduce or avoid heavily sweetened foods including diet products trying to reduce added-sugar to no more than 100–150 kcal/d.

The carbohydrate content of a diet and their relationship to the metabolic syndrome and diabetes is still not well defined. There is some evidence to suggest that a high intake of simple sugars may increase triglycerides. Low to moderate carbohydrate diets, especially diets that have complex nonstarchy or low glycemic index carbohydrates, may reduce triglycerides in some individuals. A Mediterranean-type diet or a low fat diet can also lower triglycerides.

Table 2.6 Management of the metabolic syndrome: treatment of lifestyle risk factors (adapted from [3])

Therapeutic target/goals of therapy	Therapeutic recommendations
Abdominal obesity:	
Goal – reduce body weight by 7% during first year of therapy Goal – achieve desired weight BMI < 25 kg/m^2	– Encourage weight maintenance/reduction with physical activity, reduced caloric intake, formal behavioral programs – Maintain/achieve waist circumference <40 in. in men, <35 in. in women – Initial reduction 7–10% weight from baseline
Physical inactivity:	
Goal – regular moderate-intensity physical activity, at least 30 min of continuous/intermittent (preferably 60 min) 5 day/week, preferably daily	– Patients with established CVD – assess physical activity risk (history/stress test) – Encourage 30–60 min moderate-intensity aerobic activity daily supplemented by increase in daily lifestyle activities – Encourage resistance training 2 day/week – Medically supervised programs for high-risk patients
Atherogenic diet:	
Goal – reduce saturated fat, trans fat, cholesterol	– Saturated fat <7% total calories; reduce trans fat; dietary cholesterol <200 mg/day; total fat 25–35% of total calories – Most dietary fat should be unsaturated – Simple sugars should be limited

Exercise is an essential component of any lifestyle modification program and can augment weight loss and help maintain weight reduction. Both total body weight and intraabdominal fat is reduced with regular moderate-intensity exercise [47]. Increased duration of exercise achieves a greater reduction in body fat. In addition, exercise has positive effects on all of the components of the metabolic syndrome. Moderate regular exercise can increase HDL-C 4–18% and decrease triglycerides 4–37% [48]. LDL-C tends not to change with exercise unless accompanied by diet change and weight reduction. Exercise, likely through changes in body composition, improves insulin sensitivity and lowers blood pressure. Exercise can improve endothelial function, reduce inflammation, and improved left ventricular diastolic function [49]. Guidelines for exercise training are summarized in Table 2.7.

In addition to the metabolic benefits of exercise, regular physical activity has been associated with a reduced risk for CVD, diabetes, and total mortality. The risk of death from CHD is nearly twofold in sedentary individuals compared with those that are active [50]. The total amount of physical activity and more intense activity shows the strongest reductions in CHD risk in both women and men [51, 52]. Data from the Framingham Heart Study indicate that moderate and high physical activity levels can lead to 1.3 and 3.7 more years in total life expectancy for men, and 1.5 and 3.5 more years for women aged 50 years and older compared with those who maintain a low physical activity level [53].

Table 2.7 General guidelines for exercise training (adapted from [49])

Warm-up and cool-down period (5–10 min each)	Stretching, calisthenics, low-level aerobic exercise (walking/cycling)
Types of exercise	Aerobic exercise – walking, cycling, swimming, rowing Resistance exercise – weight lifting (machines preferred for safety)
Intensity	Aerobic exercise – 55–79% of maximum heart rate (50–60% for patients with low initial level of fitness) Resistance (weight) training – 8–10 exercises at 30–50% of 1-repetition maximum. A minimum of 1 set of 12–15 repetitions; increase workload when 15 repetitions can be done without difficulty
Duration	Aerobic exercise – 30–45 min Resistance training – 20 min for 1 set each for 8–10 exercises
Frequency	Aerobic exercise – 3–4 times a week and more frequently if weight reduction is a goal Resistance exercise – twice a week

A lifestyle modification program that combines exercise and weight loss has been shown to reduce the incidence of diabetes in the Diabetes Prevention Program [54]. Over 3,000 nondiabetic individuals with an elevated fasting and postload glucose were randomized to placebo, metformin, or a lifestyle modification program with the goals of at least a 7% body weight loss and 150 min of exercise per week. After nearly 3 years of follow-up, the lifestyle modification group had a 58% reduction in the incidence of diabetes compared with the placebo group. The lifestyle program was significantly more effective than metformin which achieved only a 31% decrease in the incidence of diabetes compared with placebo. This study shows that diabetes may be prevented or at least delayed in individuals at risk for the disease by an easily performed lifestyle program. The average weight loss in the lifestyle group was 5.6 kg which is an achievable goal for most individuals. The lifestyle goal targets in this study should be the minimal goals that we recommend to all patients with the metabolic syndrome.

Pharmacological and Surgical Treatment of Obesity

Unfortunately, dietary interventions are not successful in reducing weight in many individuals who attempt a weight loss program. A number of prescription and over the counter medications are available that may have efficacy for weight loss. Pharmacological therapy for obesity is deemed appropriate for some individuals with a BMI of 30 or greater or a BMI of 27 or greater in the presence of comorbidities [5].

Appetite suppressants such as phentermine are FDA approved for short-term weight loss. These drugs are adrenergic stimulants enhancing the release of catecholamines. A meta-analysis of short-term studies with phentermine indicated an average weight loss of about 3.5 kg was achieved with this agent [55]. These drugs may significantly increase blood pressure which may be a problem in individuals who have prehypertension or are on hypertensive medications. Dependency may also be a concern with these agents. Since blood pressure is frequently elevated in patients with metabolic syndrome, these medications may not be the best choice for weight loss.

Sibutramine is approved by the FDA for induction and maintenance of weight loss as an adjunct to a comprehensive weight loss program. Sibutramine is a serotonin-norepinephrine reuptake inhibitor and appears to reduce appetite. Patients receiving subutramine alone achieved an average loss of 5 kg but those receiving sibutramine in combination with a lifestyle modification program were able to lose a mean of 12.1 kg of weight in a 1-year trial [56]. Sibutramine may also increase blood pressure and is not recommended for use in patients with cardiovascular disease. In January 2010, the European Medicine Agency's Committee for Medicinal Products for Human Use recommended that sibutramine be removed from the European market because of concern about an increase in cardiovascular events in patients with CVD and diabetes using this drug [57]. The FDA added new contraindications to the label stating that this drug should not be used in patients with a history of cardiovascular disease.

Orlistat is a medication that works in the intestine to reduce the absorption of fat. It is available as a prescription medication and over the counter at a lower dose (Alli, GlaxoSmithKline). A meta-analysis of studies using orlistat for weight loss showed only a modest 2.89 kg weight loss [58]. Orlistat has been shown to reduce the incidence of diabetes in the Xenical in the Prevention of Diabetes in Obese Subjects (XENDOS) study [59]. In this study, over 3,300 obese patients were randomized to a lifestyle program plus orlistat or placebo and followed for 4 years. After 4 years treatment, the incidence of diabetes was 9.0% with placebo and 6.2% with orlistat (37.3% risk reduction, $p=0.0032$). Greater weight loss was achieved in the orlistat group (5.8 kg vs. 3.0 kg with placebo). Gastrointestinal side effects such as fecal urgency may limit its use for some patients.

Future medications may include agents that target the endocannabinoid system which is involved in energy homeostasis. Activation of central cannabinoid receptors stimulates eating and may contribute to obesity [60]. Rimonabant is a selective cannabinoid-1 receptor blocker and has been shown to reduce body weight in obese subjects. Both the Rimonabant in Obesity-Europe study [61] and the Rimonabant in Obesity-North America study [62] showed that rimonabant induces significant weight loss that can be sustained over a 2-year period. In addition, favorable changes in cardiometabolic risk factors such as a 12.6% increase in HDL-C and a 5.3% reduction in triglycerides may make this treatment strategy useful for patients with obesity and metabolic syndrome. Unfortunately, side effects including an increase in depression and anxiety have raised concerns about rimonabant and a large outcome trial was terminated early and the drug removed from the European market because of side effects. It is unclear if other products targeting the endocannabinoid system will be developed.

Drugs that target the serotonergic system have also been used in the management of obesity and new agents in this class are in development. Fenfluramine and dexfenfluramine were removed from the market when reports of valvular heart disease were associated with these drugs [63]. Newer agents in development selectively target central 5-hydroxytryptamine (5-HT, or serotonin) 2C receptors without adverse effects on heart valves and without causing an increase in pulmonary artery pressures. A 1 year weight loss study with the selective serotonin 2 C receptor agonist lorcaserin showed an approximately 4 kg greater weight loss with this agent compared with placebo [64].

Bariatric Surgery

Weight loss surgery is an option for weight reduction in patients with severe obesity (BMI 40 or greater) or in patients with a BMI of 35 or greater and comorbidities [5]. A meta-analysis of bariatric surgery showed that the different surgical techniques are highly successful in achieving significant weight loss and that diabetes completely resolved in over 76% of the patients [65]. In addition, hyperlipidemia improved in 70% of patients and hypertension resolved in over 61% of patients. Resolution of diabetes following bariatric surgery can occur days after surgery even before marked weight loss is achieved suggesting a change in gut-related hormones may play a role [66]. Evidence is accumulating that bariatric surgery may be associated with an improvement in longevity [67].

Dyslipidemia

The National Cholesterol Education Program recommends that the LDL-C should be the primary target of therapy in individuals at cardiovascular disease risk. Patients diagnosed with the metabolic syndrome who do not fit the criteria for diabetes and do not have clinically evident atherosclerotic disease would fit the treatment guidelines for primary prevention. The LDL-C target for primary prevention is less than 130 mg/dl. For patients who are moderately high-risk defined as two or more risk factors and a 10-year risk of a cardiovascular event between 10 and 20%, an LDL-C goal of <100 mg/dl is a therapeutic option or a reasonable clinical strategy based on more recent trial evidence [68]. LDL-C lowering therapy should achieve at least a 30–40% reduction in LDL-C. Patients with the metabolic syndrome would frequently fit the moderately high-risk category based on the clustering of multiple risk factors found in this syndrome.

The NCEP guidelines recommend an LDL-C target of <100 mg/dl for secondary prevention patients. These are individuals at high CVD risk. This category includes patients with clinical atherosclerotic disease (CHD, symptomatic carotid artery disease, abdominal aortic aneurysm, or peripheral arterial disease), diabetes, or patients whose 10-year Framingham CVD risk is greater than 20% due to multiple risk factors. When the risk is considered very high, an LDL-C goal of <70 mg/dl is a therapeutic option [68]. The very high-risk category can include patients who have the metabolic syndrome in addition to the component that put them into the high-risk category.

A low HDL-C is one of the major components of the metabolic syndrome and a frequent lipid abnormality in diabetic patients. The NCEP recommends that non-HDL-C should be the second therapeutic target after LDL-C reduction. The non-HDL-C is calculated by subtracting the HDL-C from the total cholesterol value. The non-HDL-C goal is 30 mg/dl higher than the LDL-C goal. There are three strategies for further lowering the non-HDL-C; further reduction in LDL-C, raising HDL-C or reducing triglycerides.

Persons with low HDL-C levels are at increased risk of CHD. Epidemiologic studies suggest that an increase in HDL-C of 1 mg/dl is associated with a 2–3% reduction in CHD risk [69]. Strategies for raising HDL-C include lifestyle modification and pharmacological agents. The percent change in HDL-C by the different lifestyle strategies are summarized in Table 2.8. Improvement in HDL C has been associated with regular aerobic exercise, smoking cessation, weight loss, alcohol consumption, and changes in diet that replaces saturated fat and high glycemic index carbohydrates with polyunsaturated (fish oils) and monounsaturated fatty acids. The change in HDL-C with hygienic methods is dependent on the initial HDL-C level with, unfortunately, the least improvement in individuals with the lowest HDL-C levels at baseline [70].

Several classes of lipid-lowering agents can increase HDL-C including statins, niacin, and fibrates. Statins modestly increase HDL-C by about 5–15% likely through increasing levels of apolipoprotein A-I [71]. Statins are considered first line pharmacological therapy because of their ability to lower LDL-C, the primary target of treatment, and their effectiveness in improving outcomes across the risk spectrum. Statins appear to give the greatest risk reduction among patients with the lowest HDL-C both from primary prevention studies [72] and in patients with known cardiovascular disease [73].

Niacin can increase HDL-C by 20–30% as well as reduce triglycerides by 40–50% and LDL-C by 20% at doses in the 1.5–3 g per day range [71]. Niacin may be the most effective agent currently available to raise HDL-C. The main limitation to its use is tolerability. The Coronary Drug Project, using 3.0 g of short-acting niacin per day, achieved a 27% decrease in nonfatal myocardial infarction in the treatment group after 6 years [74]. The addition of niacin to a

Table 2.8 Lifestyle modification and the effect on HDL-C (from [69])

Therapeutic intervention	Increase in HDL-C levels (%)
Aerobic exercise	5–10
Tobacco cessation	5–10
Weight loss	0.35 mg/dl per kg of weight loss
Alcohol consumption	5–15
Omega 3, Omega 6, MUFA in diet	0–5

HDL-C high-density lipoprotein cholesterol, *MUFA* monounsaturated fatty acid

statin can bring about a further reduction in LDL-C and a significant increase in HDL-C. In the HDL-Atherosclerosis Treatment Study (HATS), a small group of patients with coronary artery disease and low baseline HDL-C levels achieved significant clinical and angiographic benefit from the combination of simvastatin and at least 2 g of niacin daily [75].

Niacin may be an important agent for patients with the metabolic syndrome since it can address both the low HDL-C values and elevated triglycerides that are a common pattern of dyslipidemia in these patients. However, there is concern that niacin may worsen insulin resistance and glycemic control. An early study using 4.5 g of niacin daily showed induction and aggravation of glucose intolerance in the subjects studied [76]. Longer-term studies suggest that these changes in glycemia may not lead to substantial glucose intolerance. The Arterial Disease Multiple Intervention Trial (ADMIT) studied 3.0 g of niacin daily to determine the efficacy and safety of niacin in diabetic and nondiabetic patients [77]. Glucose levels were modestly increased by niacin averaging 8.7 mg/dl in diabetics and 6.3 mg/dl in nondiabetics with no change in hemoglobin A1c from baseline. Some of the diabetic patients, however, increased their insulin during the course of the study. More analysis will need to be done to determine if the potential benefits of niacin are diminished by the modest change in glycemic control with niacin. Patients with metabolic syndrome may develop an increase in fasting sugars significant enough to change their diagnosis to diabetes. Since the increase in fasting glucose is modest, these patients are likely near the diabetic category and would likely warrant therapy for diabetes.

Hypertriglyceridemia is a common component of the dyslipidemia associated with insulin resistance and is one of the major criteria for the metabolic syndrome. High triglycerides correlate with the presence of small, dense LDL-C particles and reduced levels of HDL-C, especially the HDL_2 component of HDL-C. Because of this correlation with LDL and HDL, triglyceride levels are not usually found to be an independent predictor of coronary artery disease after adjustments for these factors are made [78].

The treatment of hypertriglyceridemia consists of a combination of lifestyle modification and pharmacological therapy when lifestyle changes alone cannot achieve the desired triglyceride goal. A diet that concentrates on reducing complex carbohydrates can lower triglyceride levels. In addition, a reduction or elimination of alcohol can be beneficial. Fish oils have been shown to reduce triglycerides although the dose needed to reduce triglycerides by about 35% are typically 3–4 g per day of a combination of eicosapentaenoic acid (EPA) and docosahexaenoic acid (DHA) [79]. Multiple brands of fish oil capsules are available over the counter and there is one branded fish oil product (Lovaza, GlaxoSmithKline) that contains 465 mg of EPA and 375 mg of DHA in each 1,000 mg capsule.

Statins, niacin, and fibrates all have triglyceride lowering effects with the fibrates having the greatest efficacy. Gemfibrozil has the most convincing outcome data. The Helsinki Heart Study was a primary prevention trial that studied 1,200 mg of gemfibrozil in over 4,000 asymptomatic men and showed a 34% reduction in the incidence of CHD compared with placebo [80]. The subgroup that achieved the greatest benefit, with a 71% lower incidence of CHD events, had an LDL-C/HDL-C ratio greater than 5 and a triglyceride level greater than 203 mg/dl [81]. This lipid pattern is commonly found in metabolic syndrome patients. The Helsinki Heart Study, however, did not find a reduction in total mortality because of a surprising and unexplained increase in noncardiac mortality that offset the fewer deaths due to CHD.

The Veterans Affairs High-Density Lipoprotein Cholesterol Intervention Trial (VA-HIT) treated over 2,500 men with coronary artery disease and lower than average HDL-C with either 1,200 mg of gemfibrozil or placebo [82]. The mean HDL-C increased 6% and the mean triglyceride level decreased 31% with no significant change in LDL-C. The gemfibrozil treated group achieved a 24% reduction in the combined outcome of death, nonfatal myocardial infarction, and stroke. In contrast, the Fenofibrate Intervention and Event Lowering in Diabetes (FIELD) study enrolled nearly 10,000 people with type 2 diabetes mellitus and only achieved a nonsignificant 11% reduction in the primary end point [83]. This disappointing finding suggests that all fibrates may not be equivalent in producing significant event reduction. It was also suggested that the high use of statins in the placebo arm of the FIELD trial may have masked the efficacy of fenofibrate in this study. Finally, combination therapy with a statin and a fibrate can be considered. There is, however, no convincing outcome data using this combination and the recent results from the Action to Control Cardiovascular Risk in Diabetes (ACCORD) study showing no reduction in cardiovascular events with the combination of simvastatin plus fenofibrate in comparison to simvastatin alone raised questions about the benefit of combination therapy in diabetics [84].

General recommendations on the treatment of dyslipidemia in the metabolic syndrome can be made based on these outcome studies. LDL-C should be the primary target of therapy and the percent reduction and treatment goal should be determined based on the risk level of the patient. If a statin drug is contraindicated, then niacin or fibrates can be considered depending on which lipid factor is most outside of the normal range. Combination therapy with a statin plus niacin or a statin plus a fibrate is a treatment option to consider in patients with an elevated non-HDL-C but there is little outcome data to support a strong recommendation. Combination therapy has the strongest appeal for the highest risk individuals. Further research is needed to better elucidate the risk reduction that can be achieved with combination therapy.

Blood Pressure

The Joint National Committee (JNC) on Prevention, Detection, Evaluation, and Treatment of High Blood Pressure seventh report recognized that the risk of CVD begins at a blood pressure of 115/75 mmHg and that this risk doubles with each 20/10 mmHg increment [85]. Individuals with blood pressure of 120–139 systolic or 80–89 diastolic are designated as having prehypertension and require a lifestyle modification program to prevent CVD. The blood pressure treatment goals are blood pressure <140/90 mmHg or <130/80 mmHg for patients with diabetes or chronic kidney disease. A blood pressure of 130/85 has been designated as one of the criteria for the metabolic syndrome so many patients with this syndrome will be in the prehypertension range. If patients are being treated with an antihypertensive agent, even if the blood pressure is at the treatment goal, they would still be classified as having hypertension. Since many individuals with the metabolic syndrome may fit the criteria for diabetes, the more aggressive treatment goal of <130/80 would apply to this group of patients.

The JNC recommends that the choice of antihypertensive is determined by compelling indications. Although all first line agents have the potential to reduce the incidence of CVD in patients with diabetes, the angiotensin-converting enzyme (ACE) inhibitor and the angiotensin receptor blocker (ARB) based treatments favorably affect the progression of renal insufficiency and reduce albuminuria [85]. Microalbuminuria is associated with the metabolic syndrome. From the NHANES III data, 34% of women and 42% of men with microalbuminuria also have the metabolic syndrome [44]. Because of the high association of microalbuminuria and metabolic syndrome, a reasonable treatment strategy would be an evaluation for the presence of microalbuminuria and institution of an ACE inhibitor or ARB if positive. A blood pressure target of <130/80 would be a therapeutic goal in such patients using the same JNC treatment goal as diabetic patients.

The use of ACE inhibitors as a preventive strategy may help delay or prevent renal disease in high-risk individuals. The Bergamo Nephrologic Diabetes Complication Trial (BENEDICT) studied over 1,200 patients with diabetes and hypertension and normal urinary albumin excretion using an ACE inhibitor treatment strategy and a target blood pressure of 120/80 [86]. The use of an ACE inhibitor significantly decreased the incidence of microalbuminuria. In addition, a number of clinical trials have suggested that the use of ACE inhibitors or ARBs may reduce the incidence of diabetes compared with placebo, diuretics, or beta-blockers. A meta-analysis of 22 clinical trials of participants who did not have diabetes at randomization showed that ACE inhibitors and ARBs were the agents the least associated with diabetes [87]. Diuretics and beta-blockers apparently increased the likelihood of diabetes compared with placebo. Finally, the use of an ARB in individuals with prehypertension may prevent or postpone the development of stage I hypertension as shown in the Trial of Preventing Hypertension (TROPHY) study [88]. In this study, over 400 individuals with prehypertension were randomized to an ARB for 2 years followed by placebo for 2 years and compared with 400 participants on placebo for the 4 years of the study. Over the 4 years of the study, stage I hypertension developed in nearly two thirds of the placebo group. The ARB significantly reduced the risk of incident hypertension during the study period.

From this analysis, it is reasonable to consider the metabolic syndrome as a compelling indication for the use of an ACE inhibitor or an ARB as first line therapy for the treatment of hypertension. If microalbuminuria is present, a treatment goal of <130/80 as indicated for diabetic patients would be recommended. For patients in the prehypertension category without microalbuminuria, there is compelling data to suggest treatment with an ACE inhibitor or ARB may prevent the development of stage I hypertension and diabetes. The role of direct renin inhibitors is being investigated as well. An aggressive lifestyle program may also be effective in preventing these conditions as well. Therefore, a reasonable strategy would be to recommend a lifestyle program and reserve the use of pharmacological agents if the lifestyle program is not successful. Further studies may help to modify these recommendations as to when to consider starting pharmacological therapy.

Insulin Resistance and Hyperglycemia

Impaired fasting glucose is one of the major criteria of the metabolic syndrome. Many patients with metabolic syndrome may fit the criteria for diabetes following a glucose tolerance test even though fasting sugars may not reach criteria (see Table 2.5 for diagnostic criteria for diabetes). Drug therapies to reduce plasma glucose or improve insulin sensitivity are FDA approved for diabetes and not for IFG. Currently, it is recommended to begin a lifestyle program with weight loss and increased physical activity to treat IFG. Drug therapy is often required once diabetes develops. How early to start hypoglycemic agents is an important question that needs further research to answer definitively.

There is emerging evidence that hypoglycemic therapy initiated in patients with IFG or metabolic syndrome can reduce the incidence of diabetes. The Diabetes Prevention Program showed that metformin reduced the incidence of diabetes by 31% compared with placebo [54]. A meta-analysis of 31 trials showed that metformin reduced BMI, improved insulin resistance, lowered triglycerides and LDL-C, and increased HDL-C compared with placebo in patients at risk for diabetes [89]. New-onset diabetes was reduced by 40% with a 6% absolute risk reduction in 1.8 years. The evidence from the Diabetes Prevention Program prompted an American Diabetes Association (ADA) consensus panel to conclude that all individuals with prediabetes should be counseled on lifestyle changes similar to those recommended in the trial [90]. The panel felt that metformin could be considered for diabetes prevention in very high-risk individuals with IFG and IGT and at least one other risk factor.

Other pharmacological agents have also been shown to reduce the incidence of diabetes. Acarbose, in the STOP-NIDDM randomized trial, was found to delay the development of diabetes by 25% in individuals with IGT although 31% discontinued therapy early most commonly due to gastrointestinal side effects [91]. In the Diabetes Reduction Assessment with Ramipril and Rosiglitazone Medication (DREAM) trial, rosiglitazone reduced the risk of diabetes or death by 60% in individuals with IFG or IGT and no previous cardiovascular disease [92]. Despite this emerging evidence, the ADA consensus panel felt that at the present time only metformin should be considered for diabetes prevention [90].

Prothrombotic and Proinflammatory Risk Factors

The metabolic syndrome is a prothrombotic and proinflammatory condition. Low-dose aspirin (75–160 mg/day) has been recommended by the American Heart Association Primary Prevention guidelines for individuals at higher CHD risk defined as a 10% 10-year risk or greater [93]. The majority of metabolic syndrome patients would fit this risk category and should be treated with aspirin unless contraindicated.

There is no specific therapy for inflammation and no current guidelines for treatment targets for the different inflammatory biomarkers. All of the treatments suggested for the treatment of the metabolic syndrome have the potential to significantly reduce inflammation and decrease levels of biomarkers such as CRP. Lifestyle modification including weight loss, dietary changes, exercise, and smoking cessation can reduce CRP levels [94]. Certain drugs including antidiabetic and antihyperlipidemic agents have also been shown to significantly reduce CRP [95]. Further research will need to be completed to determine if treatment goals for inflammatory biomarkers can further help reduce risk.

Conclusion

Metabolic syndrome is becoming increasingly more prevalent as the obesity epidemic is advancing worldwide. The designation of the metabolic syndrome can identify individuals who are at future risk for diabetes and cardiovascular events and may be an easy way for health care providers to determine a subset of patients at higher risk. Lifestyle modification is the underlying treatment and should be a strong focus of care that is discussed at every patient encounter. Individual risk factors can then be targeted with aggressiveness of therapy dependent on overall risk. The metabolic syndrome designation gives an opportunity to identify at risk individuals before the development of significant disease.

References

1. Third Report of the National Cholesterol Education Program (NCEP) Expert Panel on Detection, Evaluation, and Treatment of High Blood Cholesterol in Adults (Adult Treatment Panel III) final report. Circulation 2002;106(25):3143–21.
2. American Diabetes Association. Diagnosis and classification of diabetes mellitus. Diabetes Care. 2008;31 Suppl 1:S55–60.
3. Grundy SM, Cleeman JI, Daniels SR, et al. Diagnosis and management of the metabolic syndrome: an American Heart Association/National Heart, Lung, and Blood Institute Scientific Statement. Circulation. 2005;112(17):2735–52.
4. Alberti KG, Zimmet P, Shaw J. Metabolic syndrome–a new world-wide definition. A Consensus Statement from the International Diabetes Federation. Diabet Med. 2006;23(5):469–80.

5. Expert Panel on the Identification, Evaluation, and Treatment of Overweight in Adults. Clinical guidelines on the identification, evaluation, and treatment of overweight and obesity in adults: executive summary. Am J Clin Nutr. 1998;68(4):899–917.
6. Lean ME, Han TS, Morrison CE. Waist circumference as a measure for indicating need for weight management. BMJ. 1995;311(6998):158–61.
7. Pouliot MC, Despres JP, Lemieux S, et al. Waist circumference and abdominal sagittal diameter: best simple anthropometric indexes of abdominal visceral adipose tissue accumulation and related cardiovascular risk in men and women. Am J Cardiol. 1994;73(7):460–8.
8. Rexrode KM, Carey VJ, Hennekens CH, et al. Abdominal adiposity and coronary heart disease in women. JAMA. 1998;280(21):1843–8.
9. Janssen I, Katzmarzyk PT, Ross R. Body mass index, waist circumference, and health risk: evidence in support of current National Institutes of Health guidelines. Arch Intern Med. 2002;162(18):2074–9.
10. Carroll MD, Lacher DA, Sorlie PD, et al. Trends in serum lipids and lipoproteins of adults, 1960–2002. JAMA. 2005;294(14):1773–81.
11. McLaughlin T, Reaven G, Abbasi F, et al. Is there a simple way to identify insulin-resistant individuals at increased risk of cardiovascular disease? Am J Cardiol. 2005;96(3):399–404.
12. Bansal S, Buring JE, Rifai N, Mora S, Sacks FM, Ridker PM. Fasting compared with nonfasting triglycerides and risk of cardiovascular events in women. JAMA. 2007;298(3):309–16.
13. Nordestgaard BG, Benn M, Schnohr P, Tybjaerg-Hansen A. Nonfasting triglycerides and risk of myocardial infarction, ischemic heart disease, and death in men and women. JAMA. 2007;298(3):299–308.
14. McGavock JM, Lingvay I, Zib I, et al. Cardiac steatosis in diabetes mellitus: a 1 H-magnetic resonance spectroscopy study. Circulation. 2007;116(10):1170–5.
15. Lewington S, Clarke R, Qizilbash N, Peto R, Collins R. Age-specific relevance of usual blood pressure to vascular mortality: a meta-analysis of individual data for one million adults in 61 prospective studies. Lancet. 2002;360(9349):1903–13.
16. Ferrannini E, Buzzigoli G, Bonadonna R, et al. Insulin resistance in essential hypertension. N Engl J Med. 1987;317(6):350–7.
17. Skarfors ET, Lithell HO, Selinus I. Risk factors for the development of hypertension: a 10-year longitudinal study in middle-aged men. J Hypertens. 1991;9(3):217–23.
18. Jeppesen J, Hein HO, Suadicani P, Gyntelberg F. Low triglycerides-high high-density lipoprotein cholesterol and risk of ischemic heart disease. Arch Intern Med. 2001;161(3):361–6.
19. Sumner AE, Finley KB, Genovese DJ, Criqui MH, Boston RC. Fasting triglyceride and the triglyceride-HDL cholesterol ratio are not markers of insulin resistance in African Americans. Arch Intern Med. 2005;165(12):1395–400.
20. Nordt TK, Sawa H, Fujii S, Sobel BE. Induction of plasminogen activator inhibitor type-1 (PAI-1) by proinsulin and insulin in vivo. Circulation. 1995;91(3):764–70.
21. Wannamethee SG, Lowe GD, Shaper AG, Rumley A, Lennon L, Whincup PH. The metabolic syndrome and insulin resistance: relationship to haemostatic and inflammatory markers in older non-diabetic men. Atherosclerosis. 2005;181(1):101–8.
22. Ridker PM, Buring JE, Cook NR, Rifai N. C-reactive protein, the metabolic syndrome, and risk of incident cardiovascular events: an 8-year follow-up of 14 719 initially healthy American women. Circulation. 2003;107(3):391–7.
23. Wilson PW, D'Agostino RB, Levy D, Belanger AM, Silbershatz H, Kannel WB. Prediction of coronary heart disease using risk factor categories. Circulation. 1998;97(18):1837–47.
24. Ford ES, Giles WH, Dietz WH. Prevalence of the metabolic syndrome among US adults: findings from the third National Health and Nutrition Examination Survey. JAMA. 2002;287(3):356–9.
25. Resnick HE, Jones K, Ruotolo G, et al. Insulin resistance, the metabolic syndrome, and risk of incident cardiovascular disease in nondiabetic American Indians: the Strong Heart Study. Diabetes Care. 2003;26(3):861–7.
26. Hu G, Qiao Q, Tuomilehto J, Balkau B, Borch-Johnsen K, Pyorala K. Prevalence of the metabolic syndrome and its relation to all-cause and cardiovascular mortality in nondiabetic European men and women. Arch Intern Med. 2004;164(10):1066–76.

27. Weng X, Liu Y, Ma J, Wang W, Yang G, Caballero B. An urban-rural comparison of the prevalence of the metabolic syndrome in Eastern China. Public Health Nutr. 2007;10(2):131–6.
28. Flegal KM, Carroll MD, Ogden CL, Johnson CL. Prevalence and trends in obesity among US adults, 1999-2000. JAMA. 2002;288(14):1723–7.
29. Freedman VA, Martin LG, Schoeni RF. Recent trends in disability and functioning among older adults in the United States: a systematic review. JAMA. 2002;288(24):3137–46.
30. Ford ES, Ajani UA, Croft JB, et al. Explaining the decrease in US deaths from coronary disease, 1980–2000. N Engl J Med. 2007;356(23):2388–98.
31. Lutsey PL, Steffen LM, Stevens J. Dietary intake and the development of the metabolic syndrome: the Atherosclerosis Risk in Communities study. Circulation. 2008;117(6):754–61.
32. Dhingra R, Sullivan L, Jacques PF, et al. Soft drink consumption and risk of developing cardiometabolic risk factors and the metabolic syndrome in middle-aged adults in the community. Circulation. 2007;116(5):480–8.
33. Johnson RK, Appel LJ, Brands M, et al. Dietary sugars intake and cardiovascular health: a scientific statement from the American Heart Association. Circulation. 2009;120(11):1011–20.
34. Laaksonen DE, Lakka HM, Niskanen LK, Kaplan GA, Salonen JT, Lakka TA. Metabolic syndrome and development of diabetes mellitus: application and validation of recently suggested definitions of the metabolic syndrome in a prospective cohort study. Am J Epidemiol. 2002;156(11):1070–7.
35. Hanley AJ, Karter AJ, Williams K, et al. Prediction of type 2 diabetes mellitus with alternative definitions of the metabolic syndrome: the Insulin Resistance Atherosclerosis Study. Circulation. 2005;112(24):3713–21.
36. Wilson PW, D'Agostino RB, Parise H, Sullivan L, Meigs JB. Metabolic syndrome as a precursor of cardiovascular disease and type 2 diabetes mellitus. Circulation. 2005;112(20):3066–72.
37. Wilson PW, Meigs JB, Sullivan L, Fox CS, Nathan DM, D'Agostino Sr RB. Prediction of incident diabetes mellitus in middle-aged adults: the Framingham Offspring Study. Arch Intern Med. 2007;167(10):1068–74.
38. Ninomiya JK, L'Italien G, Criqui MH, Whyte JL, Gamst A, Chen RS. Association of the metabolic syndrome with history of myocardial infarction and stroke in the Third National Health and Nutrition Examination Survey. Circulation. 2004;109(1):42–6.
39. Lakka HM, Laaksonen DE, Lakka TA, et al. The metabolic syndrome and total and cardiovascular disease mortality in middle-aged men. JAMA. 2002;288(21):2709–16.
40. Gami AS, Witt BJ, Howard DE, et al. Metabolic syndrome and risk of incident cardiovascular events and death: a systematic review and meta-analysis of longitudinal studies. J Am Coll Cardiol. 2007;49(4):403–14.
41. Wannamethee SG, Shaper AG, Lennon L, Morris RW. Metabolic syndrome vs Framingham Risk Score for prediction of coronary heart disease, stroke, and type 2 diabetes mellitus. Arch Intern Med. 2005;165(22):2644–50.
42. Kohli P, Greenland P. Role of the metabolic syndrome in risk assessment for coronary heart disease. JAMA. 2006;295(7):819–21.
43. Watanabe H, Tanabe N, Watanabe T, et al. Metabolic syndrome and risk of development of atrial fibrillation: the Niigata preventive medicine study. Circulation. 2008;117(10):1255–60.
44. Palaniappan L, Carnethon M, Fortmann SP. Association between microalbuminuria and the metabolic syndrome: NHANES III. Am J Hypertens. 2003;16(11 Pt 1):952–8.
45. Yaffe K, Kanaya A, Lindquist K, et al. The metabolic syndrome, inflammation, and risk of cognitive decline. JAMA. 2004;292(18):2237–42.
46. Miller A, Adeli K. Dietary fructose and the metabolic syndrome. Curr Opin Gastroenterol. 2008;24(2):204–9.
47. Irwin ML, Yasui Y, Ulrich CM, et al. Effect of exercise on total and intra-abdominal body fat in postmenopausal women: a randomized controlled trial. JAMA. 2003;289(3):323–30.
48. Fletcher B, Berra K, Ades P, et al. Managing abnormal blood lipids: a collaborative approach. Circulation. 2005;112(20):3184–209.
49. Stewart KJ. Exercise training and the cardiovascular consequences of type 2 diabetes and hypertension: plausible mechanisms for improving cardiovascular health. JAMA. 2002;288(13):1622–31.

50. Berlin JA, Colditz GA. A meta-analysis of physical activity in the prevention of coronary heart disease. Am J Epidemiol. 1990;132(4):612–28.
51. Manson JE, Greenland P, LaCroix AZ, et al. Walking compared with vigorous exercise for the prevention of cardiovascular events in women. N Engl J Med. 2002;347(10):716–25.
52. Sesso HD, Paffenbarger Jr RS, Lee IM. Physical activity and coronary heart disease in men: The Harvard Alumni Health Study. Circulation. 2000;102(9):975–80.
53. Franco OH, de Laet C, Peeters A, Jonker J, Mackenbach J, Nusselder W. Effects of physical activity on life expectancy with cardiovascular disease. Arch Intern Med. 2005;165(20):2355–60.
54. Knowler WC, Barrett-Connor E, Fowler SE, et al. Reduction in the incidence of type 2 diabetes with lifestyle intervention or metformin. N Engl J Med. 2002;346(6):393–403.
55. Haddock CK, Poston WS, Dill PL, Foreyt JP, Ericsson M. Pharmacotherapy for obesity: a quantitative analysis of four decades of published randomized clinical trials. Int J Obes Relat Metab Disord. 2002;26(2):262–73.
56. Wadden TA, Berkowitz RI, Womble LG, et al. Randomized trial of lifestyle modification and pharmacotherapy for obesity. N Engl J Med. 2005;353(20):2111–20.
57. Astrup A. Drug management of obesity–efficacy versus safety. N Engl J Med. 2010;363(3): 288–90.
58. Li Z, Maglione M, Tu W, et al. Meta-analysis: pharmacologic treatment of obesity. Ann Intern Med. 2005;142(7):532–46.
59. Torgerson JS, Hauptman J, Boldrin MN, Sjostrom L. XENical in the prevention of diabetes in obese subjects (XENDOS) study: a randomized study of orlistat as an adjunct to lifestyle changes for the prevention of type 2 diabetes in obese patients. Diabetes Care. 2004;27(1):155–61.
60. Osei-Hyiaman D, DePetrillo M, Pacher P, et al. Endocannabinoid activation at hepatic CB1 receptors stimulates fatty acid synthesis and contributes to diet-induced obesity. J Clin Invest. 2005;115(5):1298–305.
61. Van Gaal LF, Rissanen AM, Scheen AJ, Ziegler O, Rossner S. Effects of the cannabinoid-1 receptor blocker rimonabant on weight reduction and cardiovascular risk factors in overweight patients: 1-year experience from the RIO-Europe study. Lancet. 2005;365(9468):1389–97.
62. Pi-Sunyer FX, Aronne LJ, Heshmati HM, Devin J, Rosenstock J. Effect of rimonabant, a cannabinoid-1 receptor blocker, on weight and cardiometabolic risk factors in overweight or obese patients: RIO-North America: a randomized controlled trial. JAMA. 2006;295(7):761–75.
63. Connolly HM, Crary JL, McGoon MD, et al. Valvular heart disease associated with fenfluramine-phentermine. N Engl J Med. 1997;337(9):581–8.
64. Smith SR, Weissman NJ, Anderson CM, et al. Multicenter, placebo-controlled trial of lorcaserin for weight management. N Engl J Med. 2010;363(3):245–56.
65. Buchwald H, Avidor Y, Braunwald E, et al. Bariatric surgery: a systematic review and meta-analysis. JAMA. 2004;292(14):1724–37.
66. Pories WJ, Swanson MS, MacDonald KG, et al. Who would have thought it? An operation proves to be the most effective therapy for adult-onset diabetes mellitus. Ann Surg. 1995;222(3): 339–50.
67. Sjostrom CD, Lissner L, Wedel H, Sjostrom L. Reduction in incidence of diabetes, hypertension and lipid disturbances after intentional weight loss induced by bariatric surgery: the SOS Intervention Study. Obes Res. 1999;7(5):477–84.
68. Grundy SM, Cleeman JI, Merz CN, et al. Implications of recent clinical trials for the National Cholesterol Education Program Adult Treatment Panel III guidelines. Circulation. 2004;110(2):227–39.
69. Gordon DJ, Probstfield JL, Garrison RJ, et al. High-density lipoprotein cholesterol and cardiovascular disease. Four prospective American studies. Circulation. 1989;79(1):8–15.
70. Williams PT. The relationships of vigorous exercise, alcohol, and adiposity to low and high-density lipoprotein-cholesterol levels. Metabolism. 2004;53(6):700–9.
71. Singh IM, Shishehbor MH, Ansell BJ. High-density lipoprotein as a therapeutic target: a systematic review. JAMA. 2007;298(7):786–98.
72. Downs JR, Clearfield M, Weis S, et al. Primary prevention of acute coronary events with lovastatin in men and women with average cholesterol levels: results of AFCAPS/TexCAPS. Air Force/Texas Coronary Atherosclerosis Prevention Study. JAMA. 1998;279(20):1615–22.

73. MRC/BHF Heart Protection Study of cholesterol lowering with simvastatin in 20,536 high-risk individuals: a randomised placebo-controlled trial. Lancet 2002;360(9326):7–22.
74. Clofibrate and niacin in coronary heart disease. JAMA 1975;231(4):360–81.
75. Brown BG, Zhao XQ, Chait A, et al. Simvastatin and niacin, antioxidant vitamins, or the combination for the prevention of coronary disease. N Engl J Med. 2001;345(22):1583–92.
76. Gaut ZN, Pocelinko R, Solomon HM, Thomas GB. Oral glucose tolerance, plasma insulin, and uric acid excretion in man during chronic administration of nicotinic acid. Metabolism. 1971;20(11):1031–5.
77. Elam MB, Hunninghake DB, Davis KB, et al. Effect of niacin on lipid and lipoprotein levels and glycemic control in patients with diabetes and peripheral arterial disease: the ADMIT study: A randomized trial. Arterial Disease Multiple Intervention Trial. JAMA. 2000;284(10): 1263–70.
78. Coughlan BJ, Sorrentino MJ. Does hypertriglyceridemia increase risk for CAD? Growing evidence suggests it plays a role. Postgrad Med. 2000;108(7):77–84.
79. Harris WS. n-3 fatty acids and serum lipoproteins: human studies. Am J Clin Nutr. 1997;65(5 Suppl):1645S–54.
80. Frick MH, Elo O, Haapa K, et al. Helsinki Heart Study: primary-prevention trial with gemfibrozil in middle-aged men with dyslipidemia. Safety of treatment, changes in risk factors, and incidence of coronary heart disease. N Engl J Med. 1987;317(20):1237–45.
81. Manninen V, Tenkanen L, Koskinen P, et al. Joint effects of serum triglyceride and LDL cholesterol and HDL cholesterol concentrations on coronary heart disease risk in the Helsinki Heart Study. Implications for treatment. Circulation. 1992;85(1):37–45.
82. Rubins HB, Robins SJ, Collins D, et al. Gemfibrozil for the secondary prevention of coronary heart disease in men with low levels of high-density lipoprotein cholesterol. Veterans Affairs High-Density Lipoprotein Cholesterol Intervention Trial Study Group. N Engl J Med. 1999;341(6):410–8.
83. Keech A, Simes RJ, Barter P, et al. Effects of long-term fenofibrate therapy on cardiovascular events in 9795 people with type 2 diabetes mellitus (the FIELD study): randomised controlled trial. Lancet. 2005;366(9500):1849–61.
84. Ginsberg HN, Elam MB, Lovato LC, et al. Effects of combination lipid therapy in type 2 diabetes mellitus. N Engl J Med. 2010;362(17):1563–74.
85. Chobanian AV, Bakris GL, Black HR, et al. The Seventh Report of the Joint National Committee on Prevention, Detection, Evaluation, and Treatment of High Blood Pressure: the JNC 7 report. JAMA. 2003;289(19):2560–72.
86. Ruggenenti P, Fassi A, Ilieva AP, et al. Preventing microalbuminuria in type 2 diabetes. N Engl J Med. 2004;351(19):1941–51.
87. Elliott WJ, Meyer PM. Incident diabetes in clinical trials of antihypertensive drugs: a network meta-analysis. Lancet. 2007;369(9557):201–7.
88. Julius S, Nesbitt SD, Egan BM, et al. Feasibility of treating prehypertension with an angiotensin-receptor blocker. N Engl J Med. 2006;354(16):1685–97.
89. Salpeter SR, Buckley NS, Kahn JA, Salpeter EE. Meta-analysis: metformin treatment in persons at risk for diabetes mellitus. Am J Med. 2008;121(2):149–57.
90. American Diabetes Association. Standards of medical care in diabetes–2008. Diabetes Care. 2008;31 Suppl 1:S12–54.
91. Chiasson JL, Josse RG, Gomis R, Hanefeld M, Karasik A, Laakso M. Acarbose for prevention of type 2 diabetes mellitus: the STOP-NIDDM randomised trial. Lancet. 2002;359(9323): 2072–7.
92. Gerstein HC, Yusuf S, Bosch J, et al. Effect of rosiglitazone on the frequency of diabetes in patients with impaired glucose tolerance or impaired fasting glucose: a randomised controlled trial. Lancet. 2006;368(9541):1096–105.
93. Pearson TA, Blair SN, Daniels SR, et al. AHA Guidelines for Primary Prevention of Cardiovascular Disease and Stroke: 2002 Update: Consensus Panel Guide to Comprehensive Risk Reduction for Adult Patients Without Coronary or Other Atherosclerotic Vascular Diseases.

American Heart Association Science Advisory and Coordinating Committee. Circulation. 2002;106(3):388–91.
94. Ridker PM. Clinical application of C-reactive protein for cardiovascular disease detection and prevention. Circulation. 2003;107(3):363–9.
95. Dandona P. Effects of antidiabetic and antihyperlipidemic agents on C-reactive protein. Mayo Clin Proc. 2008;83(3):333–42.

Chapter 3
The Role of Imaging in Cardiovascular Risk Assessment

Tamar S. Polonsky and R. Parker Ward

Keywords Calcium score • Electron beam computed tomography • Carotid intima-media thickness

Assessment of a patient's cardiovascular risk remains challenging. Cardiovascular risk assessment should always begin with office-based assessment of traditional cardiovascular risk factors, including age, hypertension, dyslipidemia, tobacco use, and family history. The Framingham risk score provides an easy to use, well-validated tool which allows physicians to readily assess the composite of these traditional risk factors. However, traditional risk factors and the Framingham risk score may not always tell the whole story. An obvious example of this comes from the Framingham study itself, where 35% of cardiovascular events occurred in patients with what have traditionally been considered normal cholesterol values (total cholesterol < 200 mg/dl) [1]. In addition, family history of coronary heart disease (CHD), a potent cardiovascular risk factor, is not reflected in the Framingham risk score. In fact, while dramatic improvements in patient outcomes have occurred over the last two decades after the diagnosis of CHD, little progress has been made in reducing the rates of initial presentation with myocardial infarction or cardiac death [2]. Thus, while traditional risk factor assessment should remain the bedrock and uniform first step in cardiovascular risk assessment, additional ways to evaluate risk and the appropriate patients in whom to employ these techniques need to be identified.

Currently, there are a variety of techniques available for physicians to assess cardiovascular risk further. Options such as exercise stress testing or ankle-brachial

T.S. Polonsky (✉)
Department of Medicine, Section of Cardiology, University of Chicago, Chicago, IL 60637, USA
e-mail: t-polonsky@northwestern.edu

M.J. Sorrentino (ed.), *Hyperlipidemia in Primary Care: A Practical Guide to Risk Reduction*, Current Clinical Practice, DOI 10.1007/978-1-60327-502-6_3,

index testing are excellent modalities to stratify risk in symptomatic patients, as these tests will identify advanced atherosclerosis which is causing obstruction to blood flow. However, they will generally not be useful for asymptomatic patients in whom initial cardiac events are frequently caused by rupture of nonobstructive atherosclerotic plaques which were not previously causing symptoms. For patients who are asymptomatic, options to assess cardiovascular risk above and beyond traditional risk factors include serologic biomarkers (e.g., high-sensitivity C-reactive protein) or imaging tests aimed at uncovering subclinical atherosclerosis. The purpose of this chapter is to review currently available noninvasive imaging tests for the identification of subclinical atherosclerosis and stratification of cardiovascular risk.

Requirements of Noninvasive Imaging Test to be Adopted for Clinical Use

For a noninvasive imaging test to be a clinically useful option for cardiovascular risk assessment, a number of requirements must be met. First, it must be available, reproducible, and not expose the patient to any significant risks. Second, it must have a proven ability to predict cardiovascular events, and thus stratify cardiovascular risk. Third, it must improve on office-based risk assessment (i.e., if an imaging test merely reflects what we know from traditional risk factors, there will be no role for the test). Finally, there must be some consensus on what represents an abnormal test result and what group of patients may benefit from the use of the imaging test for risk stratification.

Currently, there are two imaging tests that meet these criteria, and thus can be considered reasonable options for cardiovascular risk assessment: cardiac computed tomography (CT) to evaluate coronary calcium and B-mode ultrasound to determine carotid intima-media thickness (CIMT). The balance of this chapter will serve to review these imaging tests, and where they might fit into clinical practice as part of cardiovascular risk assessment in asymptomatic patients.

What Is Calcium Scoring?

Coronary calcium can be evaluated using two types of CT scanners: electron beam CT (EBCT) and multidetector CT (MDCT). An EBCT scanner obtains one image at a time, typically using 3 mm slices. This is in contrast to MDCT, which uses more advanced technology to acquire multiple parallel images simultaneously. The majority of recently published studies have evaluated coronary calcium using EBCT. Given the superior image quality and versatility of MDCT, its use is becoming more widespread in clinical practice. It should be noted that both of these CT modalities are fundamentally different than the recently popularized CT angiography.

CT angiography requires a dye injection and a substantially higher radiation dose than calcium scoring with EBCT or MDCT (discussed further below). While CT angiography is developing an expanding and exciting role in the management of symptomatic patients, for the above reasons it is not currently recommended for risk assessment in asymptomatic patients.

With both MDCT and EBCT, image acquisition typically occurs during diastole, to minimize motion artifact. A calcium score is then calculated, usually by using the Agatston method [3]. This involves multiplying the number of pixels per calcified lesion by the density of the calcification within each coronary artery. The sum of the values within each coronary artery then becomes the patient's overall calcium score. There is some variation in how studies have categorized the range of calcium scores. In general, scores have been grouped as 0, 1–100, 101–400, and greater than 400. These cutoffs provide clinically relevant risk stratification, which is discussed in detail below.

Measuring coronary calcium is useful for cardiovascular risk assessment because calcium is a marker for atherosclerosis. Early pathologic data comparing autopsy specimens with EBCT have shown a strong correlation between the total amount of calcium and the atherosclerotic burden in the coronary tree. In fact, the ratio of atherosclerotic plaque to calcium is approximately 5:1 [4]. However, sites of the most dense calcification do not necessarily match the specific sites of the most severe atherosclerosis. Thus, while the amount of coronary calcium correlates strongly with the overall burden of atherosclerosis, it is the norm for areas of noncalcified soft plaque to co-exist in the same patient.

While coronary calcium has been shown to correlate strongly with overall atherosclerotic burden, it is less reliable as a direct measure of obstructive disease. Among patients with a coronary calcium score of 0, the chance of significant obstructive disease is extremely small [5–7]. In contrast, a calcium score greater than 0 is less informative about the likelihood of obstructive disease. Several studies have shown that an elevated calcium score is a poor predictor of obstructive coronary disease on invasive angiography. For example, in a study of 2,115 symptomatic patients who had an EBCT and cardiac catheterization, the detection of any calcium was highly sensitive for at least a 50% stenosis, at 99%, but had a very low specificity of 28% [6]. When the cutoff was changed to a score of ≥100, the sensitivity decreased to 87%, but the specificity improved to 79%. In summary, an elevated calcium score can shed light on the presence of atherosclerotic disease, but should not be used to predict the location or degree of obstructive disease.

What role calcium plays in the coronary arteries is still unclear. The process of calcification is likely stimulated by damage to the vascular endothelium, which in turn stimulates a cascade of cytokine activation [8]. The cytokines lead to proliferation of cells that produce extracellular matrix and mineralization, similar to the process found in bone formation. Some have suggested that calcified plaques are less likely to rupture than soft noncalcified or mixed plaques. For example, one study using intravascular ultrasound during coronary angiography showed that the lesions in patients with stable angina had more calcium than the culprit lesions found in patients presenting with a non-ST elevation MI [9]. However, additional data suggest that calcification may act as a hinge point, and actually increase the risk of plaque rupture and dissection [10].

Does Calcium Scoring Predict Cardiovascular Events?

What is clear is that the degree of coronary calcium seen on cardiac CT scan is a potent predictor of future cardiovascular events. Large prospective studies have shown that, depending on the population studied, coronary artery calcium (CAC) scoring can significantly alter the calculation of a patient's cardiovascular risk. Results from a meta-analysis of six recently published studies showed that patients with a mildly elevated coronary calcium score of 1–112, after adjusting for traditional cardiovascular risk factors, experienced a relative risk of coronary death or myocardial infarction (MI) within 3–5 years of 1.9, when compared with patients with a calcium score of 0 [11]. The relative risk increased to 4.3 with a score of 100–400, to 7.2 with a score of 400–1,000, and to 10.8 with a score of >1,000. A more recent study, which followed more than 25,000 patients for at least 10 years, showed similar risk ratios [12]. The 10-year survival for patients with a calcium score of 0 was 99.4%, whereas survival dropped to 87.8% for those patients with a score of >1,000.

Does Calcium Scoring Improve on Office-Based Risk Assessment with Traditional Risk Factors?

While the ability of a calcium score to predict future cardiac events is compelling, CAC scoring will only be useful to clinicians as a tool for risk assessment if it adds additional information to what we already know (i.e., does it add additional prognostic information beyond traditional risk factors?). A number of studies have evaluated this question, and the answer depends on the population studied. For patients with a low Framingham risk score, the event rate is so small that few studies have shown any incremental value in obtaining a calcium score [11, 13]. For patients with a high Framingham risk score or a coronary artery disease equivalent, such as diabetes, aggressive risk-factor modification is warranted based on office-based risk assessment alone. In addition, there are no data to support the safety of treating high-risk patients less aggressively on the basis of a low calcium score. Therefore, for patients who are in high risk based on traditional risk factors, calcium scoring would not alter the patient's clinical management. As a result, the American College of Cardiology (ACC) and American Heart Association (AHA), in their consensus document published in 2007, do not recommend using CAC scoring for risk assessment in patients at low risk or high risk based on traditional risk assessment [11].

Unlike with patients who are at low or high risk, calcium scoring has shown benefit in patients who are deemed to be at intermediate risk (estimated 10-year CHD risk of 10–20%). In a secondary analysis of patients with an intermediate Framingham risk from four studies, annual CHD death or MI rates were 0.4, 1.3, and 2.4% for a CAC score of <100, 100–399, and ≥400, respectively [11]. Given that an annual event rate of 2.4% is comparable to the event rate expected for high-risk patients, a CAC score of ≥400 would increase a risk estimation based on clinical factors alone. As a result, the ACC and AHA concluded that it is reasonable to obtain a calcium score in individuals who are at intermediate risk, because patients with a CAC score of ≥400 would have their treatment modified to achieve secondary prevention treatment goals [11]. For intermediate risk patients with a CAC score of <400, the ACC guidelines would suggest it is reasonable to continue primary prevention treatment strategies.

It is important to note that in intermediate risk patients the calcium score can help determine whether to intensify or maintain a patient's treatment as is, but should not be used to reduce it. Among the cohort followed by Greenland et al., patients with a CAC score of 0 experienced a 3- to 5-year event rate of 4.4% [13]. Given the lack of prospective data to show a benefit from reduction of therapy, the ACC and AHA do not recommend reducing therapy below what would be expected based on clinical risk factors, even in the setting of a CAC score of 0 [11].

What Should Be Done with Abnormal Results?

Thus far, we have discussed recommendations for when to order a CAC score as part of cardiovascular risk assessment. In practice, patients frequently present to physicians with a previously performed CAC score in hand, often obtained on self-referral. In this setting, we can fall back on the data mentioned above. Patients with a CAC score of 400 have a 2.4% annual risk, which extrapolates to a >20% 10-year risk, of coronary events. Thus, these patients should be considered high risk. It is reasonable to intensify their medical regimen and to treat them to the same lipid and blood pressure targets as those patients who have known coronary artery disease or other CAD equivalents.

The decision about whether to pursue further testing to evaluate for obstructive CAD in patients with a calcium score of >400 is less clear. Given the poor correlation between CAC score and obstructive coronary artery disease on invasive angiography, and the lack of any evidence supporting the routine use of invasive angiography in asymptomatic patients, an elevated calcium score should not routinely prompt invasive angiography. There may, however, be a role for further noninvasive testing in patients with a high CAC score (>400). While the 2007 ACC/AHA guidelines note that there is no substantial evidence that additional noninvasive testing will result in more appropriate selection of treatments [11], other consensus documents suggest that stress testing is reasonable. The recently updated Appropriate Use Criteria for Radionuclide Imaging suggest that referral for a nuclear stress test is "Appropriate"

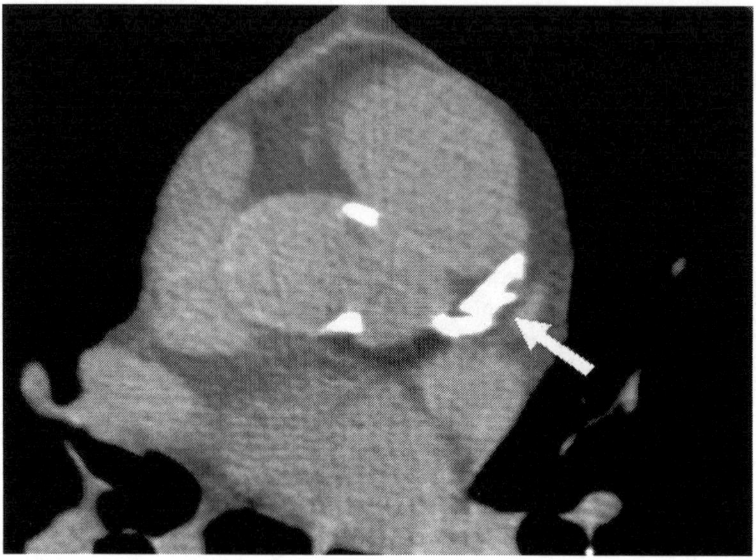

Fig. 3.1 Multidetector CT for coronary artery calcium scoring. The patient is an active 59-year-old asymptomatic male, with dyslipidemia and a strong family history of CAD. The total score, using the Agatston method, was 1,025. The majority of the calcification is seen in the proximal left anterior descending artery. Exercise nuclear stress test was normal. Aggressive risk modification with secondary prevention goals for traditional risk factors were employed

to screen for obstructive CAD in any patient with a CAC score of >400 and "Inappropriate" for any patient with a CAC score of <100 [14]. Among patients with calcium scores between 100 and 400, the appropriateness of nuclear stress testing depends on pretest Framingham risk. Patients with a CAC score of 100–400 and high Framingham risk are considered "Appropriate," while among patients with a CAC score of 100–400 who are at low-intermediate Framingham risk the value of nuclear stress testing is "Uncertain." We would agree that it is reasonable to evaluate patients with a CAC score of >400 with further noninvasive imaging options such as stress testing (see Fig. 3.1).

Is There A Role for Repeat Testing?

Another question, whose answer is not well-established, is whether there is a role for repeating a calcium score to monitor response to therapy or to look for a change in CHD prognosis. The validity of serial measurements of coronary calcium is dependent on whether changes in coronary calcium severity have prognostic relevance, and whether modification of cardiovascular risk factors modulates the progression of coronary calcium.

Observational and randomized studies have suggested that patients with a significant increase in coronary calcium over time experience higher event rates.

In one of the largest studies correlating CAC progression with event rates, Raggi et al. retrospectively examined rates of myocardial infarction (MI) among patients who had been referred for sequential EBCT, approximately 2 years apart, by their physicians [15]. Regardless of the patients' low-density lipoprotein (LDL) levels and treatment with statins, the patients who had at least a 15% increase in the amount of calcification were more likely to experience an MI. In addition, patients whose degree of calcification remained stable had lower event rates than patients whose calcification increased, even if the baseline score was higher.

A few prospective randomized trials have examined whether statin therapy affects the rate of coronary calcium progression [16–18]. The trials varied from using high-dose to low-dose statins, and focused on an array of populations, such as patients with low to intermediate risk, and postmenopausal women. Patients were re-imaged after 1–2 years of therapy. Despite a substantial lowering of LDL, none of the trials showed a significant difference between initial and subsequent calcium scores. Several potential explanations for the lack of change in calcium score have been proposed. The first is that follow-up longer than 1–2 years may be needed. Second, it is possible that statins impact structural components of calcified plaque that are not revealed by CT. Alternatively, it is possible that statins target only the degree of soft plaque, without changing calcified plaque at all, so that no change will be seen on CT.

While obtaining serial EBCTs is a potentially attractive method for evaluating risk over time, there is currently not enough evidence to recommend it, particularly given the expense and repeated radiation exposure.

Safety

A common concern regarding cardiac CT is the amount of radiation involved in each test. Radiation is measured in millisieverts (mSV), which is a standardized unit, allowing comparison between different modalities and protocols. It incorporates the amount of radiation absorbed in the organ(s) of interest, compared to total body radiation. A patient is typically exposed to 1–1.3 mSv with one EBCT. In comparison, a chest X-ray is 0.04–0.06, background radiation per year is 3.6, and a standard chest CT is 5–7 mSv.

As discussed above, it is important to distinguish between the safety profile of calcium scoring (MDCT or EBCT) and CT angiography. Obtaining a calcium score does not involve giving the patient a dye load, as is needed with CT angiography, and causes a substantially lower radiation dose – CT angiography can cause up to 21 mSv – depending on the protocol. Given the relatively small radiation dose of CT for coronary calcium, it is considered reasonable as a screening modality for appropriately selected asymptomatic patients. Because of the much higher radiation dose of CT angiography, it is currently not recommended for use as a screening tool for asymptomatic patients.

Special Populations

Several large epidemiologic studies have shown that coronary calcium scoring varies by factors such as age, gender, and ethnicity [19–22]. Coronary calcium has consistently been shown to be lower in women than in men, and to increase steadily with age, regardless of risk factors. For example, a large database of more than 35,000 patients referred for EBCT by their physicians showed that the median CAC for men aged 55–59 years was 49, compared to 1 for women [21]. Among men aged 70–74 years, the median increased to 309 and to 53 among women. Raggi et al. showed that even though the median calcium score increases significantly with age, it still provided incremental value for predicting future cardiovascular events, beyond traditional risk factors [22]. Interestingly, the difference between men and women became more attenuated with age.

There is also evidence that there are differing levels of coronary calcium among various ethnic groups. Data from the Multiethnic Study of Atherosclerosis (MESA) study showed that, when compared with Caucasians, black Hispanic, and Chinese individuals have 22, 15, and 8% less coronary calcium, even after controlling for preexisting risk factors [20]. The explanation for these differences is still being explored. Despite the differing degrees of calcification, the calcium score was still predictive of events in all four ethnic groups [23].

Given the variation of calcium scores based on demographics, Budoff et al. examined whether age- and sex-specific percentiles predicted cardiovascular events better than the absolute score [24]. The authors found that patients with an absolute calcium score of >400 experienced an increased risk of cardiovascular events, regardless of age or sex. In addition, patients with a low calcium score were at low risk of short-term events, regardless of the age- and sex-specific percentiles. It is important to note that the mean follow-up for this study was less than 4 years. Whether patients who have a low absolute score, but a high age- and sex-specific percentile experience more events over the long-term, and thus deserve an altered approach to evaluation and management, is not yet known.

Carotid Intima-Medial Thickness

What Is CIMT?

While carotid ultrasound has traditionally been used to identify obstructive plaque, it has more recently developed a broader role in further clarifying a patient's cardiovascular risk. Ultrasound can detect areas of increased thickness in the artery wall and areas of nonocclusive plaque, which represent early stages of atherosclerotic vascular disease. Imaging of the carotid wall produces two echogenic lines, which are the lumen-intima interface and the intima-media interface. The combined width of these two layers makes up the CIMT. While studies comparing findings on coronary angiography and CIMT have shown that CIMT is an independent predictor of coronary artery disease [25], the real value of CIMT is as marker of global atherosclerotic burden and as a predictor of future of cardiovascular events.

CIMT has been available for more than two decades and is a well-validated marker of cardiovascular risk. As a result, it has been the primary noninvasive imaging technique used for assessment of subclinical atherosclerosis in a wealth of large population studies evaluating coronary risk and randomized trials looking at response to therapies [26–29, 33, 35]. However, CIMT protocols have historically been time-consuming and technically challenging, thus limiting its use to research protocols in experienced centers [30]. These protocols involved imaging several sites within the carotid tree, including both the near and far walls of the common and internal carotid arteries (CCA and ICA), and the carotid bulb; analysis of the images required manual tracing along the two interfaces. While some of these protocols are still used in research studies, consensus has now emerged on simplified acquisition protocols and the use of automated border detection software [31]. As a result, CIMT is now much less time-consuming and technically challenging to obtain and analyze.

CIMT measurements obtained with these simplified protocols maintain robust prognostic value, but can be feasibly obtained in many settings, and thus are now available for clinical use for cardiovascular risk assessment. Recent guidelines by the American Society of Echocardiography (ASE) recommend CIMT measurements using widely available automated border detection software of the far wall of both the right and left CCA as the appropriate protocol for the clinical setting [31]. The CCA is preferable because of its superficial and stable location, linear shape, and high frequency of obtainable measurements. Imaging the far wall instead of the near wall minimizes artifact.

While this single site CIMT measurement is recommended, it should always be accompanied by a thorough circumferential scan along the entire length of the extracranial carotid arteries, including the ICA and the bulb, to look for nonobstructive plaque (defined as a focal thickening at least 50% greater than the adjacent wall or an absolute thickness greater than 1.5 mm). Plaque is most commonly seen in the carotid bulb, where blood flow is less laminar, and the carotid wall is subject to more sheer stress. The plaque screen serves as an alternative indication of subclinical vascular disease. The presence of plaque, regardless of a patient's CIMT, signifies subclinical atherosclerotic disease.

Does CIMT Predict Cardiovascular Events?

Several large prospective epidemiologic studies have examined the ability of CIMT to help estimate cardiovascular risk. The studies have focused primarily on asymptomatic patients without known cardiovascular disease, aged 45 and older, although one study included adults as young as 19 [26–29]. All of the studies followed at least 4,000 individuals and showed that CIMT was a potent predictor of future cardiovascular events.

For example, in the Atherosclerosis Risk in Communities (ARIC) study, which followed more than 12,000 patients for 5 years, there was a clear stepwise progression of increased CIMT thickness and increased cardiovascular risk [26]. When nonobstructive plaque is identified, the relative risk of future cardiovascular events is even higher than that based on CIMT alone [30–32].

Does CIMT Add to Traditional Office-Based Risk Assessment?

In all studies mentioned previously, increasing CIMT was associated with increased risk even after adjusting for traditional cardiovascular risk factors. Other studies have evaluated the ability of CIMT measurements to alter risk prediction above Framingham risk scoring. Baird et al. performed CIMT on 95 patients at intermediate Framingham risk and found that using absolute CIMT cutoff values (>1.0 mm = high risk, <0.8 mm = low risk), CIMT testing was able to re-classify 63% of patients into low- or high-risk categories [32]. Additional compelling evidence comes from the enrollment of the recent METEOR trial [33]. This trial was designed to evaluate the effect of rosuvastatin on atherosclerosis as measured by CIMT in a population defined as low risk based on traditional risk factors. However, to gain enrollment, patients additionally had to have a maximal CIMT measurement of >1.2 mm, which represents a high-risk CIMT result for any age and gender. Thus, the enrollment of this trial is an example of a cohort of patients with advanced subclinical atherosclerosis that would not be expected based on traditional risk factors. While these examples do not establish the role of CIMT testing in clinical practice, they do give hints as to how CIMT might be employed to improve risk stratification in certain populations.

What Is the Definition of An Abnormal CIMT Measurement?

While the prognostic value of CIMT measurements has long since been established, an additional limitation to the widespread clinical use of CIMT has been the lack of a clear definition of an abnormal result. CIMT tends to increase with age and is higher in men than women for a given age group. The ARIC study showed that CIMT also tends to be higher among African-American men than Caucasian men [26]. For example, the 75th percentile of CIMT for a 65-year-old Caucasian woman is 0.81 mm, whereas for an African-American male it is 1.0 mm. Thus, it is difficult to establish a single CIMT thickness cutoff as evidence of subclinical atherosclerosis. Recently, with the widespread availability of age- and gender-adjusted nomograms from large randomized trials, consensus has emerged on a definition of an abnormal CIMT. Regardless of clinical factors, a value of CIMT greater than the 75th percentile for age, gender, and race, or the presence of nonobstructive plaque, should be considered abnormal and evidence of advanced subclinical atherosclerosis [30–32].

What Should Be Done with Abnormal Results?

Based on the wealth of prognostic data, there is now consensus on who could benefit from CIMT testing for further stratification of cardiovascular risk. As with calcium scoring, the use of CIMT is only recommended for those patients in whom the decision about how aggressively to manage their risk factors would be altered by the results [30, 31]. According to the ASE consensus statement, CIMT is a reasonable option for further risk assessment in patients at intermediate Framingham risk (defined in this document as of 6–20% 10-year risk) and without established CVD or risk-equivalents, such as diabetes [31]. This document also suggests that CIMT could be considered in additional groups who may not have elevated Framingham risk scores, but have been shown in other studies to have higher event rates. These groups include patients with a family history of CAD in a first-degree relative, individuals younger than 60 with severe abnormalities in one risk factor, such as a genetic dyslipidemia, or women younger than 60 who have at least two CVD risk factors.

A number of ways have been proposed to incorporate the result into the clinical management of patients. The most common and widely accepted is to consider a CIMT result as normal or abnormal (>75th percentile for age, gender, race, or presence of plaque) and to consider those with an abnormal result to have advanced subclinical atherosclerosis. Using this approach, it would be reasonable to pursue more aggressive (secondary prevention) treatment goals for traditional risk factors in those with an abnormal CIMT result (see Fig. 3.2).

An alternative and more controversial approach which has been suggested to help make the CIMT result more meaningful to patients and health care professionals involves calculating a so-called "vascular age" [34]. This involves determining the

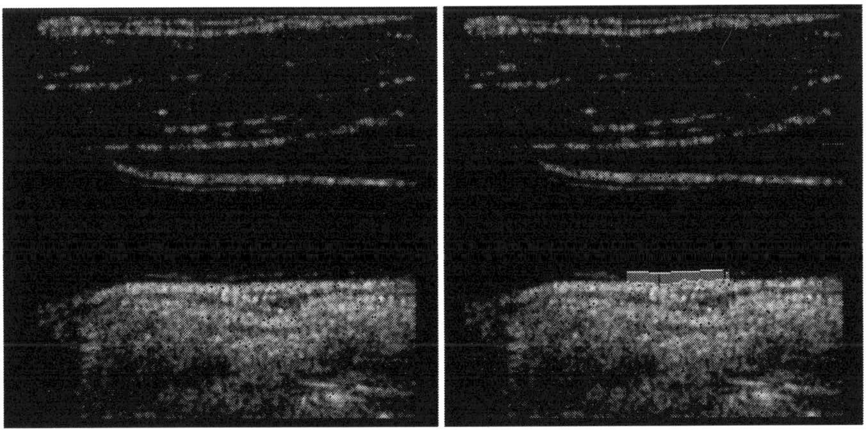

Fig. 3.2 Carotid intima-medial thickness (CIMT) measurement in a 47-year-old asymptomatic man with a strong family history of CAD. Framingham 10-year risk based on traditional risk factors = 10%. Mean common carotid CIMT = 0.81 mm, which is abnormal (86th percentile for age, gender, and race). Given this evidence of early subclinical atherosclerosis, aggressive risk modification with secondary prevention goals for traditional risk factors were employed

age at which a patient's CIMT value would be at the 50th percentile. For example, a 45-year African-American woman with a CIMT of 0.678 mm would be in the 71st percentile for her age group. This would be the 50th percentile for a woman of 55, thus giving this patient a "vascular age" of 55. When a patient's chronologic age is replaced by this "vascular age" in Framingham risk calculators, a new post-CIMT risk can be estimated. Gepner et al. examined this approach in more than 500 asymptomatic patients, aged 40–70 years [34]. The authors calculated each patient's vascular age by comparing their CIMT to race and sex-adjusted nomograms from the ARIC study. Substituting vascular age for chronological age increased the overall 10-year cardiovascular risk of Gepner's study population from 5.1 to 7.7%, and 56% of patients had a change in risk of >5%. While this strategy represents an appealing way to incorporate CIMT results into a clinical algorithm, it should be noted that this approach has not been validated or endorsed in consensus documents at this time.

Is There A Role for Repeat Testing?

Another question that has not yet been fully explored in the literature is whether to repeat CIMT to monitor progression of disease or response to therapy. A few studies have demonstrated that, depending on the population being treated, statin therapy can stop progression of CIMT or even cause regression. For example, in the METEOR trial mentioned above, the patients treated with placebo had a slight progression of their CIMT, whereas the patients treated with rosuvastatin remained stable [33]. The ARBITER trial focused on a higher risk population, and as a result had more dramatic results [35]. Only patients who already qualified for statin therapy based on risk factors alone were enrolled and randomized to either high- or low-dose statin. After 12 months, the patients on high-dose statin therapy had both a lower LDL and regression of CIMT, whereas the CIMT for patients with low-dose statin remained unchanged.

Despite data showing that it is possible to document changes in CIMT, serial CIMT imaging in the clinical arena is not currently recommended [31]. This is for a number of reasons. First, data using serial exams are only in large randomized trials using more complicated protocols. It is unclear that the findings are applicable to the more simplified protocols used in clinical practice. Second, it is still not known what degree of change in CIMT, or over what period of time, correlates with a change in outcome. As a result, it is not clear how clinicians should respond to the results of repeated images. Third, as CIMT represents a surrogate end point, it is not established that subtle changes in CIMT over time portend an improved prognosis.

Safety

Given that CIMT does not expose a patient to radiation, there is no safety risk. However, it is important that physicians and ultrasound technicians who perform and interpret CIMT testing be trained and experienced to ensure accurate and reproducible results.

Conclusion: Which Test to Choose?

Once the decision has been made to pursue imaging, there is little data to support the additional decision of which modality to use. To date, there are only two prospective studies comparing the abilities of CAC and CIMT to help predict cardiovascular event rates. The first study found that CAC was a slightly better predictor of cardiac events, while CIMT was a slightly better predictor of stroke [36]. The second study showed that the two tests were comparable [37]. As a result, availability and local expertise should be the primary consideration in choosing between CAC scoring and CIMT for further risk stratification in appropriately selected patients.

References

1. Castelli WP. Lipids, risk factors and ischaemic heart disease. Atherosclerosis. 1996; 124(Suppl):S1–9.
2. Rosamond WD, Chambless LE, Folsom AR, et al. Trends in the incidence of myocardial infarction and in mortality due to coronary heart disease, 1987 to 1994. N Engl J Med. 1998;339:861–7.
3. Agatston AS, Janowitz WR, Hildner FJ, Zusmer NR, Viamonte Jr M, Detrano R. Quantification of coronary artery calcium using ultrafast computed tomography. J Am Coll Cardiol. 1990;15(4):827–32.
4. Rumberger JA, Simons DB, Fitzpatrick LA, Sheedy PF, Schwartz RS. Coronary artery calcium area by electron-beam computed tomography and coronary atherosclerotic plaque area. A histopathologic correlative study. Circulation. 1995;92(8):2157–62.
5. Haberl R, Becker A, Leber A, et al. Correlation of coronary calcification and angiographically documented stenoses in patients with suspected coronary artery disease: results of 1,764 patients. J Am Coll Cardiol. 2001;37(2):451–7.
6. Knez A, Becker A, Leber A, et al. Relation of coronary calcium scores by electron beam tomography to obstructive disease in 2,115 symptomatic patients. Am J Cardiol. 2004;93(9):1150–2.
7. Rubinshtein R, Gaspar T, Halon DA, Goldstein J, Peled N, Lewis BS. Prevalence and extent of obstructive coronary artery disease in patients with zero or low calcium score undergoing 64-slice cardiac multidetector computed tomography for evaluation of a chest pain syndrome. Am J Cardiol. 2007;99(4):472–5.
8. Johnson RC, Leopold JA, Loscalzo J. Vascular calcification: pathobiological mechanisms and clinical implications. Circ Res. 2006;99(10):1044–59.
9. Beckman JA, Ganz J, Creager MA, Ganz P, Kinlay S. Relationship of clinical presentation and calcification of culprit coronary artery stenoses. Arterioscler Thromb Vasc Biol. 2001;21(10):1618–22.
10. Ehara S, Kobayashi Y, Yoshiyama M, et al. Spotty calcification typifies the culprit plaque in patients with acute myocardial infarction: an intravascular ultrasound study. Circulation. 2004;110(22):3424–9.
11. Greenland P, Bonow RO, Brundage BH, et al. ACCF/AHA 2007 clinical expert consensus document on coronary artery calcium scoring by computed tomography in global cardiovascular risk assessment and in evaluation of patients with chest pain: a report of the American College of Cardiology Foundation Clinical Expert Consensus Task Force (ACCF/AHA Writing Committee to Update the 2000 Expert Consensus Document on Electron Beam Computed Tomography). Circulation. 2007;115(3):402–26.
12. Budoff MJ, Shaw LJ, Liu ST, et al. Long-term prognosis associated with coronary calcification: observations from a registry of 25,253 patients. J Am Coll Cardiol. 2007;49(18):1860–70.

13. Greenland P, LaBree L, Azen SP, Doherty TM, Detrano RC. Coronary artery calcium score combined with Framingham score for risk prediction in asymptomatic individuals. JAMA. 2004;291(2):210–5.
14. Hendel RC, Berman DS, DiCarli MF, et al. ACCF/ASNC/ACR/AHA/ASE/SCCT/SCMR/SNM 2009 appropriate use criteria for cardiac radionuclide imaging: a report of the American College of Cardiology Foundation Appropriate Use Criteria Task Force, the American Society of Nuclear Cardiology, the American College of Radiology, the American Heart Association, the American Society of Echocardiography, the Society of Cardiovascular Computed Tomography, the Society for Cardiovascular Magnetic Resonance, and the Society of Nuclear Medicine: endorsed by the American College of Emergency Physicians. Circulation. 2009;119:e561–87.
15. Raggi P, Cooil B, Shaw LJ, et al. Progression of coronary calcium on serial electron beam tomographic scanning is greater in patients with future myocardial infarction. Am J Cardiol. 2003;92(7):827–9.
16. Arad Y, Spadaro LA, Roth M, Newstein D, Guerci AD. Treatment of asymptomatic adults with elevated coronary calcium scores with atorvastatin, vitamin C, and vitamin E: the St. Francis Heart Study randomized clinical trial. J Am Coll Cardiol. 2005;46(1):166–72.
17. Raggi P, Callister TQ, Shaw LJ. Progression of coronary artery calcium and risk of first myocardial infarction in patients receiving cholesterol-lowering therapy. Arterioscler Thromb Vasc Biol. 2004;24(7):1272–7.
18. Raggi P, Davidson M, Callister TQ, et al. Aggressive versus moderate lipid-lowering therapy in hypercholesterolemic postmenopausal women: beyond endorsed lipid lowering with EBT scanning (BELLES). Circulation. 2005;112(4):563–71.
19. Bild DE, Folsom AR, Lowe LP, et al. Prevalence and correlates of coronary calcification in black and white young adults: the Coronary Artery Risk Development in Young Adults (CARDIA) Study. Arterioscler Thromb Vasc Biol. 2001;21(5):852–7.
20. Bild DE, Detrano R, Peterson D, et al. Ethnic differences in coronary calcification: the Multi-Ethnic Study of Atherosclerosis (MESA). Circulation. 2005;111(10):1313–20.
21. Hoff JA, Chomka EV, Krainik AJ, Daviglus M, Rich S, Kondos GT. Age and gender distributions of coronary artery calcium detected by electron beam tomography in 35,246 adults. Am J Cardiol. 2001;87(12):1335–9.
22. Raggi P, Gongora MC, Gopal A, Callister TQ, Budoff M, Shaw LJ. Coronary artery calcium to predict all-cause mortality in elderly men and women. J Am Coll Cardiol. 2008;52(1):17–23.
23. Detrano R, Guerci AD, Carr JJ, et al. Coronary calcium as a predictor of coronary events in four racial or ethnic groups. N Engl J Med. 2008;358(13):1336–45.
24. Budoff MJ, Nasir K, McClelland RL, et al. Coronary calcium predicts events better with absolute calcium scores than age-sex-race/ethnicity percentiles: MESA (Multi-Ethnic Study of Atherosclerosis). J Am Coll Cardiol. 2009;53(4):345–52.
25. Lekakis JP, Papamichael CM, Cimponeriu AT, et al. Atherosclerotic changes of extracoronary arteries are associated with the extent of coronary atherosclerosis. Am J Cardiol. 2000;85(8):949–52.
26. Chambless LE, Heiss G, Folsom AR, et al. Association of coronary heart disease incidence with carotid arterial wall thickness and major risk factors: the Atherosclerosis Risk in Communities (ARIC) Study, 1987–1993. Am J Epidemiol. 1997;146(6):483–94.
27. Lorenz MW, von Kegler S, Steinmetz H, Markus HS, Sitzer M. Carotid intima-media thickening indicates a higher vascular risk across a wide age range: prospective data from the Carotid Atherosclerosis Progression Study (CAPS). Stroke. 2006;37(1):87–92.
28. O'Leary DH, Polak JF, Kronmal RA, Manolio TA, Burke GL, Wolfson Jr SK. Carotid-artery intima and media thickness as a risk factor for myocardial infarction and stroke in older adults. Cardiovascular Health Study Collaborative Research Group. N Engl J Med. 1999;340(1):14–22.
29. van der Meer IM, Bots ML, Hofman A, del Sol AI, van der Kuip DA, Witteman JC. Predictive value of noninvasive measures of atherosclerosis for incident myocardial infarction: the Rotterdam Study. Circulation. 2004;109(9):1089–94.
30. Roman MJ, Naqvi TZ, Gardin JM, Gerhard-Herman M, Jaff M, Mohler E. Clinical application of noninvasive vascular ultrasound in cardiovascular risk stratification: a report from the

American Society of Echocardiography and the Society of Vascular Medicine and Biology. J Am Soc Echocardiogr. 2006;19(8):943–54.
31. Stein JH, Korcarz CE, Hurst RT, et al. Use of carotid ultrasound to identify subclinical vascular disease and evaluate cardiovascular disease risk: a consensus statement from the American Society of Echocardiography Carotid Intima-Media Thickness Task Force. Endorsed by the Society for Vascular Medicine. J Am Soc Echocardiogr. 2008;21(2):93–111.
32. Bard RL, Kalsi H, Rubenfire M, et al. Effect of carotid atherosclerosis screening on risk stratification during primary cardiovascular disease prevention. Am J Cardiol. 2004;93:1030–2.
33. Crouse III JR, Raichlen JS, Riley WA, et al. Effect of rosuvastatin on progression of carotid intima-media thickness in low-risk individuals with subclinical atherosclerosis: the METEOR Trial. JAMA. 2007;297(12):1344–53.
34. Gepner AD, Keevil JG, Wyman RA, et al. Use of carotid intima-media thickness and vascular age to modify cardiovascular risk prediction. J Am Soc Echocardiogr. 2006;19(9):1170–4.
35. Taylor AJ, Kent SM, Flaherty PJ, Coyle LC, Markwood TT, Vernalis MN. ARBITER: Arterial Biology for the Investigation of the Treatment Effects of Reducing Cholesterol: a randomized trial comparing the effects of atorvastatin and pravastatin on carotid intima medial thickness. Circulation. 2002;106(16):2055–60.
36. Folsom AR, Kronmal RA, Detrano RC, et al. Coronary artery calcification compared with carotid intima-media thickness in the prediction of cardiovascular disease incidence: the Multi-Ethnic Study of Atherosclerosis (MESA). Arch Intern Med. 2008;168(12):1333–9.
37. Newman AB, Naydeck BL, Ives DG, et al. Coronary artery calcium, carotid artery wall thickness, and cardiovascular disease outcomes in adults 70 to 99 years old. Am J Cardiol. 2008;101(2):186–92.

Chapter 4
Inherited Lipoprotein Disorders

Ewa Dembowski and Michael H. Davidson

Keywords Hypertriglyceridemia • Familial combined hyperlipidemia • Familial hypercholesterolemia • Hypoalphalipoproteinemia

Abnormal lipoprotein metabolism is a major predisposing factor to atherosclerosis. Dyslipidemia is present in over 70% of patients with premature coronary heart disease (CHD), (<60 years of age in men and <65 years in women) and over 50% of these patients have a familial lipoprotein disorder [1–3]. The genetic basis for several lipoprotein disorders has been elucidated in the past two decades. The majority of these disorders result from a combination of polygenic predisposition and poor lifestyle habits, including physical inactivity, increased visceral adipose tissue, increased caloric intake, and cigarette smoking. Monogenic disorders are less common; however, important to diagnose. Unraveling the genetic basis of many lipoprotein disorders has allowed fundamental discoveries in molecular cellular physiology and has paved the way for novel therapeutic approaches for CHD. This chapter describes the known inherited lipoprotein disorders. A classification of the genetic disorders of lipoprotein metabolism and their molecular etiology is summarized in Table 4.1.

Screening for genetic lipid disorders provides an opportunity to include family members in a CHD prevention program who may have otherwise not been aware of their increased risk. A strong family history of premature CHD is often a source of much anxiety for a patient, and, if the genetic disorder can be correctly diagnosed and effectively treated, the patient is frequently relieved of the anxiety. Screening begins

---

M.H. Davidson (✉)
Department of Medicine, Section of Cardiology,
University of Chicago Pritzker School of Medicine, Chicago, IL 60637, USA
e-mail: mdavidso@medicine.bsd.uchicago.edu

M.J. Sorrentino (ed.), *Hyperlipidemia in Primary Care: A Practical Guide to Risk Reduction*, Current Clinical Practice, DOI 10.1007/978-1-60327-502-6_4,

Table 4.1 Genetic disorders of lipoprotein metabolism

Lipoprotein affected	Genetic disorder	Gene defect		Incidence	Clinical findings
↑ TG-RLPs	Lipoprotein lipase deficiency	LPL	AR	$<1/10^6$	Eruptive xanthomas, hepato splenomegaly, pancreatitis
	Familial Apo C-II deficiency	Apo C-II	AR	$<1/10^6$	Eruptive xanthomas, hepatosplenomegaly
	Familial hypertriglyceridemia (FHTG)	Polygenic	AD	1/300	Corneal arcus, xanthelasmas, eruptive xanthomas
	Familial combined hyperlipidemia (FCH)	Polygenic	AD	1/200	Premature CHD, corneal arcus, xanthelasmas
	Familial dysbetalipoproteinemia (FD)	Apo E	AR	1/10,000	Premature CHD, palmar, and tuberoeruptive xanthomas
↑ LDL	Familial hypercholesterolemia (FH)	LDLR	AD	1/500	Tendon xanthomas, xanthelas-mas, corneal arcus, premature CHD
	Familial defective Apo B-100 (FDB)	Apo B	AD	1/1,000	
	Autosomal recessive hypercholesterolemia (ARH)	ARH	AR	~50 Cases	
	Autosomal dominant hypercholesterolemia (ADH)	PCSK9	AD	~50 Cases	
	Sitosterolemia	ABCG5, ABCG8	AR	~50 Cases	
↑ Lp(a)	Familial Lp(a) hyperlipoproteinemia	Apo (a)	AD	AD	Premature CHD
↓ LDL	Abetalipoproteinemia	MTP	AR	~100 Cases	Fat malabsorption, spinocere bellar degeneration, retinopathy, possible hepatic steatosis
	Hypobetalipoproteinemia	Apo B	AD		Protection against CHD

↓ HDL	Apo A-I deficiency	Apo A1	AD	Rare	Premature CHD
	Tangier disease	ABCA1	AD	~50 Cases	Hepatosplenomegaly, enlarged orange tonsils, premature CHD
	Familial LCAT deficiency	LCAT	AD	~50 Cases	Corneal opacification, hemolytic anemia, progressive renal insufficiency
↑ HDL	CETP deficiency	CETP	AD	Rare	Possible protection against CHD

TG-RLP triglyceride-rich lipoprotein, *LDL* low-density lipoprotein, *HDL* high-density lipoprotein, *Apo* apolipoprotein, *AR* autosomal recessive, *AD* autosomal dominant, *CHD* coronary heart disease, *LCAT* lecithin:cholesterol acyltransferase, *CETP* cholesterol ester transfer protein

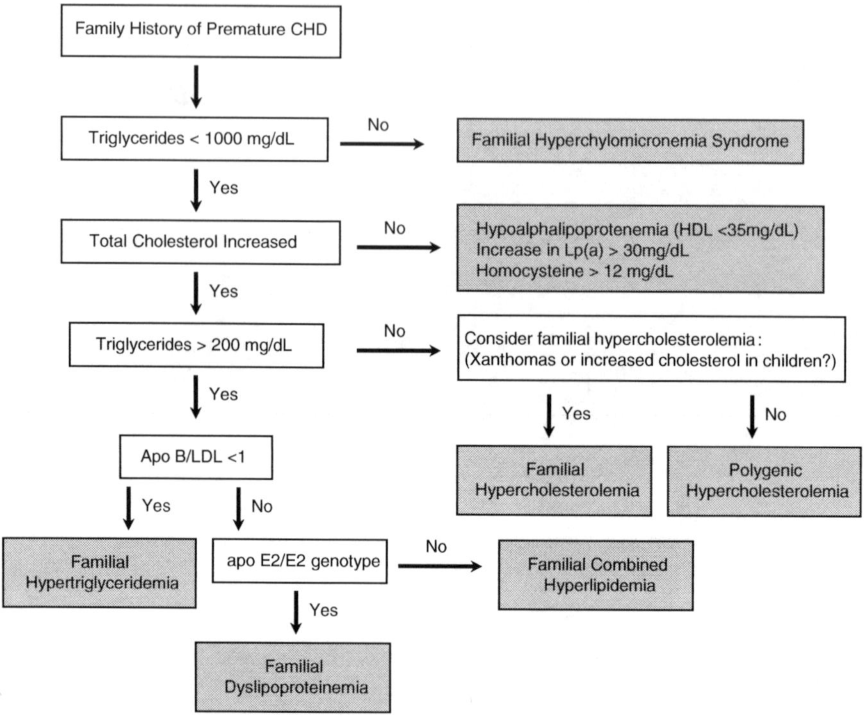

Fig. 4.1 Simplified algorithm for the diagnosis of common genetic lipoprotein disorders. *Apo* apolipoprotein, *HDL* high-density lipoprotein, *LDL* low-density lipoprotein, *Lp(a)* lipoprotein(a)

with a standard lipid profile; if this is normal, further testing should be performed with consideration paid to measurement of lipoprotein(a) and apolipoproteins (Apo) B and A-1; approximately 25% of patients with premature CHD and a normal standard profile will have an abnormality in one of these factors [4]. Figure 4.1 provides a simplified algorithm for the diagnosis of common genetic lipoprotein disorders.

Inherited Disorders of Triglyceride-Rich Lipoproteins

Almost all triglycerides are found in chylomicrons, very low-density lipoprotein (VLDL), and IDL also known as the triglyceride-rich lipoprotein particles (TG-RLPs). Genetic disorders that increase the plasma levels of TG-RLPs thus result in hypertriglyceridemia. Often, the ratio of the triglyceride to the cholesterol level in the serum can provide a clue to which TG-RLP is elevated. Chylomicrons, VLDL, and IDL have a ratio of triglycerides to cholesterol in each particle of 10:1, 5:1, and 1:1, respectively (Fig. 4.2). Thus, when chylomicrons are elevated, the serum triglycerides are usually ten times higher than the serum total cholesterol. However, if the triglycerides are only twice as high as the total cholesterol, then

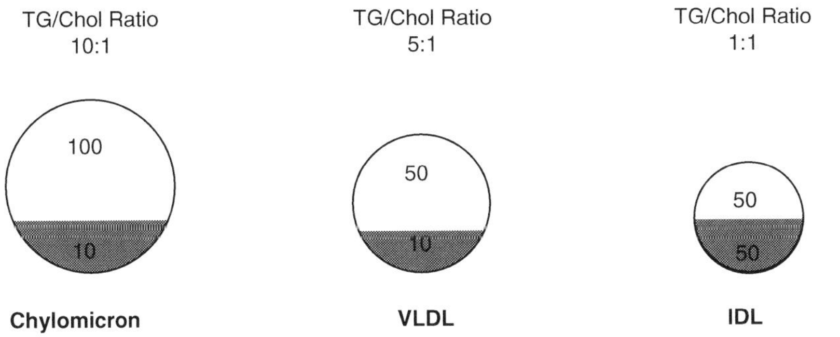

Fig. 4.2 Triglyceride (TG) and cholesterol (Chol) composition of the various classes of lipoproteins. The ratio of triglyceride to cholesterol level in the serum can provide a clue to which triglyceride-rich particles are elevated. *IDL* intermediate-density lipoprotein, *VLDL* very low-density lipoprotein

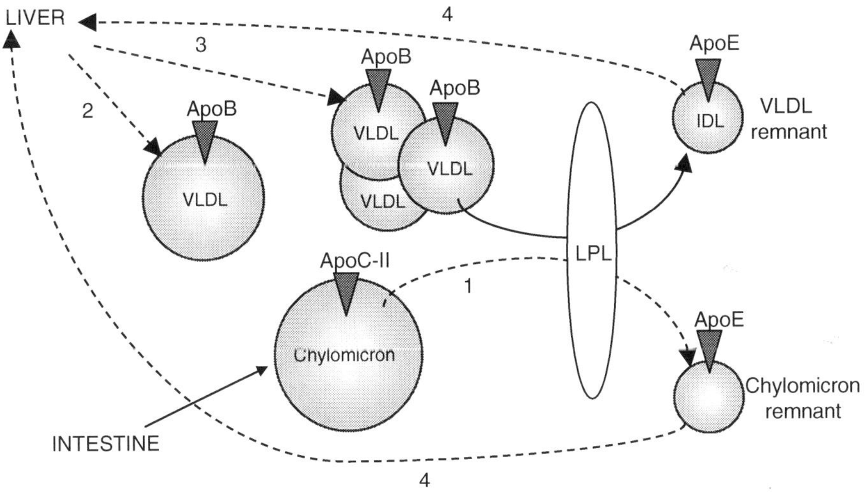

Fig. 4.3 Summary of the inherited disorders with elevated triglycerides. (1) Familial hyperchylomicronemia syndrome (FCS): deficient or impaired Apo C-II or LPL leads to accumulation of chylomicrons in the circulation. (2) Familial hypertriglyceridemia (FHTG): secretion of large VLDL particles. (3) Familial combined hyperlipidemia (FCH): overproduction of Apo B resulting in secretion of more VLDL particles. (4) Familial dysbetalipoproteinemia (Type III): Apo E2:E2 genotype causes defective removal of chylomicron and VLDL remnants (IDL). *LPL* lipoprotein lipase, *LDL* low-density lipoprotein, *IDL* intermediate-density lipoprotein, *VLDL* very low-density lipoprotein

VLDL is usually the culprit elevated lipoprotein. If both triglycerides and total cholesterol are equally elevated, the patient has an increase in IDL or a combination of high VLDL and low-density lipoprotein (LDL).

Figure 4.3 summarizes the four major genetic disorders resulting in a disorder with elevated triglycerides.

Familial Chylomicronemia Syndrome

Chylomicronemia is a rare disorder characterized by the body's inability to reduce circulating triglyceride-rich chylomicrons. Chylomicrons, formed in the intestines after absorption of dietary fat and cholesterol, account for the postprandial rise in triglycerides. Usually, fat absorption is generally complete within a few hours of food ingestion. In patients with hyperchylomicronemia, however, chylomicrons are present in plasma after a 12-h fast resulting in lipemic plasma (a creamy layer forming on the surface of the plasma).

Chylomicron metabolism requires the action of lipoprotein lipase (LPL) and the cofactor Apo C-II. Genetic causes of the familial chylomicronemia syndrome (FCS) include: deficiency of LPL, deficiency of Apo C-II, and presence of inhibitor of LPL. LPL deficiency is the most common underlying molecular defect leading to FCS [5]. This is a rare, autosomal recessive disorder affecting approximately one in one million persons. The frequency of LPL deficiency is higher in selected populations such as the French Canadians. Homozygous mutations in LPL resulting in complete loss of catalytic activity are rare, but heterozygous mutations are quite common worldwide. The clinical presentation of the obligate heterozygotes is highly variable [5]. The diagnosis of LPL deficiency can be confirmed by the measurement of LPL activity in the plasma after intravenous heparin injection (postheparin LPL activity). Apo C-II deficiency is also inherited as an autosomal recessive trait while LPL inhibitors [6] seem to have an autosomal dominant transmission. The clinical manifestations of these disorders are similar to those with LPL deficiency except that patients tend to have a milder and later onset of the chylomicronemia syndrome.

The FCS is characterized by severe fasting hypertriglyceridemia (usually greater than 1,000 mg/dL) and massive accumulations of chylomicrons in the plasma [7]. Phagocytosis of chylomicrons by macrophages in the skin results in the formation of eruptive xanthomas, small yellow papular lesions most often localized over the buttocks and extensor surfaces of the arms and legs. On fundoscopic examination, lipemia retinalis may be evident in patients with triglyceride levels greater than 4,000 mg/dL. The retinal vessels appear lipemic, and the fundus has a pale pink appearance as a result of light scattering by circulating chylomicrons. Although premature cardiovascular disease has been identified in some patients with FCS, the major morbidity associated with the disorder is recurrent episodes of pancreatitis, which, in some patients, have resulted in development of pancreatic necrosis and death.

Primary therapy for FCS is restriction of total dietary fat. Caloric supplementation with medium-chain triglycerides, which are absorbed directly into the portal vein and therefore do not promote chylomicron formation, can be used if necessary. Some patients may respond to omega-3-fatty acids (fish oils) or fibrates. The goal of therapy is to reduce plasma triglycerides to levels less than 100 mg/dL, which will reverse all of the clinical manifestations of FCS. Gene therapy with an adenovirus vector encoding human LPL is currently being studied as a treatment for those with LPL deficiency [8].

Familial Hypertriglyceridemia

Familial hypertriglyceridemia (FHTG) is a relatively common inherited disorder of unknown molecular etiology [9]. The disorder is characterized by increased levels of plasma triglycerides and VLDL, LDL, and high-density lipoprotein (HDL) cholesterol levels are usually low, and total cholesterol is normal or slightly elevated. VLDL, which is synthesized in the liver, represents the endogenous rather than exogenous source of triglycerides and cholesterol in the blood. It is assembled in the hepatocytes by microsomal transfer protein (MTP) by combining Apo B-100 with triglycerides, cholesterol, and phospholipids. In FHTG, an autosomal dominant genetic disorder, there is an abnormality in the assembly of the particle resulting in enlarged VLDL particles. Because the VLDL particles are enlarged rather than more plentiful, the Apo B level is often normal, and the ratio of Apo B to LDL is less than 1.0.

FHTG is often not associated with a significantly increased risk of CHD. Therapy for FHTG involves lifestyle management, especially weight control, and reduction in simple carbohydrates in the diet and of alcohol. Lipid-lowering drug therapy with statins, fibrates, niacin, or omega-3-fatty acids are all reasonable considerations.

Familial Combined Hyperlipidemia

The more common and potentially higher-risk VLDL disorder is familial combined hyperlipidemia (FCH) [10]. In this autosomal dominant disorder, Apo B overproduction results in secretion of more VLDL particles rather than enlarged VLDL particles. These abundant VLDL particles oversaturate the ability of LPL to break down all the triglycerides, resulting in triglyceride-enriched LDL, which are further metabolized by hepatic lipase to form dense LDL particles. Because the LDL particles are small and dense, the total LDL cholesterol (LDL-C) level may not be significantly elevated and the Apo B/LDL ratio is frequently greater than or equal to 1.0. The more prevalent VLDL particles also exchange their triglycerides for cholesterol in HDL, resulting in lower HDL cholesterol (HDL-C) levels. The net result is a combined elevation of both triglycerides and LDL, with low HDL and significantly increased risk for premature CHD.

FCH is the most common form of familial dyslipoproteinemia leading to increased risk for atherosclerosis [11]. Its prevalence is estimated to be 1 in 200 persons in the general population, and about 1 in 5 patients with CHD under the age of 60. This genetic disorder is important to diagnose because the risk of CHD is very high [9]. Among family members, the lipid profile can vary from pure hypercholesterolemia to combined hyperlipidemia to isolated hypertriglyceridemia. The disorder may not be as evident in childhood or in premenopausal women. Weight gain, especially visceral fat increase, usually worsens the condition, and the patients are at much higher risk for insulin resistance leading to the metabolic syndrome and type 2 diabetes. Patients with FCHL should be treated aggressively with lifestyle management and drug therapy. Statins, fibrates, niacin, and cholesterol absorption inhibitors are all used, often in different combinations, to achieve adequate control of lipids.

Familial Dysbetalipoproteinemia (Type III Hyperlipoproteinemia)

Familial dysbetalipoproteinemia (FD), also known as Type III hyperlipidemia, is a rare genetic lipoprotein disorder characterized by tuberoeruptive xanthomas (clusters of small papules on the elbows, knees, and buttocks) and palmar xanthomas (orange-yellow discoloration in the creases of the palms) [12]. The disorder is caused by mutations in the gene for apolipoprotein E (Apo E). Apo E is present on chylomicron and VLDL remnants, and mediates their removal from the plasma by binding to receptors in the liver. Defective Apo E is impaired in its ability to bind to these receptors, resulting in the accumulation of remnant lipoprotein or IDL [13]. The biochemical profile shows elevated cholesterol and triglycerides often to a similar degree as well as elevated Apo E levels and low HDL-C. Premature atherosclerotic CHD is often seen in this disorder, making aggressive drug therapy mandatory.

There are three different Apo E alleles (E2, E3, and E4), with the most prevalent being the Apo E3 allele [13]. FD is most commonly caused by the Apo E2 allele. Apo E2 differs from Apo E3 by a single amino acid. Although the prevalence of the Apo E2/2 genotype occurs at a population frequency of less than 1%, it is estimated that the prevalence of type III dysbetalipoproteinemia is less than 1 in 10,000 in the population. A second genetic "hit" is postulated to be necessary for expression of the lipid disorder. Obesity, diabetes mellitus, hypothyroidism, renal disease, and alcohol use are all associated with an increased probability of FD in Apo E2/E2 patients, but many patients with FD do not have an obvious second hit.

Inherited Disorders of LDL Metabolism

Disorders of Elevated LDL

Plasma levels of LDL-C are directly related to the incidence of CHD and cardiovascular deaths. Approximately 50% of the variation in plasma levels of LDL-C is attributable to genetic variation [14]. The major portion of this genetic variation is polygenic, reflecting the multiple variables in any given individual. A subset of patients with very high plasma LDL-C levels have monogenic forms of hypercholesterolemia, which are associated with the deposition of cholesterol in tissues, producing xanthomas and xanthelasmas, as well as premature coronary atherosclerosis. Figure 4.4 summarizes the two most common inherited disorders of elevated LDL-C.

Familial Hypercholesterolemia

Familial hypercholesterolemia (FH) is the most common and most severe form of monogenic hypercholesterolemia. It is the first genetic disease of lipid metabolism to be clinically and molecularly characterized [15]. The disorder has an autosomal

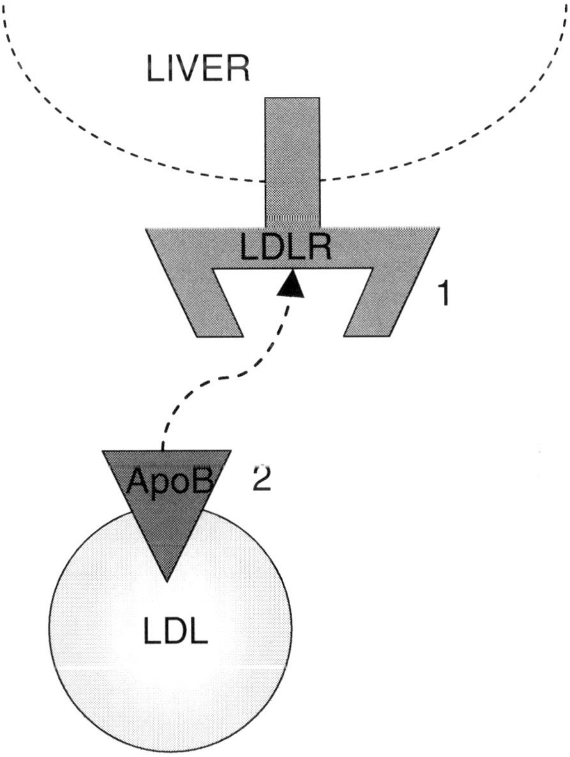

Fig. 4.4 Schematic of the most common inherited disorders with elevated LDL-C. (1) Familial hypercholesterolemia (FH): reduction in functional hepatic LDLR leads to reduced clearance of plasma LDL by the liver. (2) Familial defective apolipoprotein B-100 (FDB): defective Apo B, the ligand for LDLR, results in impaired binding and reduced clearance of LDL. *LDL* low-density lipoprotein, *LDLR* low-density lipoprotein receptor, *Apo B* apolipoprotein B

co-dominant pattern of inheritance and is caused by mutations in the LDL receptor gene (*LDLR*) leading to impairment or absence of the LDL receptor, reduced clearance of plasma LDL by the liver, and substantial elevations in LDL-C [16–19].

Homozygous FH patients (1 in 1,000,000) are severely affected with plasma levels of LDL-C that are uniformly very high, irrespective of diet, medications, or lifestyle. The LDL levels often exceed 1,000 mg/dL at birth, and these children develop coronary atherosclerosis at an early age. Atherosclerosis develops initially in the aortic root, causing supravalvular aortic stenosis, and then extends into the coronary ostia. The severity of atherosclerosis is proportional to the extent and duration of elevated plasma LDL-C levels (calculated as the cholesterol-year score) [20]. If the LDL-C level is not effectively reduced, FH homozygotes die prematurely of atherosclerotic cardiovascular disease. Optimization of other cardiovascular risk factors has little impact on the clinical course of the disease.

Patients with homozygous FH are classified into one of two major groups based on the amount of LDL receptor activity measured in their skin fibroblasts: patients with less than 2% of normal LDL receptor activity (receptor-negative) and patients with 2–25% of normal LDL receptor activity (receptor-defective). In general, plasma levels of LDL-C are inversely related to the level of residual LDL receptor activity. Untreated, receptor-negative patients with homozygous FH rarely survive beyond the second decade; receptor-defective patients have a better prognosis but, with few exceptions, develop clinically significant atherosclerotic vascular disease by the age of 30, and often sooner.

The much more common heterozygous FH patients have one-half the number of normal LDL receptors and develop LDL levels between 200 and 400 mg/dL. Although the nature of the molecular defect has some impact on the severity of hypercholesterolemia, FH heterozygotes with the same *LDLR* mutation can have widely different plasma levels of LDL-C. The clinical prognosis of FH heterozygotes is related not only to the magnitude of the elevation in plasma LDL-C, but also to the presence of other coronary risk factors. Heterozygous FH occurs in approximately 1 in 500 persons worldwide, making it one of the most common monogenic disorders. Over 900 mutations in the *LDLR* gene cause FH [15]. Most mutations are unique, making the molecular diagnosis difficult, except in patients from populations where a limited number of mutations predominate. However, to date, there is no evidence that molecular diagnosis of the disease has important therapeutic implications.

Heterozygous FH patients are usually responsive to medical management. Medical management, however, has only modest effects on plasma levels of LDL-C in FH homozygotes, even when drugs are administered at high doses [21]. While some FH homozygotes with receptor-defective mutations may retain sufficient LDLR activity to respond to these potent lipid-lowering agents, drug therapy alone is never adequate treatment for these patients. The current treatment of choice for homozygous FH (and for heterozygotes whose plasma LDL-C remains elevated with drug therapy) is LDL apheresis [22]. This process, in which the LDL particles are selectively removed from the circulation through extracorporeal binding to either dextran sulfate or heparin, can promote regression of xanthomas and may slow the progression of atherosclerosis [23]. However, although LDL apheresis retards the development of atherosclerosis, it does not prevent it, because of the recurrent hypercholesterolemia between procedures. Therefore, new therapies are urgently being investigated to treat the hypercholesterolemia of individuals suffering from homozygous FH. Liver transplantation is effective in decreasing LDL levels but is associated with substantial risks. Inhibition of MTP, which is required for the synthesis of Apo B-containing lipoproteins, is therapeutic target in development. Liver-directed gene transfer of the LDLR is also a promising area for the future [24].

Familial Defective Apolipoprotein B-100

A subset of individuals with a clinical presentation similar to FH and reduced rates of LDL metabolism have normal LDL receptor activity. These patients, instead, have mutations in the receptor binding region of Apo B-100, the ligand for the LDL receptor, which impairs its binding and delays the clearance of LDL. Familial defective apolipoprotein B-100 (FDB) occurs with a frequency of about 1 in 1,000 in Central Europe but is much less common in other populations [25]. Like FH, FDB is characterized by elevated plasma LDL-C levels with normal triglycerides, tendon xanthomas, and premature atherosclerosis. The mean concentration of LDL-C is about 100 mg/dL higher in patients with FDB than in age-matched controls.

The most common mutation causing FDB is a substitution of glutamine for arginine at position 3,500 in Apo B-100 [26]. Other mutations have also been reported that have a similar effect on Apo B binding to the LDL receptor. FDB is a dominantly inherited disorder and cannot be clinically distinguished from heterozygous FH, although patients with FDB tend to have lower levels of plasma LDL-C and fewer xanthomas. The clinical management of FDB and heterozygous FH is similar; thus, it is not necessary to establish the molecular diagnosis of FDB.

Rare Disorders of Elevated LDL

Two other very rare disorders have been described with clinical features similar to FH and FDB. Both of these disorders cause elevations in LDL-C and clinically manifest with xanthomas and premature coronary artery disease. There are however no abnormalities in the *LDLR* or *APOB* genes.

Autosomal recessive hypercholesterolemia (ARH), described in the island of Sardinia (Italy), clinically resembles receptor-defective homozygous FH and is caused by mutations in the *ARH* gene [27]. In this disorder, LDL receptor function in cultured fibroblasts is relatively normal; however, LDL receptor function in the liver is markedly reduced, leading to reduced LDL metabolism. The ARH protein appears to be involved in the regulation of LDL receptor-mediated endocytosis in the liver. In contrast to FH, the condition is recessive and heterozygotes have normal cholesterol levels. Patients sometimes respond partially to treatment with statins but often require LDL apheresis.

Autosomal dominant hypercholesterolemia (ADH) is another rare disorder caused by gain-of-function mutations in the proprotein convertase subtilisin/kexin type 9 (*PCSK9*) gene [28]. The function of *PCSK9* and its role in cholesterol metabolism are unclear; however, experimental data suggest that *PCSK9* may regulate the density of functional LDL receptors in the liver.

Sitosterolemia is a rare autosomal recessive disorder characterized by hyperabsorption and decreased biliary excretion of dietary sterols leading to hypercholestero lemia, xanthomas, and premature CHD. The molecular defect is caused by mutations in one of two members of ATP-binding cassette (ABC) transporter family, ABCG5 and ABCG8, which are expressed in the intestine and liver [29]. The hypercholesterolemia in subjects with sitosterolemia in unusually responsive to reductions in dietary cholesterol content and sitosterolemia should be suspected in patients in whom LDL-C falls more than 50% on a low cholesterol diet or on bile acid sequestrants.

Familial Hyperlipoproteinemia (a)

Lipoprotein(a) excess is one of the most common lipid disorders among patients with a family history of premature CHD [4]. Lp(a) is a modified form of LDL in which a large glycoprotein, apolipoprotein (a), is covalently bound to Apo B by a disulfide bridge. The Apo (a) chain contains five cysteine-rich domains known as "kringles" resulting in a structure with significant homology to plasminogen. Because of this, Lp(a) interferes with fibrinolysis by competing with plasminogen binding to molecules and cells. Lp(a) also binds to macrophages promoting foam cell formation and the deposition of cholesterol in the atherosclerotic plaque [30]. The majority of observational trials support the association of Lp(a) with enhanced cardiovascular risk [31]. Serum Lp(a) levels are primarily genetically determined. Elevated Lp(a) is more common in the Asian Indian and Turkish populations. Therapeutically modifying Lp(a) is controversial, and only two pharmacologic treatments, niacin and estrogen, modestly lower Lp(a) [32]. There have been no clinical outcome trials to date that support targeting Lp(a) levels.

Hypobetalipoproteinemia: Disorders of Low LDL

Inherited syndromes of low levels of LDL-C are termed familial hypobetalipoproteinemia. These syndromes historically have been determined to be due to a range of missense mutations in Apo B resulting in reduced secretion or accelerated metabolism of LDL-C [33]. More recently, loss-of-function mutations in *PCSK9* have been shown to cause low LDL-C levels (usually less than 80 mg/dL) [34]. The mechanism of these mutations is uncertain but may results in the upregulation of the hepatic LDL receptor and therefore increased uptake of LDL by the liver. Gain-of-function mutations in *PCSK9* result in an ADH.

Individuals with familial hypobetalipoproteinemia appear to be protected from the development of atherosclerotic vascular disease. In fact, studies of these patients provide the opportunity to demonstrate that the effects of lifelong low LDL levels are a substantial reduction in CHD with no other adverse consequences [35]. This strongly supports the concept that aggressive LDL-C reduction is associated with a long-term substantial reduction in cardiovascular risk.

Abetalipoproteinemia

Abetalipoproteinemia is a rare autosomal recessive disorder caused by defective MTP, a protein that transfers lipids to chylomicrons in the intestine and to VLDL in the liver [36]. This defect results in decreased plasma levels of cholesterol and triglycerides, and no beta-lipoproteins (chylomicrons, VLDL, and LDL) in the plasma. Heterozygotes have normal plasma lipid and Apo B levels. Abetalipoproteinemia causes severe malabsorption of dietary fats and fat-soluble vitamins (vitamins A, D, E, and K) from the digestive tract into the bloodstream. The clinical manifestations begin in childhood with steatorrhea, failure to thrive, spinocerebellar degeneration, pigmented retinopathy, and acanthocytosis. The initial neurological manifestations are loss of deep tendon reflexes, followed by decreased distal lower extremity vibratory and proprioceptive sense, dysmetria, ataxia, and the development of spastic gait, often by the third or fourth decade of life. The pigmented retinopathy begins with decreased night and color vision, followed by reductions in daytime visual acuity and ultimately progresses to near blindness. It is imperative that treatment be initiated as soon as possible to prevent the neurological sequela. Treatment consists of a low-fat, high caloric, vitamin-enriched diet accompanied by large supplemental doses of vitamin E.

Inherited Disorders of HDL-C Metabolism

HDL-C is positively associated with a decreased risk of CHD. As defined by the US National Cholesterol Education Program Adult Treatment Panel III guidelines, an HDL C level of 60 mg/dL or greater is protective against CHD [37]. On the other hand, a high-risk HDL-C level is described as one that is below 40 mg/dL. Randomized, controlled clinical trials have demonstrated that interventions to raise HDL-C levels are associated with reduced CHD events.

There is significant interest in understanding the genetic basis of HDL-C metabolism. Modulating this metabolism has significant potential in the treatment and prevention of coronary disease. Although several environmental factors are known to affect HDL levels, most of the variation in HDL is genetically determined. A large number of proteins, enzymes, and receptors are involved in HDL metabolism, and mutations in the genes encoding these factors are associated with marked alterations in plasma HDL-C levels. Mutations in Apo A-I, ATP-binding cassette A1 (ABCA1), and lecithin:cholesterol acyltransferase (LCAT) have all been shown to underlie familial hypoalphalipoproteinemia (low HDL), whereas cholesteryl ester transfer protein (CETP) gene defects underlie familial hyperalphalipoproteinemia (high HDL).

Studying these genetic disorders has given crucial insight into the proteins involved in HDL metabolism and in the role of reverse cholesterol transport. Yet to date only a few of the genes responsible for inherited syndromes have been identified. Furthermore, it remains unclear whether cardiovascular risk increases, decreases, or remains unchanged with many of these disorders. For example, in the general population, lower-than-normal HDL-C levels are closely correlated with CHD; the risk of a coronary event is thought to increase 2% for every 1% decrease in HDL-C. However, extreme HDL deficiencies caused by rare autosomal recessive disorders, including familial hypoalphalipoproteinemia (HA), familial LCAT deficiency, and Tangier disease, do not always correlate with more frequent CHD. Furthermore, it has been suggested, in single case descriptions and small family studies, that some monogenetic disorders of HDL-C metabolism result in "paradoxical phenotypes"; that is, low HDL-C but unaltered CAD risk, as well as high HDL-C associated with increased risk. The following section reviews the known monogenic disorders of HDL metabolism. Figure 4.5 summarizes the disorders associated with HDL metabolism.

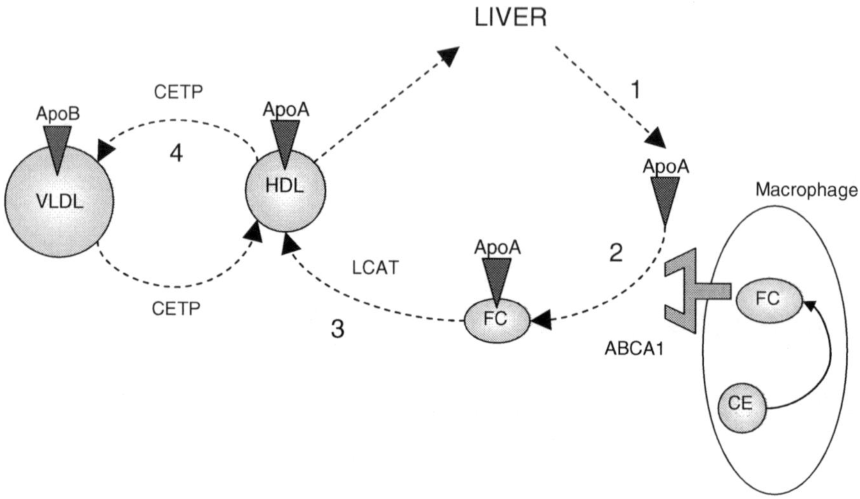

Fig. 4.5 Schematic of inherited disorders of HDL metabolism. (1) Deficient Apo A: deficient or functionally abnormal Apo A results in nonfunctional HDL. (2) Tangier disease: deficiency of ABCA1, the ligand to Apo A, prevents association of FC with Apo A. (3) LCAT deficiency: prevents maturation of HDL particles resulting in rapid clearance of circulating Apo A. (4) CETP deficiency: prevents transfer of CE from HDL to VLDL resulting in high levels of HDL. *VLDL* very low-density lipoprotein, *Apo B* apolipoprotein B, *HDL* high-density lipoprotein, *Apo A* apolipoprotein A, *CETP* cholesteryl ester transfer protein, *LCAT* lecithin:cholesterol acyltransferase deficiency, *ABCA1* ATP-binding cassette protein A1, *FC* free cholesterol, *CE* cholesteryl ester

Hypoalphalipoproteinemia: Disorders of Low HDL

Low levels of HDL-C or hypoalphalipoproteinemia include a variety of conditions in which concentrations of alpha lipoproteins or HDL are reduced. The etiology of HDL deficiencies ranges from secondary causes, such as smoking, to specific genetic mutations. Hypoalphalipoproteinemia is usually defined as HDL-C levels in the tenth percentile.

A low HDL-C level is thought to accelerate the development of atherosclerosis because of impaired reverse cholesterol transport and possibly because of the absence of other protective effects of HDL, such as decreased oxidation of other lipoproteins. Patients may have premature coronary heart or peripheral vascular disease, as well as a family history of low HDL-C levels and premature CHD. In fact, hypoalphalipoproteinemia is frequently found in patients with CHD. Research indicates that 58% of patients with CHD have HDL-C levels below the tenth percentile of normal values.

Apo A-I Deficiency and Structural Abnormalities

Complete deficiency of Apo A-I either from *APOA1* gene deletion or from nonsense mutations results in virtually absent plasma HDL-C [38, 39]. Cases of Apo A-I deficiency are rare and are associated with premature CHD.

Structurally abnormal or truncated Apo A-I proteins, caused by missense or nonsense mutations, are also rare causes of low HDL-C. The best known of these mutations is Apo A-I_{Milano}, where a single amino acid substitution results in the mutant protein [40]. This mutation is inherited as an autosomal dominant trait and results in increased turnover of the mutant Apo A-I_{Milano} protein, as well as of the wild-type Apo A-I, resulting in a substantial reduction in HDL-C. The low HDL-C levels associated with Apo A-I_{Milano}, however, are not associated with an increased risk of atherosclerosis. In fact, animal studies with intravenous infusion of recombinant Apo A-I_{Milano} exhibit less atherosclerosis. In addition, a small trial of intravenous infusion of Apo A-I_{Milano} in humans demonstrated a reduction from baseline coronary atheroma volume as measured by intravascular ultrasound [41]. The mechanism of these observations is not well understood.

There have been several other Apo A-I structural mutations described that cause low HDL-C but these mutations are rare [42]. In the general population, Apo A-I mutations are not thought to be a common source of variation in HDL-C levels.

Tangier Disease (ABCA1 Deficiency)

Tangier disease is an autosomal co-dominant disorder that causes a complete absence or extreme deficiency of HDL. The disease was first described as a rare disorder in which individuals had cholesterol accumulation in the reticuloendothelial system causing enlarged orange tonsils, hepatosplenomegaly, intestinal mucosal abnormalities, and peripheral neuropathy, in association with a markedly low HDL-C level lower than 5 mg/dL [43].

Tangier disease is caused by homozygous mutations in the ABCA1 [44]. ABCA1 is involved in the efflux of unesterified cholesterol and phospholipids from cells to Apo A-I. When ABCA1 is nonfunctional or absent, Apo A-I is not appropriately lipidated and is rapidly cleared from the circulation HDL-C levels which are usually lower than 5 mg/dL. The impaired cholesterol efflux from tissues results in cholesterol accumulation leading to many of the clinical characteristics.

Both patients with Tangier disease and heterozygotes for ABCA1 mutations are at some increased risk for premature CHD. Several large studies also suggest that common genetic variation in the *ABCA1* gene may be an important contributor to the variation in HDL-C levels in the general population and may be associated with low HDL-C levels and increased CHD risk [45].

Familial LCAT Deficiency

LCAT deficiency is a very rare autosomal recessive disorder characterized by corneal opacities, normochromic anemia, and renal failure in young adults [46]. LCAT deficiency results in decreased esterification of cholesterol to cholesteryl esters on HDL particles. This in turn results in an accumulation of free cholesterol on lipoprotein particles and in peripheral tissues, such as the cornea, red blood cells, renal glomeruli, and vascular walls. Although LCAT clearly has important effects on HDL metabolism, its relationship to atherosclerosis remains unclear. At present, no effective method has been found to increase plasma LCAT levels; therefore, therapy is limited to dietary restriction of fat to prevent the development of complications.

Two kinds of genetic LCAT deficiencies have been described: complete deficiency known as classic LCAT deficiency and partial deficiency known as fish-eye disease [47]. Both types are characterized by corneal opacification from deposition of free cholesterol, low HDL-C (usually <10 mg/dL), and variable hypertriglyceridemia. Partial deficiency has no clinical sequela. Individuals with complete LCAT deficiency also have low-grade hemolytic anemia and progressive renal insufficiency that eventually leads to end-stage renal disease. Neither is associated with premature coronary disease despite reduced HDL-C and Apo A-I levels.

Familial Hypoalphalipoproteinemia

Familial hypoalphalipoproteinemia is the most common inherited form of low HDL-C [48]. Criteria for the definition of familial hypoalphalipoproteinemia are (1) HDL-C levels below the tenth percentile in the presence of normal VLDL cholesterol and LDL cholesterol levels, (2) an absence of diseases or factors to which hypoalphalipoproteinemia may be secondary, and (3) the presence of a similar lipoprotein pattern in a first-degree relative. This condition is autosomal dominant and although the molecular etiology is unknown, accelerated metabolism of Apo A-I and HDL-C appears to be the final common pathway [49]. Some families with familial hypoalphalipoproteinemia have an increased incidence of CHD and others do not.

Hyperalphalipoproteinemia: Disorders of High HDL-C

An elevated concentration of Apo A-I and Apo AII, the major apolipoproteins of HDL, is called hyperalphalipoproteinemia. Familial hyperalphalipoproteinemia is defined as an inherited condition of HDL-C level greater than the 90th percentile. Elevated HDL levels are also associated with low levels of VLDL and TG levels while LDL levels may be within the reference range or elevated. Hyperalphalipoproteinemia does not have any unusual clinical features, and the condition should not be considered a disease entity but rather a fortuitous condition that can increase longevity because of the associated decreased incidence of CHD.

CETP Deficiency

CETP is a key plasma protein that influences circulating levels of HDL-C by facilitating the transfer of esterified cholesterol from HDL to VLDL and the transfer of triacylglycerol from VLDL particles to HDL [50]. In conditions where hypertriglyceridemia exists, the efficiency of transfer of triacylglycerol is enhanced leading to triacylglycerol enrichment and cholesterol depletion of HDL. This cholesterol-poor HDL particle is cleared more rapidly from the kidney, and thereby leads to lower circulating HDL-C levels.

CETP deficiency in humans is associated with markedly elevated plasma HDL-C levels, usually greater than 120 mg/dL. CETP deficiency is common in Japan, where it explains almost half of all hyperalphalipoproteinemia cases. In Caucasians, however, CETP deficiency is rare. Multiple different mutations in the gene encoding for CETP have been described [51, 52]. Individuals homozygous for these mutations have differing levels of CETP mass or activity, ranging from complete absence to only partial CETP deficiency and HDL-C levels that are less markedly elevated. Heterozygous individuals have 60–70% normal CETP activity, but only a modest increase in HDL-C levels.

The relationship between CETP defects and CHD is confusing [53]. Initially, CETP-deficient patients were thought to have a reduced CHD risk, but, in contrast, more recent studies reveal an increased CHD risk. Some investigators have suggested that despite the elevations in plasma HDL-C levels, these particles are dysfunctional and may not be cardioprotective.

References

1. Genest Jr JJ, Martin-Munley SS, McNamara JR, et al. Familial lipoprotein disorders in patients with premature coronary artery disease. Circulation. 1992;85(6):2025–33.
2. Roncaglioni MC, Santoro L, D'Avanzo B, et al. Role of family history in patients with myocardial infarction. An Italian case-control study. GISSI-EFRIM Investigators. Circulation. 1992;85(6):2065–72.
3. Yusuf S, Hawken S, Ounpuu S, et al. Effect of potentially modifiable risk factors associated with myocardial infarction in 52 countries (the INTERHEART study): case-control study. Lancet. 2004;364(9438):937–52.
4. Davidson, MH. Lipoprotein metabolism and the pathogenesis of atherosclerosis. In: The mobile lipid clinic: a companion guide. 2nd ed. New York: Lippincott Williams & Wilkins; 2005. p. 45–69.
5. Hayden MR, Ma Y. Molecular genetics of human lipoprotein lipase deficiency. Mol Cell Biochem. 1992;113(2):171–6.
6. Brunzell JD, Miller NE, Alaupovic P, et al. Familial chylomicronemia due to a circulating inhibitor of lipoprotein lipase activity. J Lipid Res. 1983;24(1):12–9.
7. Santamarina-Fojo S. The familial chylomicronemia syndrome. Endocrinol Metab Clin North Am. 1998;27(3):551–67. viii.
8. Stroes ES, Nierman MC, Meulenberg JJ, et al. Intramuscular administration of AAV1-lipoprotein lipase S447X lowers triglycerides in lipoprotein lipase-deficient patients. Arterioscler Thromb Vasc Biol. 2008;28(12):2303–4.
9. Hopkins PN, Heiss G, Ellison RC, et al. Coronary artery disease risk in familial combined hyperlipidemia and familial hypertriglyceridemia: a case-control comparison from the National Heart, Lung, and Blood Institute Family Heart Study. Circulation. 2003;108(5):519–23.
10. Ayyobi AF, Brunzell JD. Lipoprotein distribution in the metabolic syndrome, type 2 diabetes mellitus, and familial combined hyperlipidemia. Am J Cardiol. 2003;92(4A):27J–33J.
11. Shoulders CC, Jones EL, Naoumova RP. Genetics of familial combined hyperlipidemia and risk of coronary heart disease. Hum Mol Genet 2004;13 Spec No 1:R149–60.

12. Mahley RW, Huang Y, Rall Jr SC. Pathogenesis of type III hyperlipoproteinemia (dysbetalipoproteinemia). Questions, quandaries, and paradoxes. J Lipid Res. 1999;40(11):1933–49.
13. Mahley RW, Rall Jr SC. Apolipoprotein E: far more than a lipid transport protein. Annu Rev Genomics Hum Genet. 2000;1:507–37.
14. Heller DA, de Faire U, Pedersen NL, Dahlen G, McClearn GE. Genetic and environmental influences on serum lipid levels in twins. N Engl J Med. 1993;328(16):1150–6.
15. Rader DJ, Cohen J, Hobbs HH. Monogenic hypercholesterolemia: new insights in pathogenesis and treatment. J Clin Invest. 2003;111(12):1795–803.
16. Austin MA, Hutter CM, Zimmern RL, Humphries SE. Familial hypercholesterolemia and coronary heart disease: a HuGE association review. Am J Epidemiol. 2004;160(5):421–9.
17. Ishibashi S, Brown MS, Goldstein JL, Gerard RD, Hammer RE, Herz J. Hypercholesterolemia in low density lipoprotein receptor knockout mice and its reversal by adenovirus-mediated gene delivery. J Clin Invest. 1993;92(2):883–93.
18. Hobbs HH, Russell DW, Brown MS, Goldstein JL. The LDL receptor locus in familial hypercholesterolemia: mutational analysis of a membrane protein. Annu Rev Genet. 1990;24:133–70.
19. Grossman M, Rader DJ, Muller DW, et al. A pilot study of ex vivo gene therapy for homozygous familial hypercholesterolaemia. Nat Med. 1995;1(11):1148–54.
20. Hoeg JM, Feuerstein IM, Tucker EE. Detection and quantitation of calcific atherosclerosis by ultrafast computed tomography in children and young adults with homozygous familial hypercholesterolemia. Arterioscler Thromb. 1994;14(7):1066–74.
21. Gagne C, Gaudet D, Bruckert E. Efficacy and safety of ezetimibe coadministered with atorvastatin or simvastatin in patients with homozygous familial hypercholesterolemia. Circulation. 2002;105(21):2469–75.
22. Sachais BS, Katz J, Ross J, Rader DJ. Long-term effects of LDL apheresis in patients with severe hypercholesterolemia. J Clin Apher. 2005;20(4):252–5.
23. Thompson GR. LDL apheresis. Atherosclerosis. 2003;167(1):1–13.
24. Cuchel M, Qasim A, Rader DJ. Genetic disorders of lipoprotein metabolism. In: Davidson M, Toth P, Maki K, editors. Therapeutic lipodology. New Jersey: Humana Press; 2007. p. 23–35.
25. Myant NB. Familial defective apolipoprotein B-100: a review, including some comparisons with familial hypercholesterolaemia. Atherosclerosis. 1993;104(1–2):1–18.
26. Tybjaerg-Hansen A, Humphries SE. Familial defective apolipoprotein B-100: a single mutation that causes hypercholesterolemia and premature coronary artery disease. Atherosclerosis. 1992;96(2–3):91–107.
27. Garcia CK, Wilund K, Arca M, et al. Autosomal recessive hypercholesterolemia caused by mutations in a putative LDL receptor adaptor protein. Science. 2001;292(5520):1394–8.
28. Abifadel M, Varret M, Rabes JP, et al. Mutations in PCSK9 cause autosomal dominant hypercholesterolemia. Nat Genet. 2003;34(2):154–6.
29. Berge KE, Tian H, Graf GA, et al. Accumulation of dietary cholesterol in sitosterolemia caused by mutations in adjacent ABC transporters. Science. 2000;290(5497):1771–5.
30. Marcovina SM, Koschinsky ML. Lipoprotein(a) as a risk factor for coronary artery disease. Am J Cardiol. 1998;82(12A):57U–66U. discussion 86U.
31. Stubbs P, Seed M, Lane D, Collinson P, Kendall F, Noble M. Lipoprotein(a) as a risk predictor for cardiac mortality in patients with acute coronary syndromes. Eur Heart J. 1998;19(9):1355–64.
32. Angelin B. Therapy for lowering lipoprotein (a) levels. Curr Opin Lipidol. 1997;8(6):337–41.
33. Schonfeld G, Lin X, Yue P. Familial hypobetalipoproteinemia: genetics and metabolism. Cell Mol Life Sci. 2005;62(12):1372–8.
34. Kotowski IK, Pertsemlidis A, Luke A, et al. A spectrum of PCSK9 alleles contributes to plasma levels of low-density lipoprotein cholesterol. Am J Hum Genet. 2006;78(3):410–22.
35. Cohen JC, Boerwinkle E, Mosley Jr TH, Hobbs HH. Sequence variations in PCSK9, low LDL, and protection against coronary heart disease. N Engl J Med. 2006;354(12):1264–72.
36. Sharp D, Blinderman L, Combs KA, et al. Cloning and gene defects in microsomal triglyceride transfer protein associated with abetalipoproteinaemia. Nature. 1993;365(6441):65–9.

37. Executive Summary of The Third Report of the National Cholesterol Education Program (NCEP) Expert Panel on Detection, Evaluation, and Treatment of High Blood Cholesterol in Adults (Adult Treatment Panel III). JAMA 2001;285(19):2486–97.
38. Norum RA, Lakier JB, Goldstein S, et al. Familial deficiency of apolipoproteins A-I and C-III and precocious coronary-artery disease. N Engl J Med. 1982;306(25):1513–9.
39. Schaefer EJ, Heaton WH, Wetzel MG, Brewer Jr HB. Plasma apolipoprotein A-1 absence associated with a marked reduction of high density lipoproteins and premature coronary artery disease. Arteriosclerosis. 1982;2(1):16–26.
40. Chiesa G, Sirtori CR. Apolipoprotein A-I(Milano): current perspectives. Curr Opin Lipidol. 2003;14(2):159–63.
41. Nissen SE, Tsunoda T, Tuzcu EM, et al. Effect of recombinant ApoA-I Milano on coronary atherosclerosis in patients with acute coronary syndromes: a randomized controlled trial. JAMA. 2003;290(17):2292–300.
42. von Eckardstein A. Differential diagnosis of familial high density lipoprotein deficiency syndromes. Atherosclerosis. 2006;186(2):231–9.
43. Fredrickson DS. The inheritance of high density lipoprotein deficiency (tangier disease). J Clin Invest. 1964;43:228–36.
44. Rust S, Rosier M, Funke H, et al. Tangier disease is caused by mutations in the gene encoding ATP-binding cassette transporter 1. Nat Genet. 1999;22(4):352–5.
45. Clee SM, Zwinderman AH, Engert JC, et al. Common genetic variation in ABCA1 is associated with altered lipoprotein levels and a modified risk for coronary artery disease. Circulation. 2001;103(9):1198–205.
46. Asztalos BF, Schaefer EJ, Horvath KV, et al. Role of LCAT in HDL remodeling: investigation of LCAT deficiency states. J Lipid Res. 2007;48(3):592–9.
47. Kuivenhoven JA, Pritchard H, Hill J, Frohlich J, Assmann G, Kastelein J. The molecular pathology of lecithin:cholesterol acyltransferase (LCAT) deficiency syndromes. J Lipid Res. 1997;38(2):191–205.
48. Chien KL, Chen MF, Hsu HC, et al. Genetic association study of APOA1/C3/A4/A5 gene cluster and haplotypes on triglyceride and HDL cholesterol in a community-based population. Clin Chim Acta. 2008;388(1–2):78–83.
49. Lewis GF, Rader DJ. New insights into the regulation of HDL metabolism and reverse cholesterol transport. Circ Res. 2005;96(12):1221–32.
50. Brown ML, Inazu A, Hesler CB, et al. Molecular basis of lipid transfer protein deficiency in a family with increased high-density lipoproteins. Nature. 1989;342(6248):448–51.
51. Inazu A, Brown ML, Hesler CB, et al. Increased high-density lipoprotein levels caused by a common cholesteryl-ester transfer protein gene mutation. N Engl J Med. 1990;323(18):1234–8.
52. Inazu A, Jiang XC, Haraki T, et al. Genetic cholesteryl ester transfer protein deficiency caused by two prevalent mutations as a major determinant of increased levels of high density lipoprotein cholesterol. J Clin Invest. 1994;94(5):1872–82.
53. Rader DJ. Inhibition of cholesteryl ester transfer protein activity: a new therapeutic approach to raising high-density lipoprotein. Curr Atheroscler Rep. 2004;6(5):398–405.

Chapter 5
Advanced Lipid Testing

Matthew J. Sorrentino

Keywords Direct LDL • LDL phenotyping • Apolipoprotein B • Lipoprotein(a) • High-sensitivity C-reactive protein • Lp-PLA_2

A high serum cholesterol is a well-established major risk factor for coronary heart disease (CHD). Evidence that supports the lipid hypothesis includes research in animal models, epidemiological studies, studies of genetic forms of hyperlipidemia, and laboratory and clinical trials of cholesterol-lowering therapy. Low-density lipoprotein cholesterol (LDL-C) is the major atherogenic lipoprotein and has been designated the primary target of therapy by the National Cholesterol Education Program (NCEP) [1].

The first step in considering LDL-C-lowering therapy is to assess a person's risk status. Risk assessment requires measurement of a lipid panel that includes a measurement of the LDL-C. The NCEP recommends that all adults aged 20 years or older should have a fasting lipoprotein profile that would include a total cholesterol, high-density lipoprotein cholesterol (HDL-C), triglyceride, and LDL-C [1]. In the typical lipid panel, the LDL-C is a calculated number. If the profile is normal, it is recommended that it should be re-measured every 5 years.

There are a large number of lipoproteins and associated biomarkers that can be measured to help modify an individual's risk assessment. Even with effective LDL-C-lowering therapy, cardiac events still occur. This is referred to as the residual risk; the number of events that occur despite the introduction of effective preventive therapies. Additional biomarkers may offer a way to further evaluate this residual

M.J. Sorrentino (✉)
Department of Medicine, Section of Cardiology,
University of Chicago Pritzker School of Medicine, Chicago, IL 60637, USA
e-mail: msorrent@medicine.bsd.uchicago.edu

M.J. Sorrentino (ed.), *Hyperlipidemia in Primary Care: A Practical Guide to Risk Reduction*, Current Clinical Practice, DOI 10.1007/978-1-60327-502-6_5,

risk and become secondary treatment targets to further lower risk. This chapter will explore some of the available lipoprotein, inflammatory, and thrombotic biomarkers that are available for measurement, and discuss when they can be considered in your patients.

Low-Density Lipoprotein

Lipid Panel with a Calculated LDL-C

Most laboratories measure serum total and HDL-C and triglycerides and calculate the LDL-C by the Friedewald formula [2]:

$$\text{LDL-C} = \text{Total cholesterol} - [\text{HDL-C} - \text{Triglycerides}/5].$$

One-fifth of the triglyceride level gives an estimate of the very low-density lipoprotein (VLDL) level. This formula is thought to be fairly accurate as long as the triglycerides are below 400 mg/dl. For individuals who have a triglyceride value between 400 and 600 mg/dl, the triglycerides can be divided by 6 to improve accuracy [3] or direct measurement of LDL-C can be performed. The lipid panel is best measured in the fasting state to eliminate the presence of chylomicrons that make the LDL calculation less accurate. The calculated LDL-C will contain other cholesterol containing lipoproteins in the serum such as lipoprotein(a) [Lp(a)], intermediate-density lipoprotein (IDL), and chylomicron and VLDL remnants. These other lipoproteins typically add only 5–10 mg/dl to the LDL-C, but in some patients very high levels of these additional lipoproteins will make the LDL-C value inaccurate. The Friedewald LDL-C may be less accurate in type 2 diabetes although the discrepancy may be due to elevated triglyceride levels commonly found in this condition [4].

When to Use a Calculated LDL-C

The lipid panel with the Friedewald calculated LDL-C is the standard test for assessing hyperlipidemia and is recommended by the NCEP for screening and setting treatment goals. This is an easily obtained inexpensive automated test. It is also the method most commonly used in many clinical trials. Ideally, this lipid panel should be ordered after a 9–12 h fast to clear chylomicrons for an accurate estimate of the LDL-C. The LDL-C level should not be relied on when triglycerides are greater than 400 mg/dl. In addition, it may be less accurate in individuals with greatly increased total cholesterol levels as seen in familial hypercholesterolemia [5].

Direct LDL

Assays have been developed that measure LDL-C directly. Initial methods used chemical precipitation or immunoseparation techniques but these methods did not achieve the accuracy desired. Newer generation homogeneous methods use techniques to dissolve the lipoproteins to expose and directly measure the associated cholesterol. These newer methods have been shown to be reasonably specific and free from major endogenous interferences [6]. The homogeneous methods are less susceptible to interference from increased triglycerides than the Friedewald equation and can be used reliably in postprandial samples. The homogeneous methods are fully automated and are now available in most laboratories. In comparison to the Friedewald equation, the direct LDL-C should be about 5–10 mg/dl lower than the calculated LDL-C since the direct LDL-C typically does not include IDL and Lp(a). If the difference is significantly higher, this may indicate abnormally high levels of these particles. Some of the direct LDL-C assays, however, may have some interaction with IDL-C and Lp(a) which may affect accuracy [7]. NCEP treatment goals are based on the calculated LDL-C so goals may need to be set slightly lower if using a direct LDL-C.

When to Use a Direct LDL-C

The direct LDL-C measurement is a reliable way to measure LDL in nonfasting individuals. In these patients, a direct LDL-C and HDL-C can be measured for monitoring. Most laboratories run a lipid panel with the Freidewald calculated LDL-C so the direct LDL-C measurement would be an additional test and cost. It is important to recall that guidelines and most clinical trials used the calculated LDL-C as a treatment target.

LDL Subfractions

LDL particles are heterogeneous in respect to size, density, and composition. Each LDL particle consists of a single molecule of apolipoprotein B_{100} (apoB), the protein component of the LDL particle. The lipid content of LDL helps to determine the particle's density which ranges from 1.019 to 1.063 g/ml. The triglyceride content of the LDL is one of the key determinants of its density and hydrolysis of triglycerides can lead to smaller and denser particles. A number of different measurement techniques can identify multiple subfractions of LDL. The LDL-C measurement is the sum of the cholesterol contained in all of the particles but if the sample shows significant heterogeneity it will not be an accurate measure of the number of LDL particles. Since each LDL particle contains a single apoB molecule, measuring apoB can be used as an estimate of the number of LDL particles. The higher the apoB, the more LDL particles are present.

Early studies used density gradient ultracentrifugation to isolate LDL subfractions [8]. Some patients with coronary artery disease were found to have an elevated apoB to cholesterol ratio in the LDL fraction even when total LDL-C levels were in the normal range [9]. These patients were termed "hyperapobetalipoproteinemia" to indicate this elevated apoB to LDL-C ratio. An elevated apoB to cholesterol ratio identifies individuals with an increased number of particles and if the cholesterol levels are normal they must have smaller and denser particles.

The smaller and denser LDL particles are thought to be more highly atherogenic than larger particles. Smaller LDL particles are more likely to become oxidized, bind poorly to the LDL receptor, and have delayed clearance from the plasma [10]. Small, dense LDL particles are associated with elevated triglyceride levels and decreased HDL-C [11]. Investigators began characterizing the distribution of LDL particle size using polyacrylamide gradient gel electrophoresis and have simplified the analysis by dividing the LDL particles into two size distributions called LDL phenotypes; pattern A is characterized by a predominance of large, buoyant LDL particles and pattern B has a predominance of small, dense LDL particles (the typical cut point used is a diameter of 25.5 nm or less) [12]. The triglyceride level can predict which pattern is likely present. In one study, 83% of individuals with pattern A had a triglyceride level below 95 mg/dl, whereas only 17% of pattern B individuals had triglyceride levels below this cutoff [12].

Certain patient types are known to more likely to have a pattern B phenotype. Small, dense LDL is a common feature of insulin resistance, metabolic syndrome, and diabetes mellitus [13, 14]. Small, dense LDL particles are elevated in metabolic syndrome and increases with the number of metabolic syndrome components [13]. Since it has been known that small, dense LDL is associated with elevated triglyceride and low HDL-C, it is not surprising that small, dense LDL is elevated in conditions that tend to have this dyslipidemic pattern.

Evidence from prospective epidemiological studies of LDL particle size indicated that small, dense LDL particles predict CHD risk. In the prospective Stanford Five-City Project, LDL particle size was significantly smaller in individuals with CHD than in controls [15]. In the Physician's Health Study, small LDL particles were associated with the risk of myocardial infarction but not after adjustment for triglyceride level [16]. The prospective Quebec Cardiovascular Study found that the presence of small, dense LDL particles was associated with developing CHD in men [17]. A meta-analysis of the above three studies showed that small, dense LDL was statistically associated with an increased CHD risk [18]. When adjusted for triglyceride and HDL-C, the summary odds ratio was 1.3 which remained statistically significant indicating that small, dense LDL was associated with a 30% increased risk of CHD. A study from Japan found that small, dense LDL is strongly associated with CHD and after multiple logistic regression analysis, it was independently associated with CHD in both men and women [19]. The European EPIC-Norfolk prospective population study showed higher concentrations of small, dense LDL particles in cases of CHD matched to controls free of CHD, but after adjustment for confounding variables, the association between small, dense LDL and CHD was no longer significant [20].

It remains to be determined if knowledge of LDL size improves risk determination compared with traditional measurements of LDL and if treatments directed to changing LDL phenotype will lead to further risk reduction beyond LDL-lowering alone. The presence of small, dense LDL is associated with CHD, but in many studies, it is not an independent risk factor when other factors are taken into account. Some small intervention studies suggest that small, dense LDL may be a therapeutic target. The Stanford Coronary Risk Intervention Project suggested that the rate of atherosclerosis progression was reduced in patients receiving risk reduction therapy and a pattern B phenotype.[21] The Familial Atherosclerosis Treatment Study showed that an increase in LDL particle size was associated with CAD regression [22]. These preliminary findings need to be verified in larger outcome trials before treatments targeted at changing LDL particle size can be recommended as a standard therapeutic approach.

When to Use LDL Phenotyping

Small, dense LDL particles are associated with CHD and more commonly found in patients with insulin resistance. Most studies have shown, however, that the phenotype is not an independent risk factor so for most patients it will not change a risk assessment based on traditional risk factor analysis. Studies need to be completed to determine if targeting the LDL phenotype and instituting therapy that can change a predominantly pattern B to pattern A will add an incremental benefit to LDL-lowering alone. Most therapeutic intervention studies have shown a reduction in risk that correlates with a reduction in LDL-C particles.

A number of therapies can bring about a change in LDL phenotype including diet [23, 24], bariatric surgery [25], intensive glycemic control with insulin [26] and thiazolidinediones [27], and hyperlipidemic therapy with niacin [28], fibrates [29, 30], and some statins [31, 32]. Most of the studies that demonstrate a beneficial effect on small, dense LDL show an overall reduction in particle number. Studies in which shifting LDL subfraction from pattern B to pattern A and increasing particle size appear to be dependent on baseline triglycerides and achieving a reduction in triglycerides usually to the normal range. Since many of these agents have multiple effects on a number of risk factors, it is unknown if shifting the LDL subclass to the more buoyant particles adds any further risk reduction. Until larger long-term trials assessing LDL subfraction profiles are completed, treatment should continue to focus on reducing the number of particles. If a number of therapies can achieve the same LDL-C goal, medications that also improve LDL subclass can be chosen in patients known to have predominantly pattern B. If a patient is at their LDL-C goal and pattern B subfraction persists, more aggressive risk-lowering therapy may be considered although outcome studies are not available to prove that this strategy leads to further benefit.

Vertical Auto Profile Method

The vertical auto profile (VAP) method simultaneously determines the cholesterol content of all the lipoprotein particles in the blood. The technique separates the lipoprotein classes according to their density by using vertical spin density gradient ultracentrifugation. Following separation, an enzymatic reagent reacts with the cholesterol in the sample to form a colored product which can be detected and measured. This method directly measures the VLDL, IDL, LDL, and HDL-C concentration as well as a number of lipoprotein subfractions. The newer VAP methods (VAP-II) are highly sensitive and include direct measurements of lipoprotein(a) and IDL cholesterol [33].

The VAP lipid analysis has been commercially marketed as the VAP cholesterol test by Atherotech. The company reports 15 separate components of blood cholesterol as summarized in Table 5.1. With the newer VAP-II methodology, the direct LDL-C, termed the "real" LDL by Atherotech, is less likely to have interference from IDL and Lp(a). In addition, the real LDL-C can be further evaluated and five subclasses based on density (LDL-1 most buoyant through LDL-5 most dense) can be identified [34]. Patients can be classified as having mostly large buoyant LDL (pattern A), small dense LDL (pattern B), or a combination of both (pattern A/B).

When to Use the VAP Test

The VAP cholesterol test is a relatively inexpensive analysis of a number of lipoproteins. It gives a reliable direct LDL-C and Lp(a) cholesterol. The direct LDL-C in

Table 5.1 VAP cholesterol test components (Atherotech)

Total LDL-C, direct	Includes IDL and Lp(a)
Total HDL-C, direct	
Total VLDL-C, direct	
Sum of total cholesterol	Sum of the above three direct measurements
Triglycerides, direct	
Total non-HDL-C	LDL + VLDL
Total apolipoprotein B_{100}	Calculated
Lp(a) cholesterol	
IDL-C	
Real LDL-C	LDL-C minus IDL and Lp(a)
Sum of total LDL-C	Real LDL-C + Lp(a) + IDL-C
Real LDL-C size pattern	Patterns B, A/B, A
Remnant lipoprotein	IDL + $VLDL_3$
Metabolic syndrome	Constellation of small, dense LDL, elevated triglyceride, low HDL
HDL_2	Large buoyant
HDL_3	Small dense
$VLDL_3$	Small remnant

the VAP method may be more accurate than some of the direct LDL-C assays available because of better separation of IDL and Lp(a). This test may be useful in certain patient populations such as metabolic syndrome and diabetic patients who may not have a markedly elevated LDL-C but may have a preponderance of small, dense LDL particles. More research will need to be done to determine if the additional pattern information gives further risk prediction for a patient above and beyond the total cholesterol level. In addition, more research is needed to determine if therapy that can change a patient's LDL pattern will give further risk reduction beyond that achieved by aggressive LDL lowering. Until that is determined, the test gives some further risk analysis but there are currently no guidelines on how to use the values as targets to optimize patient outcomes.

Gradient Gel Electrophoresis (Berkeley Heartlab, Inc.)

Analytic ultracentrifugation was the original technique used to separate lipoprotein subclasses. This method is highly accurate and reproducible but a complicated technique and has been limited to research laboratories. Gradient gel electrophoresis (GGE) [8] was developed as a more practical and reproducible method of lipoprotein subclass analysis and is commercially available through the University of California by Berkeley Heartlab, Inc. LDL-segmented GGE (LDL-S_3GGE) identifies seven subclasses of LDL and therefore measures more subclasses than techniques that report pattern A/B phenotypes. Subclasses IIIa, IIIb, and IVb make up the small, dense LDL particles. In addition, apoB levels are measured and Berkeley is able to separate $apoB_{48}$ (the particle associated with chylomicrons) from $apoB_{100}$ (associated with LDL) and report apoB-ultra which is thought to be a more accurate measurement of LDL particle number. The Berkeley technique measures the relative percent distribution of LDL particles using S_3GGE, determines total LDL particle amount by measuring apoB-ultra, and then integrates size-adjusted relative LDL particle distribution and the apoB-ultra derived particle number to generate quantitative LDL particle amount in each LDL subclass. The laboratory then reports Q-LDL which is the quantitative LDL particle amount of the small, dense LDL subclasses (IIIa+b and IVb). Table 5.2 lists the recommended ideal goals for percent and quantitative amount of small, dense LDL subfractions.

There are additional companies that use gel electrophoresis to subfractionate LDL particles. The LipoPrint system (Quantimetrix) is an electrophoresis kit that can be purchased by a laboratory and will give subfractions of LDL in about 3 h. A computer printout gives a visual display of the LDL subclasses, quantifies the

Table 5.2 Berkeley Heartlab, Inc. recommended percent and quantitative amount of small, dense LDL subclasses

	Goal (%)	Goal (mg/dl)
LDL IIIa+b	≤15	≤13
LDL IVb	≤5	≤4

subclasses in mg/dl, and determines if the pattern is high risk (predominantly pattern B). Other companies sell electrophoresis kits to laboratories such as the SPIFE cholesterol profile (Helena Laboratories) that use gel electrophoresis and can determine if small, dense LDL is present. These companies have not developed a commercial profile as detailed as the Berkeley test.

When to Use LDL-S_3GGE (Berkeley Heartlab) Test

The Berkeley Heartlab test gives both the percent small, dense LDL and small, dense LDL particle amount. Residual cardiovascular risk may be associated with an excess number of atherogenic particles even when the cholesterol value is treated to goal. Treatment outcome studies will need to be completed to determine if targeting the percent of small, dense LDL and particle amount will further reduce risk. This test is one method that accurately gives the percent and amount of small, dense LDL and is a reasonable alternative to other tests that offer similar information.

Nuclear Magnetic Resonance

Nuclear magnetic resonance (NMR) spectroscopy has been developed to give direct measurements of LDL particle number (LDL-P) and size of LDL particles. HDL and VLDL subclasses are measured as well. The test is based on the observation that different size particles produce a slightly different methyl lipid NMR signal with a distinct shape. A total of 15 subpopulations of particle diameter can be extracted; five HDL, three LDL, one IDL, and six VLDL subpopulations. An NMR lipid profile test is marketed by LipoScience and reports LDL-P in nanomoles per liter with an LDL-P <1,000 nmol/l thought to be optimal. Ranges of LDL particles are determined by population studies. The LipoScience profile usually combines some of the subpopulations and typically reports nine subclasses of particles displaying the results against a reference population.

Population studies have shown a frequent discrepancy between LDL-C and LDL-P. LDL-C may under represent the number of LDL particles. A number of clinical studies have used NMR LDL-P as a marker for CVD risk. In the Cardiovascular Health Study, LDL-P was related to incident myocardial infarction and angina in women [35]. In the Pravastatin Limitation of Atherosclerosis in the Coronary Arteries (PLAC-1) trial, LDL-P related to CAD progression [36]. In the primary prevention Women's Health Study, LDL-P predicted CVD risk in the women in this study [37]. In comparison to other markers, however, LDL-P was not substantially different than the total cholesterol:HDL ratio in predicting CVD risk. In the Veterans Affairs High-Density Lipoprotein Intervention (VA-HIT) trial, gemfibrozil significantly reduced LDL-P (although LDL-C was unchanged) and this was independently associated with a reduction in CHD events [30]. Finally, in the

Framingham Offspring study, LDL-P was a more sensitive indicator of CVD risk than LDL-C [38]. In this study, for participants with LDL-P or LDL-C below the population 25th percentile, those with a low LDL-P had a lower CVD rate than those with a low LDL-C.

When to Use the NMR Test

The NMR test gives an accurate measure of LDL particle number. An LDL-C may be in the therapeutic range but still contain an excessive number of LDL particles that may correlate with increased risk. This may account for the residual risk seen in studies in which the LDL-C is treated to goal. LDL-P may be considered a potential treatment target once the LDL-C is at goal. This may be especially important in individuals with a high incidence of smaller denser LDL particles such as diabetics, patients with metabolic syndrome, and individuals with high triglyceride levels [39]. Individuals with high particle number may benefit from additional LDL targeted therapy. Treatment studies that target LDL-P will need to be completed to determine if reducing LDL-P once LDL-C is at goal can achieve further risk reduction before LDL-P can be recommended as a standard test.

Non-HDL-Cholesterol

The non-HDL-cholesterol (non-HDL-C) is simply calculated by subtracting the HDL-C from the total cholesterol. In a fasting state, the non-HDL-C is the sum of all the potentially atherogenic particles including VLDL, IDL, LDL, remnant lipoproteins, and Lp(a). The National Cholesterol Education Program Adult Treatment Panel III has recommended using the non-HDL-C as a secondary target in patients with fasting triglycerides ≥200 mg/dl after achieving the LDL-C goal [1]. In general, the non-HDL-C goal is set at 30 mg/dl higher than the LDL-C goal.

Non-HDL-C has been shown to be predictive of heart disease in many studies and may be a better marker than LDL-C. The Lipid Research Clinics Program Follow-up Study found that non-HDL-C was a better predictor for CVD mortality in men and women with a high incidence of hyperlipidemia [40]. Non HDL C was a better predictor of future CVD events for women in the Women's Health Study [41] and for men in the Health Professionals Follow-up Study [42] as well. Data from the Framingham Study found the same association [43]. Non-HDL-C may be an important marker for risk in diabetic populations. Non-HDL-C was a strong predictor of CVD events in diabetic American Indians in the Strong Heart Study [44] as well as in diabetics from pooled data sets of individuals [45]. Non-HDL-C is also a strong and independent predictor of nonfatal myocardial infarction and angina in a coronary artery disease population as reported in the Bypass Angioplasty Revascularization Investigation (BARI) group [46]. In the BARI study, HDL-C and LDL-C did not predict events during follow-up.

Non-HDL-C may have advantage over measurement of other lipoproteins because it is readily derived from the standard lipid panel. Using non-HDL-C as a secondary therapeutic target after LDL-C is at goal in individuals with elevated triglyceride levels may help identify groups of patients with significant residual risk such as metabolic syndrome and diabetic populations. Non-HDL-C is a good surrogate measure of atherogenic particle concentration and has a high correlation with apolipoprotein B_{100} [47].

When to Use Non-HDL-C

The NCEP ATP III recommends that the non-HDL-C be used as a secondary therapeutic target in patients with fasting triglycerides ≥200 mg/dl. The non-HDL-C goal is set at 30 mg/dl above the LDL-C goal. Since this is an easily calculated number from the standard lipid panel, a non-HDL-C should be readily available for all patients. It remains to be proven if apoB rather than non-HDL-C would be a better treatment target. Since measurement of apoB is not as readily available, non-HDL-C is generally the preferred target. Non-HDL-C treatment goals are summarized in Table 5.3.

Apolipoprotein B_{100} (ApoB)

Apolipoprotein B_{100} is present on LDL, IDL, and VLDL particles. Each of these atherogenic particles contains one molecule of apoB. ApoB, therefore, represents the total atherogenic particle number in circulation. Since LDL particles account for approximately 90% of all atherogenic particles in most people, apoB is an estimate of the number of LDL particles.

Table 5.3 LDL-C and non-HDL-C goals according to risk categories

Risk category	LDL-C goal (mg/dl)	Non-HDL-C goal (triglycerides ≥ 200 mg/dl) (mg/dl)
Very high risk	<70 Optional goal	<100 Optional goal
High risk (CHD or CHD risk equivalent, 10-year risk >20%)	<100	<130
Moderate high risk (≥2 risk factors, 10–20% 10-year risk)	<130 (<100 optional goal)	<160 (<130 optional goal)
Moderate risk (≥2 risk factors, <10% 10-year risk)	<130	<160
Low risk (0 or 1 risk factor)	<160	<190

Adapted from NCEP ATPIII guidelines [1] and the National Heart, Lung, and Blood Institute update [105]

ApoB may be a better marker of cardiovascular risk than the LDL-C and a better guide to the success of lipid-lowering therapy. Epidemiological studies have suggested that apoB is a better predictor of CVD risk, although some studies have found that apoB did not add appreciably to a traditional risk assessment. The Apolipoprotein-related Mortality Risk (AMORIS) study recruited 175,553 Swedish men and women to determine if apolipoproteins predicted the risk of fatal myocardial infarction [48]. ApoB and the apoB/apoA-I ratio were strongly and positively related to the increased risk of fatal myocardial infarction and apoB was a stronger predictor of risk than LDL-C in both men and women. Likewise, the Quebec Cardiovascular Study of 2,155 men showed that apoB was strongly associated with the onset of clinical ischemic heart disease and was the strongest correlate of all the variables measured [49]. The Health Professionals Follow-up study also concluded that apoB was more predictive of CHD than LDL-C or non-HDL-C [42]. In contrast, the Atherosclerosis Risk in Communities (ARIC) study of 12,339 participants followed for 10 years failed to show that apoB enhanced risk prediction when considered with LDL-C, HDL-C, and triglycerides. The subset of patients with an excess apoB compared with LDL-C also did not show an increased CHD risk when adjusted for diabetes and other risk factors [50]. This study has been criticized, however, because a nonstandardized assay with unacceptable error was used to measure apoB [51]. The Framingham Offspring study, however, also did not find an incremental advantage to measuring lipoproteins when total cholesterol and HDL-C were available [43].

Treatment studies have also studied the relationship between lipoproteins and cardiovascular risk both using the placebo and on-treatment arms of the studies. In the primary prevention Air Force/Texas Coronary Atherosclerosis Prevention Study, on-treatment apoB was predictive of subsequent risk [52]. In the secondary prevention Treating to New Targets (TNT) and Incremental Decrease in End Points through Aggressive Lipid Lowering (IDEAL) studies, on-treatment levels of non-HDL-C and apoB were more closely related to CVD events than LDL-C supporting the use of non-HDL-C and apoB as treatment targets [53].

The data from epidemiologic and clinical trials mostly support the finding that apoB is at least as good and probably a better index of risk for CHD than LDL-C and non-HDL-C. ApoB may add information regarding risk in individuals who have achieved an LDL-C goal but still have an elevated apoB. These patients will have an increased number of smaller denser LDL particles. As with LDL particle number and measurement of pattern B LDL, an increased apoB is associated with hypertriglyceridemia, metabolic syndrome, and diabetes. A consensus statement on lipoprotein management in patients with cardiometabolic risk was published in 2008 by the American Diabetes Association (ADA) and the American College of Cardiology Foundation (ACCF) [54]. They concluded that patients with cardiometabolic risk should measure apoB as well as LDL-C and non-HDL-C to help guide therapy. Table 5.4 lists the suggested treatment goals for LDL-C, non-HDL-C, and apoB in patients with cardiometabolic risk. Population studies have shown that an apoB level of 120 mg/dl represents the 75th percentile [55]. An apoB of <90 mg/dl is a recommended goal for high-risk individuals and an apoB <80 mg/dl for the highest risk patients.

Table 5.4 Treatment goals in patients with cardiometabolic risk and lipoprotein abnormalities [54]

	Goals		
	LDL-C (mg/dl)	Non-HDL-C (mg/dl)	Apolipoprotein B (mg/dl)
Highest risk patients:			
Known CVD or diabetes plus one additional risk factor	<70	<100	<80
High-risk patients:			
No diabetes or known clinical CVD but two or more risk factors or diabetes but no other CVD risk factors	<100	<130	<90

Other risk factors beyond dyslipoproteinemia include smoking, hypertension, and family history of CAD

When to Use ApoB

The ADA/ACCF consensus statement recommends apoB as the third treatment goal in patients with cardiometabolic risk [54]. Even in the best clinical trials, a number of patients continue to have CVD events. The goal is to try to identify which patients on standard therapy are still at residual risk. Measurement of apoB, an estimate of LDL particle number, may help identify this higher-risk cohort. Because of the heterogeneity of particles, achieving an LDL-C and non-HDL-C goal does not guarantee that apoB is optimally reduced as well. In the Measuring Effective Reductions in Cholesterol Using Rosuvastatin Therapy (MERCURY) II trial, less than half of the patients who could achieve the dual LDL-C and non-HDL-C targets were able to meet the apoB target of <90 mg/dl [56]. Clinical trials are needed to determine if targeting apoB once LDL-C and non-HDL-C are at goal can bring about an incremental reduction in risk in a safe and cost-effective manner. In addition, for apoB to be widely accepted, the assay will need to be universally available and standardized and offered at a reasonable cost. An apoB measurement through our laboratory currently costs 95 dollars and is less expensive than other methods that estimate particle number or LDL patterns.

Summary Recommendations for Advanced LDL Testing

The National Cholesterol Education Program recommends that the LDL-C be the primary target of therapy and the Non-HDL-C the secondary target of therapy. By using these guidelines, there is good evidence that significant cardiovascular risk reduction can be achieved. There remains residual cardiovascular risk even in patients who have achieved these goals. It is reasonable to continue a lipoprotein targeted approach to risk reduction in high-risk individuals. Both the size and number of LDL particles can be used as an additional treatment target. At this point in time, further lowering the number of LDL particles is likely the best approach for further risk reduction. The different commercial tests offered can give information about the percent and amount of small, dense LDL. No one test appears to be superior to another to prefer any particular method. Cost and availability may determine which test is preferred. A relatively inexpensive test would be measurement of apoB in addition to the standard lipid panel and using the goals set by the ADA/ACCF as listed in Table 5.4. This may be the most practical target at the present time until more research is generated to determine if there is a better target than apoB. Therefore, for high-risk cardiometabolic patients, the additional measurement of apoB is reasonable and a recommended target to consider.

Lipoprotein(a)

Lipoprotein(a) is a variant of LDL. The lipoprotein moiety is very similar to LDL and contains apoB. In addition, Lp(a) contains a unique glycoprotein [apolipoprotein(a) or apo(a)] which is covalently linked to apoB. Apo(a) has a structural similarity to plasminogen and may represent a link between the development of atherosclerosis and thrombosis.

Lp(a) levels can vary over 1,000-fold in the human population from undetectable to an Lp(a) cholesterol of greater than 100 mg/dl. The variability in Lp(a) is largely genetic; therefore, there is very little change in Lp(a) concentration during lifetime or by environmental factors [57]. There can be a marked difference in Lp(a) levels between ethnic populations. African American patients tend to have Lp(a) levels that are two to three times higher than Caucasians [58], although this increase may not correlate with an increased cardiovascular risk. Lp(a) levels have also been shown to be higher in individuals from the Indian subcontinent compared with Europeans [59] and may be associated with a higher CHD [60] and ischemic stroke risk [61] in this population.

Lp(a) shows a marked heterogeneity in density and size in large part due to different isoforms of apo(a) that can vary between 300 and 800 kDa due to differences in the number of kringle repeats of the molecule [62]. The size variation of apo(a) leads to poor correlation of Lp(a) values obtained by different measurement methods. More recently, a specific monoclonal antibody technique was developed to allow measurement of Lp(a) levels that are not influenced by the size heterogeneity of apo(a) [63]. Use of this method showed that immunochemical methods can give highly variable results that can lead to misclassification of CHD risk. Most laboratories report Lp(a) cholesterol levels. Lp(a), like LDL particles, can exist as multiple subclasses from smaller denser particles to larger more buoyant particles. The cholesterol content of the particles may be dependent in part by the size of the apo(a) molecule. Lp(a) cholesterol values will not be an accurate measurement of the number of particles that are present. Table 5.5 gives the recommended ranges for interpreting Lp(a) values and cardiovascular risk.

Table 5.5 Lipoprotein(a) values and cardiovascular risk

	Lp(a) cholesterol value (mg/dl)
Desirable	<14
Borderline risk	14–30
High risk	31–50
Very high risk	>50

When to Measure Lp(a)

A number of epidemiologic studies have shown an association between high Lp(a) levels and CVD risk [64]. In addition, there is evidence to support high Lp(a) levels as a thrombotic risk factor as well [65]. Knowledge of Lp(a) values may help to determine CVD risk especially in certain subpopulations where Lp(a) may be a genetic trait. Therefore, it is reasonable to consider measuring Lp(a) in high-risk populations. This would include Caucasians and South Asians with a family history of CVD. It is not likely useful to measure Lp(a) in African American populations until we have more information about apo(a) isoforms that may be linked to CVD. In addition, occasionally a patient may be treated with an LDL-lowering therapy and not achieve the expected reduction in LDL-C. Since the Friedewald LDL-C includes Lp(a), this individual may have a high Lp(a) making up a large portion of the calculated LDL-C. An increased Lp(a) may also account for a large discrepancy between a calculated LDL-C and some direct LDL assays that are able to separate out the Lp(a). Measurement of Lp(a) would be useful in these groups. Many of the advanced lipid testing commercial products (VAP, Berkeley) include Lp(a) as a part of the lipid testing.

HDL Subfractions

HDL-C has long been known to inversely correlate with the development of coronary artery disease. High levels of HDL-C may have an antiatherogenic role. High-density lipoproteins are the smallest and densest of the lipoproteins and contain a number of apolipoproteins. Apolipoprotein A-I (apoA-I) and apolipoprotein A-II (apoA-II) are the two main HDL lipoproteins. HDL, as with LDL, is a heterogeneous lipoprotein consisting of several distinct subfractions that differ in size and density. Ultracentrifugation can separate HDL into two major subfractions designated HDL_2 (density 1.063–1.125 g/ml) and HDL_3 (density 1.125–1.21 g/ml) [66]. Gradient gel electrophoresis separates HDL on the basis of particle size into five subpopulations (HDL 2b, 2a, 3a, 3b, and 3c in decreasing size from 10.6 to 7.6 nm) [67].

The clinical correlation of the individual HDL subfractions and CVD has generated conflicting results. It was generally believed that the larger HDL_2 particles would be protective but multiple studies have indicated that *both* HDL_2 and HDL_3

are strong predictors of coronary artery disease [68]. Indeed, a recent post hoc analysis of the Incremental Decrease in End-Points through Aggressive Lipid Lowering (IDEAL) study and the European Prospective Investigation into Cancer and Nutrition (EPIC)-Norfolk case–control study showed the surprising finding that very high plasma HDL-C and very large HDL particles may correlate with increased CHD risk [69]. Some of the discrepancy between studies may be due to different separation techniques employed in these studies. Second, HDL function may be a more important parameter of risk than measurement of HDL-C or particle size.

When to Measure HDL Subfractions

The NCEP recognizes that HDL is a risk factor for CVD. HDL-C is indirectly included as a treatment target when non-HDL-C is used as a secondary target after LDL-C. Because of the conflicting results regarding HDL subfractions, it is unclear how to use HDL subfractions as a risk marker and it is premature to consider HDL subfractions as a treatment target. Further emerging research evaluating the function of HDL may be useful in future development of alternative biomarkers and treatment targets. Until that time, there does not appear to be an important role in determining HDL subfractions.

Apolipoprotein A-I

Apolipoprotein A-I (apoA-I) is one of the main structural proteins for HDL. It is involved in reverse cholesterol transport and mediates the transfer of cholesterol from cells to lipoprotein particles and activates the enzyme responsible for cholesterol esterification. ApoA-I correlates with HDL-C and, like HDL-C, is inversely related to CHD. Early retrospective studies showed that patients with CHD have substantially lower apoA-I than healthy controls [70]. Prospective studies have likewise shown that there is an approximately 60% increased risk of CHD for individuals in the bottom tercile for apoA-I compared with the top third [71].

ApoA-I has appeal as a CHD biomarker because it does not require a fasting sample for accurate measurement. This can avoid the errors that occur using calculated lipid values such as the Friedewald LDL-C. In addition, internationally standardized methods and reagents are used in measuring apoA-I, making the results accurate and reproducible across laboratories.

Many investigators have argued that the apolipoproteins are better than lipoprotein cholesterol measurements for risk prediction because of heterogeneity of particles, the need for fasting samples, and better standardization of assays. A ratio of apoB (the atherogenic particles) to apoA-I (particles involved in reverse cholesterol transport) could ideally be the one best value to correlate with risk. The INTERHEART study was designed to determine whether lipoproteins were better markers than lipids for CHD [72]. The INTERHEART study was a large case–control study of acute myocardial infarction in 12,461 cases and 14,637 age-matched and sex-matched controls in 52 countries. The apoB/apoA-I ratio was superior to any cholesterol ratios for the estimation of risk. This study verified the results of the AMORIS study also showing that the apoB/apoA-I ratio was highly predictive of CHD risk [48]. In contrast, both the Women's Health Study [41] and the Framingham Offspring Study [43] showed that the apoB/apoA-I ratio did not offer additional prognostic data beyond what was conveyed by the total cholesterol/HDL-C ratio.

When to Use Apolipoprotein A-I

The NCEP recommends that LDL-C should be the primary target of therapy. Non-HDL-C is the secondary target and is indirectly taking HDL-C into account. ApoA-I is likely a more accurate measure of HDL-C avoiding the heterogeneity of HDL particles and the confusion that exists between studies measuring HDL subfractions. There are no clear studies recommending an apoA-I target and few treatment studies showing improved outcomes based on apoA-I therapies. Most of the predictive information conveyed by the apoB/apoA-I ratio is present in the total cholesterol/HDL ratio which in a sense is a similar measurement. Since the cholesterol values are readily available, measuring all of the apolipoproteins to obtain the apoB/apoA-I ratio is not likely to further discriminate risk or change therapy in many patients. ApoB as a third treatment target is gaining acceptance as noted above. There is less compelling data supporting apoA-I at this time.

Inflammatory Markers

High-Sensitivity C-Reactive Protein

Atherosclerosis has an inflammatory component that may contribute to progression of disease and vascular events. C-reactive protein (CRP) is an inflammatory cytokine that has been extensively studied in vascular disease. CRP binds to the C-polysaccharide of the pneumococcal cell wall and to phospholipids of damaged cells activating the complement system [73]. CRP is a nonspecific biomarker of inflammation and may be involved in progression of atherosclerosis by activating endothelial cells to express adhesion molecules and activate macrophages to take up LDL. During acute inflammation, CRP levels can increase as much as 500-fold. In the absence of acute inflammation, CRP levels can be nearly undetectable. This has led to the development of more precise assays termed high-sensitivity C-reactive protein (hs-CRP) that are able to detect CRP down to levels of 0.3 mg/l or below. CRP levels within this low range have been found to correlate with cardiovascular risk.

hs-CRP can be used as a marker of risk assessment that may give additional information about risk beyond traditional risk factors. CRP levels correlate with the Framingham risk score [74] and in a cohort of men aged 45–74 years, gave a significant contribution to CHD event prediction independent of the Framingham score [75]. The measurement of CRP may be most useful in individuals determined to be in the intermediate risk group (between 10 and 20% 10-year risk) since it may lead to a reclassification of risk or lead to more aggressive risk reduction therapy if elevated. Not all studies, however, have shown that measurement of CRP gives further prognostic information. An investigation of a Framingham cohort [76] and findings from the Atherosclerosis Risk in Communities (ARIC) study [77] found that elevated CRP levels added no further prognostic information beyond traditional risk factor assessment. Critics of CRP point out that a risk assessment using established risk factors provide a remarkably good ability to discriminate individuals at risk for CHD and that routine measurement of novel biomarkers rarely adds further predictive power [78].

Primary prevention trials have attempted to verify the use of hs-CRP in predicting CVD risk. Analysis of two primary prevention trials (Air Force/Texas Coronary Atherosclerosis Prevention Study [79] and the Physicians Health Study [80]) showed that coronary events increased significantly with increased hs-CRP. CRP may be a stronger predictor of risk than LDL-C [81]. Specific risk groups tend to have elevated CRP levels. CRP levels are higher in obese or overweight individuals [82], especially if insulin resistance is present [83]. Metabolic syndrome is associated with a high-risk level of hs-CRP [84]. The combination of metabolic syndrome and a high-risk hs-CRP may identify a higher-risk cohort of individuals.

Secondary prevention studies have shown that CRP is associated with an increased risk for subsequent events. In the Cholesterol and Recurrent Events (CARE) trial, the highest risk for recurrent events occurred in the individuals with the highest CRP levels [85]. CRP may be useful in patients admitted to the hospital with an acute coronary syndrome. Patients with unstable angina and elevated CRP levels had more ischemic episodes and were more likely to have a myocardial infarction or require revascularization [86, 87]. CRP levels that remain elevated at hospital discharge after an acute coronary syndrome were associated with recurrent unstable angina or a new myocardial infarction [88]. Treatment with intense lipid-lowering therapy can reduce CRP levels and may be associated with clinical benefit [89] and less progression of coronary disease compared with standard dose therapy [90].

hs-CRP can be divided into three tercile risk levels (Table 5.6). hs-CRP >3.0 mg/l is designated the high-risk group and has a twofold increase in relative risk for CHD

Table 5.6 hs-CRP risk levels

hs-CRP (mg/l)	Risk level
<1.0	Low risk
1.0–3.0	Average risk
>3.0	High risk

compared with the low-risk tercile (<1.0 mg/l) [91]. CRP is a nonspecific inflammatory marker and acute inflammation typically increases CRP levels well beyond the levels measured by the hs-CRP assay. Values >10 mg/l are usually secondary to other sources of inflammation or infection and are not exclusively the result of atherosclerotic inflammation.

When to Measure hs-CRP

hs-CRP may be a useful biomarker to help define CVD risk. hs-CRP will not likely add additional prognostic information in the lowest or highest risk individuals. hs-CRP may not change risk categories for an individual patient but as an additional marker of risk may suggest the need for more aggressive risk reduction therapy. For example, the NCEP would recommend that a patient determined to be in the intermediate risk group have an LDL treatment target of <130 mg/dl. The addition of a high-risk hs-CRP may suggest a change of therapy to the optional goal of <100 mg/dl. The early termination of the JUPITER trial which studied lipid lowering in primary prevention patients with low levels of LDL-C and elevated hs-CRP suggests that this strategy may be useful for a subset of intermediate risk patients [92]. As a treatment target, however, CRP cannot be used as a reliable treatment goal since many noncardiac conditions influence the level.

Lipoprotein-Associated Phospholipase A_2

Lipoprotein-associated phospholipase A_2 (Lp-PLA_2) is a member of a superfamily of enzymes that hydrolyzes phospholipids. Lp-PLA_2 is produced and secreted by macrophages and foam cells where it preferentially binds to apoB containing particles [93]. Lp-PLA_2 degrades phopholipids present in oxidized LDL releasing further inflammatory products. Lp-PLA_2 has been found to accumulate in atherosclerotic plaque and concentrates in the shoulder region and necrotic core of fibrous caps. Its presence in lipid laden plaques may contribute to instability of the plaque and plaque rupture. Unlike other inflammatory biomarkers, Lp-PLA_2 is not usually elevated in systemic inflammatory conditions such as rheumatoid arthritis [94]. Therefore, Lp-PLA_2 is thought to be a more specific marker for inflammation due to atherosclerosis than hs-CRP.

A number of primary prevention trials have found that Lp-PLA_2 predicts coronary events. The West of Scotland Coronary Prevention Study showed that patients with the highest levels of Lp-PLA_2 had close to a doubling of the risk for cardiovascular events [95]. In the Atherosclerosis Risk in Communities (ARIC) study, Lp-PLA_2 was associated with CHD in over 12,000 healthy individuals although the risk was not statistically significant when adjusted for traditional risk factors [96]. Individuals with LDL-C <130 mg/dl, however, and both Lp-PLA_2 and CRP in the highest tercile were at the greatest risk for a CHD event. This suggests that these biomarkers may be useful in identifying individuals at higher CHD risk who have lipoprotein values in the desirable range. Secondary prevention trials have shown a similar relationship between high levels of Lp-PLA$_2$ and cardiovascular events. Over 25 prospective primary and secondary epidemiologic studies have shown an association between Lp-PLA$_2$ and cardiovascular events with a hazard ratio of 1.5–2.0 for Lp-PLA$_2$ in the top quintile compared with the bottom quintile [97]. Some studies in patients with CHD have shown that Lp-PLA$_2$ remains an independent predictor of risk after controlling for traditional risk factors and other biomarkers [98].

Lp-PLA$_2$ may become a novel treatment target in addition to a biomarker of risk. Darapladib is a selective inhibitor of Lp-PLA$_2$ and has been shown to produce sustained inhibition of Lp-PLA$_2$ activity. In addition, treatment with darapladib lowers inflammatory biomarkers such as interleukin-6 and hs-CRP [99]. In an intravascular coronary ultrasound study, darapladib prevented expansion of the necrotic core, whereas the necrotic core continued to expand in patients on placebo [100]. Necrotic core expansion could be responsible for future cardiovascular events. Clinical outcome studies are now underway to determine if this therapeutic approach may lead to a reduction in cardiovascular events.

Lp-PLA$_2$ is available as a turbidimetric immunoassay or an ELISA format from diaDexus and is FDA-cleared for determination of Lp-PLA$_2$ (PLAC test). A blood sample can be sent to the company since many laboratories do not run the test in house. The test is currently covered by Medicare (approximately $47) but not by all insurance carriers.

From the epidemiologic studies, an Lp-PLA$_2$ <200 ng/ml is considered low risk, 200–235 ng/ml borderline high risk, and >235 ng/ml high risk. It has been suggested that levels >235 ng/ml in an intermediate risk patient should move the patient into the high-risk category. An algorithm proposing how to use Lp-PLA$_2$ to determine LDL-C treatment goals for moderate- and high-risk individuals is shown in Fig. 5.1.

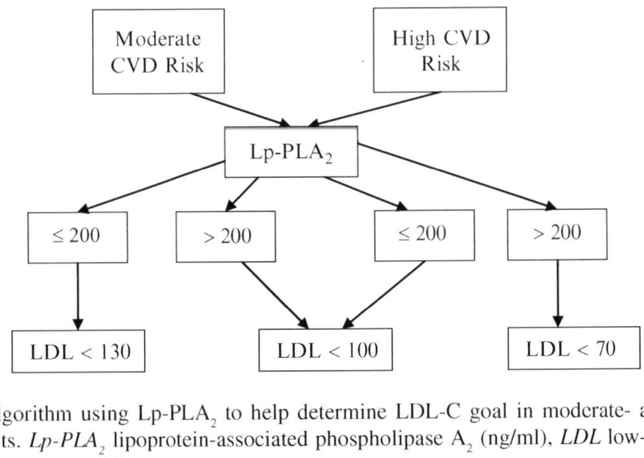

Fig. 5.1 Algorithm using Lp-PLA$_2$ to help determine LDL-C goal in moderate- and high-risk CVD patients. *Lp-PLA$_2$* lipoprotein-associated phospholipase A$_2$ (ng/ml), *LDL* low-density lipoprotein cholesterol (mg/dl)

When to Measure Lp-PLA$_2$

As with other inflammatory markers, Lp-PLA$_2$ usually does not add a significant change in risk prediction beyond traditional risk factor assessment. Measuring inflammatory markers may be most useful in intermediate risk patients if an elevated value would lead to a more aggressive treatment. For most intermediate risk patients, an option to choose the more aggressive LDL-C goal can be made by simply counting the number of risk factors. Inflammatory markers may also prove useful in evaluating patients who are thought to be at the optimal lipoprotein goal. Elevated markers in these individuals may suggest further aggressive therapy or combination therapy to target residual risk. Outcome trials need to be completed to determine if this strategy will lead to further clinical event reduction. Finally, Lp-PLA$_2$ may prove to be a treatment target. Outcome studies will need to be completed to determine if targeting Lp-PLA$_2$ will lead to incremental reduction in events. Until these studies are completed, Lp-PLA$_2$ cannot be recommended as a routine screening test.

Thrombotic Markers – Homocysteine

Homocystinuria is a rare genetic disease that causes significantly elevated levels of homocysteine and is associated with serious thromboembolic complications including myocardial infarction, pulmonary embolism, and stroke. Studies of individuals with this rare disorder led to speculation that elevated homocysteine levels in the general population may be a cause of thrombotic events. An association between elevated plasma homocysteine levels was first noted in retrospective case–control studies. A summary of 11 series with more than 2,000 patients showed that homocysteine values were higher in patients with CVD [101]. A subsequent meta-analysis determined that hyperhomocysteinemia was an independent risk factor for vascular disease with an odds ratio of 1.7 for CHD for a 5 μmol/l homocysteine increment [102]. Prospective studies have been less conclusive about the association between homocysteine and vascular thrombotic events. After adjustment for traditional risk factors, the Atherosclerosis Risk in Communities (ARIC) study did not find an independent association with homocysteine and CHD [103].

Since homocysteine levels can be reduced by dietary or supplemental folic acid, a number of treatment trials were designed to determine if homocysteine as a treatment target can lead to a reduction in clinical events. A summary of these trials to date indicate that there are no sufficient data to show that lowering plasma homocysteine concentrations prevents vascular events [104]. One possible explanation for the failure of the initial trials of homocysteine lowering to prevent CVD events may be that the fortification of foods with B vitamins has had a population impact on homocysteine levels making it difficult to show a treatment benefit with further supplementation. The results of these trials has led to the conclusion that B vitamin supplements cannot be recommended for the prevention of CVD events and that routine screening of homocysteine is not justified.

When to Measure Homocysteine

Routine screening of homocysteine levels is not recommended. However, there may be some patients in whom the measurement of homocysteine may be considered. Very high levels of homocysteine can lead to thrombotic complications. Therefore, homocysteine should be measured as part of a hypercoagulable work-up. It can be considered in individuals with a strong family history of premature atherosclerosis or in someone with significant disease out of proportion to their traditional risk factors.

Conclusions

The measurement of lipoproteins remains the mainstay for determining cardiovascular risk. For routine screening, a fasting lipid panel that includes a total cholesterol, HDL-C, triglyceride, and a calculated LDL-C is recommended. If triglyceride levels are elevated above 400 mg/dl, a direct LDL can be measured. From this analysis, a non-HDL-C and a total cholesterol/HDL-C ratio can be calculated. In addition, these values can then be used to determine treatment targets for LDL-C and non-HDL-C.

For patients with multiple cardiometabolic risk factors or high-risk individuals, more aggressive therapy is warranted and consideration of further biomarker measurements can be made with the goal of reducing further residual risk. Treatment studies with documented further risk reduction beyond what can be achieved by reaching LDL-C and non-HDL-C goals have not yet proven that this strategy will lead to clinically significant benefit. The measurement of apoB appears the most promising biomarker since it is a measure of the number of LDL particles. The addition of an inflammatory marker may identify a cohort of individual still at risk despite achievement of lipoprotein goals. More specific atherosclerosis inflammatory markers are needed. Lp-PLA_2 is a promising marker and possible treatment target, but further data are required before it can be recommended as a routine measurement.

References

1. Third Report of the National Cholesterol Education Program (NCEP) Expert Panel on Detection, Evaluation, and Treatment of High Blood Cholesterol in Adults (Adult Treatment Panel III) final report. Circulation 2002;106(25):3143–421.
2. Friedewald WT, Levy RI, Fredrickson DS. Estimation of the concentration of low-density lipoprotein cholesterol in plasma, without use of the preparative ultracentrifuge. Clin Chem. 1972;18(6):499–502.
3. DeLong DM, DeLong ER, Wood PD, Lippel K, Rifkind BM. A comparison of methods for the estimation of plasma low- and very low-density lipoprotein cholesterol. The Lipid Research Clinics Prevalence Study. JAMA. 1986;256(17):2372–7.

4. Branchi A, Rovellini A, Torri A, Sommariva D. Accuracy of calculated serum low-density lipoprotein cholesterol for the assessment of coronary heart disease risk in NIDDM patients. Diabetes Care. 1998;21(9):1397–402.
5. Wilson PW, Zech LA, Gregg RE, et al. Estimation of VLDL cholesterol in hyperlipidemia. Clin Chim Acta. 1985;151(3):285–91.
6. Nauck M, Warnick GR, Rifai N. Methods for measurement of LDL-cholesterol: a critical assessment of direct measurement by homogeneous assays versus calculation. Clin Chem. 2002;48(2):236–54.
7. Friday KE. Specialized lipid profiles. Curr Atheroscler Rep. 2002;4(5):359–62.
8. Krauss RM, Burke DJ. Identification of multiple subclasses of plasma low density lipoproteins in normal humans. J Lipid Res. 1982;23(1):97–104.
9. Sniderman A, Shapiro S, Marpole D, Skinner B, Teng B, Kwiterovich Jr PO. Association of coronary atherosclerosis with hyperapobetalipoproteinemia [increased protein but normal cholesterol levels in human plasma low density (beta) lipoproteins]. Proc Natl Acad Sci USA. 1980;77(1):604–8.
10. Roheim PS, Asztalos BF. Clinical significance of lipoprotein size and risk for coronary atherosclerosis. Clin Chem. 1995;41(1):147–52.
11. Campos H, Blijlevens E, McNamara JR, et al. LDL particle size distribution. Results from the Framingham Offspring Study. Arterioscler Thromb. 1992;12(12):1410–9.
12. Austin MA, King MC, Vranizan KM, Krauss RM. Atherogenic lipoprotein phenotype. A proposed genetic marker for coronary heart disease risk. Circulation. 1990;82(2):495–506.
13. Kathiresan S, Otvos JD, Sullivan LM, et al. Increased small low-density lipoprotein particle number: a prominent feature of the metabolic syndrome in the Framingham Heart Study. Circulation. 2006;113(1):20–9.
14. Selby JV, Austin MA, Newman B, et al. LDL subclass phenotypes and the insulin resistance syndrome in women. Circulation. 1993;88(2):381–7.
15. Gardner CD, Fortmann SP, Krauss RM. Association of small low-density lipoprotein particles with the incidence of coronary artery disease in men and women. JAMA. 1996;276(11):875–81.
16. Stampfer MJ, Krauss RM, Ma J, et al. A prospective study of triglyceride level, low-density lipoprotein particle diameter, and risk of myocardial infarction. JAMA. 1996;276(11):882–8.
17. Lamarche B, Tchernof A, Moorjani S, et al. Small, dense low-density lipoprotein particles as a predictor of the risk of ischemic heart disease in men. Prospective results from the Quebec Cardiovascular Study. Circulation. 1997;95(1):69–75.
18. Austin MA. Triglyceride, small, dense low-density lipoprotein, and the atherogenic lipoprotein phenotype. Curr Atheroscler Rep. 2000;2(3):200–7.
19. Koba S, Hirano T, Kondo T, et al. Significance of small dense low-density lipoproteins and other risk factors in patients with various types of coronary heart disease. Am Heart J. 2002;144(6):1026–35.
20. Arsenault BJ, Lemieux I, Despres JP, et al. Cholesterol levels in small LDL particles predict the risk of coronary heart disease in the EPIC-Norfolk prospective population study. Eur Heart J. 2007;28(22):2770–7.
21. Miller BD, Alderman EL, Haskell WL, Fair JM, Krauss RM. Predominance of dense low-density lipoprotein particles predicts angiographic benefit of therapy in the Stanford Coronary Risk Intervention Project. Circulation. 1996;94(9):2146–53.
22. Zambon A, Hokanson JE, Brown BG, Brunzell JD. Evidence for a new pathophysiological mechanism for coronary artery disease regression: hepatic lipase-mediated changes in LDL density. Circulation. 1999;99(15):1959–64.
23. Azadbakht L, Mirmiran P, Hedayati M, Esmaillzadeh A, Shiva N, Azizi F. Particle size of LDL is affected by the National Cholesterol Education Program (NCEP) step II diet in dyslipidaemic adolescents. Br J Nutr. 2007;98(1):134–9.
24. Goulet J, Lamarche B, Charest A, et al. Effect of a nutritional intervention promoting the Mediterranean food pattern on electrophoretic characteristics of low-density lipoprotein particles in healthy women from the Quebec City metropolitan area. Br J Nutr. 2004;92(2):285–93.

25. Barakat HA, Carpenter JW, McLendon VD, et al. Influence of obesity, impaired glucose tolerance, and NIDDM on LDL structure and composition. Possible link between hyperinsulinemia and atherosclerosis. Diabetes. 1990;39(12):1527–33.
26. Caixas A, Ordonez-Llanos J, de Leiva A, Payes A, Homs R, Perez A. Optimization of glycemic control by insulin therapy decreases the proportion of small dense LDL particles in diabetic patients. Diabetes. 1997;46(7):1207–13.
27. Goldberg RB, Kendall DM, Deeg MA, et al. A comparison of lipid and glycemic effects of pioglitazone and rosiglitazone in patients with type 2 diabetes and dyslipidemia. Diabetes Care. 2005;28(7):1547–54.
28. Superko HR, Krauss RM. Differential effects of nicotinic acid in subjects with different LDL subclass patterns. Atherosclerosis. 1992;95(1):69–76.
29. Guerin M, Bruckert E, Dolphin PJ, Turpin G, Chapman MJ. Fenofibrate reduces plasma cholesteryl ester transfer from HDL to VLDL and normalizes the atherogenic, dense LDL profile in combined hyperlipidemia. Arterioscler Thromb Vasc Biol. 1996;16(6):763–72.
30. Otvos JD, Collins D, Freedman DS, et al. Low-density lipoprotein and high-density lipoprotein particle subclasses predict coronary events and are favorably changed by gemfibrozil therapy in the Veterans Affairs High-Density Lipoprotein Intervention Trial. Circulation. 2006;113(12):1556–63.
31. Caslake MJ, Stewart G, Day SP, et al. Phenotype-dependent and -independent actions of rosuvastatin on atherogenic lipoprotein subfractions in hyperlipidaemia. Atherosclerosis. 2003;171(2):245–53.
32. Sirtori CR, Calabresi L, Pisciotta L, et al. Effect of statins on LDL particle size in patients with familial combined hyperlipidemia: a comparison between atorvastatin and pravastatin. Nutr Metab Cardiovasc Dis. 2005;15(1):47–55.
33. Kulkarni KR, Garber DW, Marcovina SM, Segrest JP. Quantification of cholesterol in all lipoprotein classes by the VAP-II method. J Lipid Res. 1994;35(1):159–68.
34. Kulkarni KR, Garber DW, Jones MK, Segrest JP. Identification and cholesterol quantification of low density lipoprotein subclasses in young adults by VAP-II methodology. J Lipid Res. 1995;36(11):2291–302.
35. Kuller L, Arnold A, Tracy R, et al. Nuclear magnetic resonance spectroscopy of lipoproteins and risk of coronary heart disease in the cardiovascular health study. Arterioscler Thromb Vasc Biol. 2002;22(7):1175–80.
36. Rosenson RS, Otvos JD, Freedman DS. Relations of lipoprotein subclass levels and low-density lipoprotein size to progression of coronary artery disease in the Pravastatin Limitation of Atherosclerosis in the Coronary Arteries (PLAC-I) trial. Am J Cardiol. 2002;90(2):89–94.
37. Blake GJ, Otvos JD, Rifai N, Ridker PM. Low-density lipoprotein particle concentration and size as determined by nuclear magnetic resonance spectroscopy as predictors of cardiovascular disease in women. Circulation. 2002;106(15):1930–7.
38. Cromwell WC, Otvos JD, Keyes MJ, et al. LDL particle number and risk of future cardiovascular disease in the Framingham Offspring Study – implications for LDL management. J Clin Lipidol. 2007;1:583–92.
39. Cromwell WC, Otvos JD. Heterogeneity of low-density lipoprotein particle number in patients with type 2 diabetes mellitus and low-density lipoprotein cholesterol <100 mg/dl. Am J Cardiol. 2006;98(12):1599–602.
40. Cui Y, Blumenthal RS, Flaws JA, et al. Non-high-density lipoprotein cholesterol level as a predictor of cardiovascular disease mortality. Arch Intern Med. 2001;161(11):1413–9.
41. Ridker PM, Rifai N, Cook NR, Bradwin G, Buring JE. Non-HDL cholesterol, apolipoproteins A-I and B100, standard lipid measures, lipid ratios, and CRP as risk factors for cardiovascular disease in women. JAMA. 2005;294(3):326–33.
42. Pischon T, Girman CJ, Sacks FM, Rifai N, Stampfer MJ, Rimm EB. Non-high-density lipoprotein cholesterol and apolipoprotein B in the prediction of coronary heart disease in men. Circulation. 2005;112(22):3375–83.
43. Ingelsson E, Schaefer EJ, Contois JH, et al. Clinical utility of different lipid measures for prediction of coronary heart disease in men and women. JAMA. 2007;298(7):776–85.

44. Lu W, Resnick HE, Jablonski KA, et al. Non-HDL cholesterol as a predictor of cardiovascular disease in type 2 diabetes: the strong heart study. Diabetes Care. 2003;26(1):16–23.
45. Liu J, Sempos C, Donahue RP, Dorn J, Trevisan M, Grundy SM. Joint distribution of non-HDL and LDL cholesterol and coronary heart disease risk prediction among individuals with and without diabetes. Diabetes Care. 2005;28(8):1916–21.
46. Bittner V, Hardison R, Kelsey SF, Weiner BH, Jacobs AK, Sopko G. Non-high-density lipoprotein cholesterol levels predict five-year outcome in the Bypass Angioplasty Revascularization Investigation (BARI). Circulation. 2002;106(20):2537–42.
47. Abate N, Vega GL, Grundy SM. Variability in cholesterol content and physical properties of lipoproteins containing apolipoprotein B-100. Atherosclerosis. 1993;104(1–2):159–71.
48. Walldius G, Jungner I, Holme I, Aastveit AH, Kolar W, Steiner E. High apolipoprotein B, low apolipoprotein A-I, and improvement in the prediction of fatal myocardial infarction (AMORIS study): a prospective study. Lancet. 2001;358(9298):2026–33.
49. Lamarche B, Moorjani S, Lupien PJ, et al. Apolipoprotein A-I and B levels and the risk of ischemic heart disease during a five-year follow-up of men in the Quebec cardiovascular study. Circulation. 1996;94(3):273–8.
50. Sharrett AR, Ballantyne CM, Coady SA, et al. Coronary heart disease prediction from lipoprotein cholesterol levels, triglycerides, lipoprotein(a), apolipoproteins A-I and B, and HDL density subfractions: The Atherosclerosis Risk in Communities (ARIC) Study. Circulation. 2001;104(10):1108–13.
51. Sniderman AD. How, when, and why to use apolipoprotein B in clinical practice. Am J Cardiol. 2002;90(8A):48i–54i.
52. Gotto Jr AM, Whitney E, Stein EA, et al. Relation between baseline and on-treatment lipid parameters and first acute major coronary events in the Air Force/Texas Coronary Atherosclerosis Prevention Study (AFCAPS/TexCAPS). Circulation. 2000;101(5): 477–84.
53. Kastelein JJ, van der Steeg WA, Holme I, et al. Lipids, apolipoproteins, and their ratios in relation to cardiovascular events with statin treatment. Circulation. 2008;117(23):3002–9.
54. Brunzell JD, Davidson M, Furberg CD, et al. Lipoprotein management in patients with cardiometabolic risk: consensus statement from the American Diabetes Association and the American College of Cardiology Foundation. Diabetes Care. 2008;31(4):811–22.
55. Contois JH, McNamara JR, Lammi-Keefe CJ, Wilson PW, Massov T, Schaefer EJ. Reference intervals for plasma apolipoprotein B determined with a standardized commercial immunoturbidimetric assay: results from the Framingham Offspring Study. Clin Chem. 1996;42(4):515–23.
56. Ballantyne CM, Bertolami M, Hernandez Garcia HR, et al. Achieving LDL cholesterol, non-HDL cholesterol, and apolipoprotein B target levels in high-risk patients: measuring Effective Reductions in Cholesterol Using Rosuvastatin therapY (MERCURY) II. Am Heart J. 2006;151(5):975.e1–9.
57. Koschinsky ML. Lipoprotein(a) and atherosclerosis: new perspectives on the mechanism of action of an enigmatic lipoprotein. Curr Atheroscler Rep. 2005;7(5):389–95.
58. Sorrentino MJ, Vielhauer C, Eisenbart JD, Fless GM, Scanu AM, Feldman T. Plasma lipoprotein (a) protein concentration and coronary artery disease in black patients compared with white patients. Am J Med. 1992;93(6):658–62.
59. Bhatnagar D, Anand IS, Durrington PN, et al. Coronary risk factors in people from the Indian subcontinent living in west London and their siblings in India. Lancet. 1995;345(8947): 405–9.
60. Geethanjali FS, Jose VJ, Kanagasabapathy AS. Lipoprotein (a) phenotypes in south Indian patients with coronary artery disease. Indian Heart J. 2002;54(1):50–3.
61. Sharobeem KM, Patel JV, Ritch AE, Lip GY, Gill PS, Hughes EA. Elevated lipoprotein (a) and apolipoprotein B to AI ratio in South Asian patients with ischaemic stroke. Int J Clin Pract. 2007;61(11):1824–8.
62. Scanu AM. Lp(a) lipoprotein–coping with heterogeneity. N Engl J Med. 2003;349(22): 2089–90.

63. Marcovina SM, Albers JJ, Scanu AM, et al. Use of a reference material proposed by the International Federation of Clinical Chemistry and Laboratory Medicine to evaluate analytical methods for the determination of plasma lipoprotein(a). Clin Chem. 2000;46(12):1956–67.
64. Danesh J, Collins R, Peto R. Lipoprotein(a) and coronary heart disease. Meta-analysis of prospective studies. Circulation. 2000;102(10):1082–5.
65. Marcovina SM, Koschinsky ML. Evaluation of lipoprotein(a) as a prothrombotic factor: progress from bench to bedside. Curr Opin Lipidol. 2003;14(4):361–6.
66. Chapman MJ, Goldstein S, Lagrange D, Laplaud PM. A density gradient ultracentrifugal procedure for the isolation of the major lipoprotein classes from human serum. J Lipid Res. 1981;22(2):339–58.
67. Anderson DW, Nichols AV, Forte TM, Lindgren FT. Particle distribution of human serum high density lipoproteins. Biochim Biophys Acta. 1977;493(1):55–68.
68. Kontush A, Chapman MJ. Functionally defective high-density lipoprotein: a new therapeutic target at the crossroads of dyslipidemia, inflammation, and atherosclerosis. Pharmacol Rev. 2006;58(3):342–74.
69. van der Steeg WA, Holme I, Boekholdt SM, et al. High-density lipoprotein cholesterol, high-density lipoprotein particle size, and apolipoprotein A-I: significance for cardiovascular risk: the IDEAL and EPIC-Norfolk studies. J Am Coll Cardiol. 2008;51(6):634–42.
70. Rader DJ, Hoeg JM, Brewer Jr HB. Quantitation of plasma apolipoproteins in the primary and secondary prevention of coronary artery disease. Ann Intern Med. 1994;120(12):1012–25.
71. Thompson A, Danesh J. Associations between apolipoprotein B, apolipoprotein AI, the apolipoprotein B/AI ratio and coronary heart disease: a literature-based meta-analysis of prospective studies. J Intern Med. 2006;259(5):481–92.
72. McQueen MJ, Hawken S, Wang X, et al. Lipids, lipoproteins, and apolipoproteins as risk markers of myocardial infarction in 52 countries (the INTERHEART study): a case-control study. Lancet. 2008;372(9634):224–33.
73. Yeh ET, Willerson JT. Coming of age of C-reactive protein: using inflammation markers in cardiology. Circulation. 2003;107(3):370–1.
74. Albert MA, Glynn RJ, Ridker PM. Plasma concentration of C-reactive protein and the calculated Framingham Coronary Heart Disease Risk Score. Circulation. 2003;108(2):161–5.
75. Koenig W, Lowel H, Baumert J, Meisinger C. C-reactive protein modulates risk prediction based on the Framingham Score: implications for future risk assessment: results from a large cohort study in southern Germany. Circulation. 2004;109(11):1349–53.
76. Wilson PW, Nam BH, Pencina M, D'Agostino Sr RB, Benjamin EJ, O'Donnell CJ. C-reactive protein and risk of cardiovascular disease in men and women from the Framingham Heart Study. Arch Intern Med. 2005;165(21):2473–8.
77. Folsom AR, Chambless LE, Ballantyne CM, et al. An assessment of incremental coronary risk prediction using C-reactive protein and other novel risk markers: the atherosclerosis risk in communities study. Arch Intern Med. 2006;166(13):1368–73.
78. Lloyd-Jones DM, Tian L. Predicting cardiovascular risk: so what do we do now? Arch Intern Med. 2006;166(13):1342–4.
79. Ridker PM, Rifai N, Clearfield M, et al. Measurement of C-reactive protein for the targeting of statin therapy in the primary prevention of acute coronary events. N Engl J Med. 2001;344(26):1959–65.
80. Ridker PM, Cushman M, Stampfer MJ, Tracy RP, Hennekens CH. Inflammation, aspirin, and the risk of cardiovascular disease in apparently healthy men. N Engl J Med. 1997;336(14):973–9.
81. Ridker PM. Clinical application of C-reactive protein for cardiovascular disease detection and prevention. Circulation. 2003;107(3):363–9.
82. Visser M, Bouter LM, McQuillan GM, Wener MH, Harris TB. Elevated C-reactive protein levels in overweight and obese adults. JAMA. 1999;282(22):2131–5.
83. McLaughlin T, Abbasi F, Lamendola C, et al. Differentiation between obesity and insulin resistance in the association with C-reactive protein. Circulation. 2002;106(23):2908–12.

84. Ridker PM, Buring JE, Cook NR, Rifai N. C-reactive protein, the metabolic syndrome, and risk of incident cardiovascular events: an 8-year follow-up of 14 719 initially healthy American women. Circulation. 2003;107(3):391–7.
85. Ridker PM, Rifai N, Pfeffer MA, et al. Inflammation, pravastatin, and the risk of coronary events after myocardial infarction in patients with average cholesterol levels. Cholesterol and Recurrent Events (CARE) Investigators. Circulation. 1998;98(9):839–44.
86. Liuzzo G, Biasucci LM, Gallimore JR, et al. The prognostic value of C-reactive protein and serum amyloid a protein in severe unstable angina. N Engl J Med. 1994;331(7):417–24.
87. Rebuzzi AG, Quaranta G, Liuzzo G, et al. Incremental prognostic value of serum levels of troponin T and C-reactive protein on admission in patients with unstable angina pectoris. Am J Cardiol. 1998;82(6):715–9.
88. Biasucci LM, Liuzzo G, Grillo RL, et al. Elevated levels of C-reactive protein at discharge in patients with unstable angina predict recurrent instability. Circulation. 1999;99(7):855–60.
89. Kinlay S, Schwartz GG, Olsson AG, et al. High-dose atorvastatin enhances the decline in inflammatory markers in patients with acute coronary syndromes in the MIRACL study. Circulation. 2003;108(13):1560–6.
90. Nissen SE, Tuzcu EM, Schoenhagen P, et al. Effect of intensive compared with moderate lipid-lowering therapy on progression of coronary atherosclerosis: a randomized controlled trial. JAMA. 2004;291(9):1071–80.
91. Pearson TA, Mensah GA, Alexander RW, et al. Markers of inflammation and cardiovascular disease: application to clinical and public health practice: a statement for healthcare professionals from the Centers for Disease Control and Prevention and the American Heart Association. Circulation. 2003;107(3):499–511.
92. Ridker PM. Rosuvastatin in the primary prevention of cardiovascular disease among patients with low levels of low-density lipoprotein cholesterol and elevated high-sensitivity C-reactive protein: rationale and design of the JUPITER trial. Circulation. 2003;108(19):2292–7.
93. Zalewski A, Macphee C. Role of lipoprotein-associated phospholipase A2 in atherosclerosis: biology, epidemiology, and possible therapeutic target. Arterioscler Thromb Vasc Biol. 2005;25(5):923–31.
94. Lerman A, McConnell JP. Lipoprotein-associated phospholipase A2: a risk marker or a risk factor? Am J Cardiol. 2008;101(12A):11F–22F.
95. Packard CJ, O'Reilly DS, Caslake MJ, et al. Lipoprotein-associated phospholipase A2 as an independent predictor of coronary heart disease. West of Scotland Coronary Prevention Study Group. N Engl J Med. 2000;343(16):1148–55.
96. Ballantyne CM, Hoogeveen RC, Bang H, et al. Lipoprotein-associated phospholipase A2, high-sensitivity C-reactive protein, and risk for incident coronary heart disease in middle-aged men and women in the Atherosclerosis Risk in Communities (ARIC) study. Circulation. 2004;109(7):837–42.
97. Corson MA, Jones PH, Davidson MH. Review of the evidence for the clinical utility of lipoprotein-associated phospholipase A2 as a cardiovascular risk marker. Am J Cardiol. 2008;101(12A):41F–50F.
98. Khuseyinova N, Imhof A, Rothenbacher D, et al. Association between Lp-PLA2 and coronary artery disease: focus on its relationship with lipoproteins and markers of inflammation and hemostasis. Atherosclerosis. 2005;182(1):181–8.
99. Mohler III ER, Ballantyne CM, Davidson MH, et al. The effect of darapladib on plasma lipoprotein-associated phospholipase A2 activity and cardiovascular biomarkers in patients with stable coronary heart disease or coronary heart disease risk equivalent: the results of a multicenter, randomized, double-blind, placebo-controlled study. J Am Coll Cardiol. 2008;51(17):1632–41.
100. Serruys PW, Garcia-Garcia HM, Buszman P, et al. Effects of the direct lipoprotein-associated phospholipase A(2) inhibitor darapladib on human coronary atherosclerotic plaque. Circulation. 2008;118(11):1172–82.
101. Malinow MR. Hyperhomocyst(e)inemia. A common and easily reversible risk factor for occlusive atherosclerosis. Circulation. 1990;81(6):2004–6.

102. Boushey CJ, Beresford SA, Omenn GS, Motulsky AG. A quantitative assessment of plasma homocysteine as a risk factor for vascular disease. Probable benefits of increasing folic acid intakes. JAMA. 1995;274(13):1049–57.
103. Folsom AR, Nieto FJ, McGovern PG, et al. Prospective study of coronary heart disease incidence in relation to fasting total homocysteine, related genetic polymorphisms, and B vitamins: the Atherosclerosis Risk in Communities (ARIC) study. Circulation. 1998;98(3): 204–10.
104. Kaul S, Zadeh AA, Shah PK. Homocysteine hypothesis for atherothrombotic cardiovascular disease: not validated. J Am Coll Cardiol. 2006;48(5):914–23.
105. Grundy SM, Cleeman JI, Merz CN, et al. Implications of recent clinical trials for the National Cholesterol Education Program Adult Treatment Panel III guidelines. Circulation. 2004; 110(2):227–39.

Chapter 6
Therapeutic Lifestyle Change for the Prevention and Treatment of Hyperlipidemia and Coronary Artery Disease

Rajesh Gupta, Bashar Almadani, and Neil Stone

Keywords Diet • Exercise • Hyperlipidemia • Coronary artery disease • Coronary heart disease • Prevention • Lifestyle • Treatment • Metabolic syndrome • Omega-3-fatty acids • Weight loss

Since the earliest experimental and epidemiologic studies on the pathogenesis of atherosclerosis, diet composition and level of physical activity have been recognized as important etiological factors [1]. Despite advances from major programs on cholesterol, hypertension, obesity, and physical activity from the National Heart Lung Blood Institutes, more remains to be done. Indeed, in a recent analysis of the decline in CHD deaths from 1980 through 2000, approximately 44% of the decline was attributed to changes in risk factors such as total cholesterol, systolic blood pressure (BP), smoking prevalence, and physical inactivity. However, these reductions were partially offset by increases in the body mass index (BMI) and the prevalence of diabetes (DM) [2]. Although CHD with rare exceptions is an adult disease, we are reminded that the precursors of atherosclerosis are present in the young. Data from the Pathobiological Determinants of Atherosclerosis in Youth (PDAY) study, an autopsy study of individuals aged 15–34 years, showed that early atherosclerosis can be found in the abdominal aorta just proximal to the bifurcation and in the coronary arteries [3]. Metabolic risk factors such as triglycerides, smoking, low high-density lipoprotein cholesterol (HDL C), high non HDL C, blood pressure, and BMI are associated with this initial atherosclerosis and are also predictive of early intimal thickening in the aorta and carotid arteries in adolescents [4]. In addition, a recent report from the Coronary Artery Risk Development in Young Adults (CARDIA) study demonstrated that elevated low-density lipoprotein cholesterol

N. Stone (✉)
Division of Cardiology, Feinberg School of Medicine,
Northwestern Memorial Hospital, Chicago, IL 60611, USA
e-mail: nstonemd1@gmail.com

M.J. Sorrentino (ed.), *Hyperlipidemia in Primary Care: A Practical Guide to Risk Reduction*, Current Clinical Practice, DOI 10.1007/978-1-60327-502-6_6,

(LDL-C) and other lipid abnormalities in young age are associated with greater coronary calcium in middle age [5]. With an increased prevalence of metabolic syndrome and diabetes seen in the young [6], it makes sense to target lifestyle change recommendations to all members of the family instead of just adult patients.

Indeed, if all Americans would heed the American Heart Association's "Life's Simple 7," a "to do" list for cardiovascular health, the metabolic syndrome, and obesity epidemic would likely be at an end [7].

1. Do not smoke
2. Maintain a healthy weight
3. Engage in regular physical activity
4. Eat a healthy diet
5. Manage blood pressure
6. Take charge of cholesterol
7. Keep blood sugar, or glucose, at healthy levels

Understanding Diet's Role in Cholesterol Lowering

A large body scientific evidence links cholesterol (and more precisely LDL-C) with CHD. Insightful studies of the cardioprotective effect of a genetic mutation in PCSK9, which results in lifelong reductions in LDL levels, has led Nobel Prize winners Michael Brown and Joseph Goldstein to an important conclusion [8]. Carriers of mutations in this gene have much greater reductions in CHD events than would be predicted based on the extent of LDL lowering [9]. Brown and Goldstein reasoned that the more impressive reduction in CHD outcomes in subjects with mutations in the PCSK9 gene compared with subjects in statin therapy clinical trials was most likely due to the early age of onset and lifelong duration of the cholesterol lowering seen with the genetic mutation.

They further argued that the consistent epidemiologic data, informative experimental studies, and most recently, double-blind, randomized clinical trial (RCT) intervention studies were sufficiently persuasive to justify an aggressive public health program aimed at keeping LDL-C levels low before the atherosclerotic process became advanced. Moreover, dietary change to lower LDL-C can also play an important role in the overall management of high-risk patients who require statin therapy. Although the degree of LDL-C lowering with dietary changes varies, even smaller reductions in LDL-C attained with diet can be beneficial in reducing the total dose of statin required to reach goal levels for LDL. This is due to the observation that for each doubling of the statin dose, LDL-C is reduced only 6–8% more. Thus, diet can prevent one doubling of the statin dosage [10]. Since common side effects of statins are often dose-dependent, this "statin-sparing" effect of diet can be a useful clinical tactic.

After focusing on achieving LDL targets, therapeutic lifestyle change (TLC) coupling diet and physical activity can be shown to be associated with modest weight loss and improvement in all five of the clinical determinants of the metabolic syndrome – increased waist circumference, elevated triglycerides (TG), low HDL-C, elevated BP, and elevated blood sugar [11]. The National Cholesterol Education Program (NCEP) Adult Treatment Panel III (ATP III) suggested that the initial focus should be on regular exercise. This has been shown to help the patient avoid gaining weight that has been lost.

This chapter focuses on those lifestyle interventions that lower LDL-C and metabolic risk factors with an emphasis both on the components (macronutrients) and dietary patterns (e.g., Portfolio, Mediterranean, and Ornish diets) that are helpful to patients with lipid disorders who are at risk for cardiovascular disease (CVD). We conclude with a helpful approach to lifestyle counseling that is useful in the busy clinic/doctor's office.

Lowering LDL-C

A critical review of nutritional studies suggests that when saturated fats are replaced with healthier fats such as monounsaturated fatty acids (MUFAs) or polyunsaturated fatty acids (PUFAs) or whole grains, fruits, and vegetables, there is a net beneficial effect on CHD [12]. In contrast, there is concern about exchanging easily digested carbohydrates for saturated fat (such as in some versions of a low-fat diet) due to the associated negative metabolic effects of raising TG and lower HDL-C [13]. As with any diet, many factors can affect the success of an LDL-lowering diet (Table 6.1).

Examples of dietary interventions designed primarily to reduce LDL include the Portfolio diet, the Pritikin diet, and the Ornish diet. The Portfolio diet [14, 15] is a vegetarian or largely vegetarian diet with four main LDL-lowering food groups: almonds, viscous fibers, soy protein, and plant sterols. Viscous fibers are soluble fibers in oats, barley, beans, certain fruits and vegetables (such as okra, eggplant, strawberries, prunes, and apples), and psyllium. Plant sterols were provided in margarines enriched with these compounds. The Portfolio diet was compared with a diet low in saturated fat in a randomized controlled trial. After approximately 4 weeks, LDL-C was reduced by 30.9% in subjects randomized to the Portfolio diet, which was similar to reductions achieved with low-dose statin therapy in another arm of this study. Subjects randomized to the control low-saturated fat had an LDL-C reduction of 8.0%. Some have criticized this "Portfolio diet" as difficult to follow in the real world because it is vegetarian. However, elements of this Portfolio diet, such as daily almond intake, replacement of fatty meats with soy or vegetable

Table 6.1 Factors affecting responsiveness to an LDL-C-lowering diet

Favors LDL-C lowering	Reduces likelihood of LDL-C lowering
Maximum dietary adherence	Poor dietary adherence
More plant-based foods	Inherited LDL-receptor deficiency/absence
Weight loss	Elevated hs-CRP
Exercise component	

proteins, and addition of fruits and vegetables high in viscous fibers, could be added to modify a conventional diet. Although this less strict interpretation of the Portfolio diet may not result in a 30% reduction in LDL-C, it will likely be applicable to a wider group of patients.

The Ornish [16] and Pritikin [17] diets are very low-fat diets aimed at preventing and treating coronary artery disease. In the Lifestyle Heart Trial, Ornish and colleagues randomized 28 patients to an experimental group which included a very low-fat (<10% of total calories from fat) vegetarian diet, smoking cessation counseling, stress management training, and moderate exercise while 20 patients were randomized to a usual-care group. The experimental group had a 37% reduction in LDL-C at 1 year and a 20% reduction in LDL-C at 5 years. A striking finding was the 10 kg weight loss that occurred in the intervention group. Although a small group, those assigned to the intervention regimen were found to have regression of coronary artery disease lesions as measured by quantitative coronary angiography in the experimental group contrasted with progression in the control group. Similarly, a very low-fat diet (<10% of total calories from fat) combined with exercise and lifestyle changes in the Pritikin Lifestyle Program resulted in a 23% reduction in LDL-C. The degree of LDL-C lowering with very low-fat diets has been debated in the literature. In addition, the degree of changes in HDL-C and triglyceride levels as well as the significance of these findings has been controversial. However, despite this ongoing debate, we believe that common sense recommendations can be made to patients to improve their diet, lower their LDL-C, and improve cardiovascular health. We believe limiting saturated fat intake, replacing saturated fats with MUFAs or PUFAs, and incorporating aspects of the Portfolio diet such as increased intake of almonds, fruits and vegetables high in viscous fibers, and vegetable protein sources are all reasonable recommendations.

A word about HDL-C is necessary since lowering saturated fat reduces HDL-C as well as LDL-C [18]. The ratios of total cholesterol or LDL-C to HDL-C may not correctly estimate atherosclerotic risk in the setting of dietary saturated fat restriction since saturated fat intake impairs the functionality of HDL-C [19]. Thus, behaviors that are "healthy" and raise HDL-C such as quitting tobacco smoking, losing weight, aerobic activity, and reducing excess carbohydrates such as sweetened foods and drinks [20] are clinically more important than behaviors such as high-saturated fat intake that raise HDL-C. HDL biology is an emerging area of medical science and it appears that there is great diversity in HDL function [21]. Not all things that raise HDL can be considered "good" and not all things that lower HDL can be considered "bad." In the coming years, we expect greater insights into the functionality of HDL will allow a more fine tuned approach to interpreting the significance of HDL levels and changes in HDL with dietary manipulations.

Reducing Metabolic Risk Factors

One of the strengths of the metabolic syndrome concept is that it alerts physicians to the relationship among insulin resistance, weight gain, and risk factors such as elevated blood sugar, dyslipidemia (low HDL-C and high TG), and hypertension. Moreover, a common source of confusion is to assume that the only benefit from weight reducing diets is measured in how many pounds are lost. A further advantage of the metabolic syndrome concept is the understanding that effective TLC can achieve measurable improvement in metabolic risk factors with only a moderate amount (about 7% of total weight) of weight loss [22]. We would argue that goals of a healthy lifestyle should include not just weight loss, but also the ability to achieve and maintain desirable life habits such as healthier eating and increased physical activity. This section discusses macronutrients such as carbohydrates and omega-3, -6, and -9 fatty acids and then considers popular diets such as the Mediterranean diets and very low carbohydrate diets.

Improving Triglycerides and HDL-C

Once LDL-C is at goal, attention turns to improving the TG and HDL parameters. Rather than a risk target, ATP III recommended that non-HDL-C (Non-HDL-C = Total cholesterol − HDL-C) be the secondary treatment target if TG was ≥200 mg/dl once the LDL-C goal was obtained. The non-HDL-C goal is 30 mg/dl higher than the LDL goal. For example, if the LDL goal is <100 mg/dl, then the non-HDL-C goal is <130 mg/dl. The importance of non-HDL-C as a risk marker cannot be emphasized enough in the population with metabolic syndrome and/or diabetes. In these patients, the LDL-C that is calculated by the Friedewald formula (LDL = total cholesterol − HDL-C − TG/5) may be <100 mg/dl and yet the very high TG and low HDL-C indicate that there is a population of small, dense LDL that can be estimated by either non-HDL-C (no further testing needed) or by measurements of apolipoprotein B_{100} or LDL particle number [23]. Aggressive prevention and treatment measures should include not only reaching LDL goals, but also reaching the secondary target of non-HDL-C goal.

The advantage of lifestyle change in improving progression to diabetes and hence long-term risk of CHD was seen in the Finnish Diabetes Program [24] and the Diabetes Prevention Program (DPP) [25]. In both studies, middle-aged men and women with impaired glucose tolerance were randomized to intervention groups that lost a moderate amount of weight, had reductions in saturated fat and increased fiber intake, and were more active. The progression to diabetes was reduced by almost 60% in these studies. In the DPP, lifestyle change was even more effective than that seen with metformin treatment.

Glycemic Index

Carbohydrate-containing foods elicit a wide range of postprandial glucose responses. To capture this variability, a concept called glycemic index (GI) has been proposed and advocates claim that it improves TG/HDL-C as well as CHD risk. GI is defined as the measure of how much a standard quantity of food raises blood glucose compared with that seen with either glucose or white bread. It is expressed as the difference in percentage from the baseline fasting glucose value [26]. Critics of the GI concept note that GI fails to account for the total amount of carbohydrate in a typical food serving or meal, even though both the type and amount of carbohydrate do affect the postprandial glucose and insulin responses to a given food. Moreover, when response to white bread is carefully determined, the within-individual variability can be greater than the between-person variability [27]. To avoid the pitfall of being concerned by the GI of carrots or watermelon, since the amount of carbohydrate per serving is small, the glycemic load (GL) of a food is calculated by multiplying the GI by the amount of carbohydrate (in grams) provided by a food and dividing the total by 100. As a rule of thumb, most refined starchy foods in the US diet have a high GI, whereas nonstarchy vegetables, fruits, and legumes can be regarded as having a low GI.

Despite numerous provocative observational studies and meta-analyses, the role of glycemic index/load in affecting lipids and CVD risk remains controversial. From a practical standpoint, although many healthy foods have a low GI, less desirable foods for a heart-healthy diet such as soft drinks and candies fall into the moderate GI categories. Indeed, the cutoffs for GI vary from study to study. Thus, it is not clear that this concept is a useful one over and above recommending healthy food choices and restricting excess carbohydrates.

Fatty Acids: Focus on Omega-3-Fatty Acids and the Mediterranean-Style Diet

Fatty acids (FAs) serve several functions in addition to providing energy. Linoleic acid (an omega-6-fatty acid) is an essential nutrient and the longer-chain fatty acids are structural components of cell membranes. The fatty acids are essential building blocks for triglycerides. Those fatty acids that have no double bonds are known as saturated fatty acids (SFAs). When a pair of hydrogen atoms is removed, a double bond exists and the more double bonds, the more unsaturated the fatty acid. Fatty acids with one double bond, such as oleic acid, are known as monounsaturated fatty acids (MUFAs). Those with two or more double bonds are considered PUFAs. In addition to being recognized by their chain length and number of double bonds, the location of the first double bond from the methyl end creates the distinction among omega-9 (olive oil and canola), omega-6 (corn oil), and omega-3 (fish oil) fatty acids. Unsaturated fatty acids are the preferred substitution in the diet for SFAs over carbohydrates. A detailed analysis showed evidence that consuming PUFA in place of SFA reduces CHD events in RCTs [28]. This is consistent with the ATP III guidelines that recommend total fat to range from 25 to 35% of calories and yet limit SFA in the diet.

Two good choices to replace carbohydrates are MUFA and PUFA. Most know olive oil as a good source of oleic acid (omega-9) and an essential part of the Mediterranean-style diet. Seed oils (omega-6-fatty acids) are useful in the diet and a good source of an essential fatty acid, linoleic acid. Omega-3-fatty acids, however, appear to effect CHD event rates and hence will be considered in greater detail.

The marine omega-3-fatty acids are eicosapentanoic acid (EPA) and docosahexanoic acid (DHA). Sources rich in these fatty acids are fatty fish such as salmon, trout, mackerel, herring, and sardines, and sea bass. The nonmarine omega-3-fatty acid is alpha-linolenic acid (ALA) found in flax, canola oil, walnuts, and soybean oil [29]. Omega-3-fatty acids have a variety of potentially beneficial effects but are used clinically for two purposes: (1) Treat hypertriglyceridemia to prevent the increased risk of pancreatitis in those with TG > 500 mg/dl or as part of the treatment regimen for those with hypertriglyceridemic pancreatitis. It is important to note that marine omega-3-fatty acids are used for this purpose, not ALA fatty acids such as those found in flax seed oil. (2) Reduce the likelihood of fatal CHD in those with CHD as seen in clinical trials discussed below.

The TG reduction seen with EPA and DHA is due to their favorable effects in reducing hepatic production and secretion of triglyceride-rich very low-density lipoprotein (VLDL) and VLDL apolipoprotein B particles, along with improvement in lipid disposal through lipoprotein lipase-mediated clearance, as well as the stimulation of beta-oxidation of other fatty acids in the liver [30]. Their hypotriglyceridemic properties are related to both the dose of omega-3-FAs used and the baseline TG concentrations of the population. Thus, for those with TG > 1,000 mg/dl, the TG lowering seen with marine omega-3-fatty acids can be up to 50% in contrast to only a 25% lowering at lower TG concentrations.

In the Diet and Reinfarction Trial (DART), male myocardial infarction (MI) survivors who were randomized to receive dietary advice to increase fatty fish consumption had a 29% reduction in all-cause mortality at 2-year follow-up which was strikingly improved over more usual dietary advice [31]. Italian survivors (men and women) of myocardial infarction (MI) randomized to receive omega-3-fatty acid supplements (1 g/day) in the GISSI Prevenzione trial had a significant 10–15% reduction in the combined primary end point of death, nonfatal myocardial infarction, and stroke [32]. This effect seemed especially focused on preventing CHD death and was not related to the minor lipid changes, mainly in triglycerides, seen with the dose of omega-3-fatty acids used in this study.

In the Lyon Diet Heart Study, patients randomized to receive a Mediterranean-type diet enriched in canola oil (participants were given a special margarine) had significant reductions at a mean of 27 months follow-up in the combined primary end point of death from cardiovascular causes or nonfatal acute MI (73%) as well as in cardiac mortality (76%) and total mortality (70%) [33, 34]. What was the composition of the diet that produced these striking effects? Subjects randomized to the Mediterranean-style diet in this trial averaged 30% of calories from fat, 8% from saturated fat, 13% from mono-unsaturated fat, 5% from polyunsaturated fat, and 203 mg/day of dietary cholesterol [35]. Moreover, these subjects consumed more oleic acid, ALA, and dietary fiber and less linoleic acid. Plasma fatty acid analysis conducted on a representative sample after 52 weeks of follow-up confirmed these changes. Those critical of the remarkable trial results pointed to methodological problems where the diet of the control group was only assessed at the end of the trial. Moreover, only 30% of the total control cohort and <50% of the total experimental group providing dietary data at the conclusion of the study so there is concern that the results may be difficult to reproduce.

An important primary prevention clinical trial was conducted in Japan where fish intake is much higher than in the USA on average. The investigators compared a regimen of 1,800 mg of EPA, a long-chain omega-3-marine fatty acid, added to statin therapy versus statin therapy alone. They found a significant reduction in the relative and absolute risk for combined CHD outcomes for those who had their statin therapy augmented by omega-3-fatty acids [36]. Interestingly, sudden death was not improved in this study, suggesting that the beneficial effect of omega-3-fatty acid supplementation may depend on the baseline fish consumption and omega-3-fatty acid levels of the population studied.

Although there have been many prospective cohort trials, there has been a much smaller number of the more definitive RCTs. Nonetheless recent pooled analysis of dietary RCTs showed that increased consumption of omega-3-fatty acids and a Mediterranean dietary pattern were each associated with a significantly lower risk of CHD [37]. Mediterranean-style diets are characterized by vegetables, legumes, fruits and nuts, fish and seafoods, and are typically low in fatty cuts of meat, butter, and full-fat milk products. Greek investigators reported on their prospective follow-up of 23,349 healthy men and women that were rated on a Mediterranean diet scale at entry [38]. This 9-point scale looked at vegetables, legumes, fruits and nuts, dairy products, cereals, meat and meat products, fish and seafood, monounsaturated to saturated lipid ratio, and ethanol. They considered a higher ratio of monounsaturated fat to saturate fat to be beneficial and reflective of the high olive oil consumption that characterizes the traditional Mediterranean diet. They used the ethanol category to reflect consumption of alcoholic beverages, which in the Mediterranean countries are mostly consumed during meals and mainly in the form of wine. In this cohort, the components of the Mediterranean diet score that predicted lower mortality were moderate consumption of alcohol, low consumption of meat and meat products, and high consumption of vegetables, fruits and nuts, olive oil, and legumes. Fish and seafood were not significant predictors. This is in contrast to the Lyon Diet trial where omega-3-fatty acids were clearly increased in the intervention group, whereas alcohol was not different between the two groups. Owing to informative studies of omega-3-fatty acids and the Mediterranean-style diet such as the Lyon Diet Heart Study, we have incorporated many of these principles in our overall "dietary prescription" (Table 6.3).

Trans Fats

Trans fats are commonly found in margarines, commercially processed baked goods, and fried foods such as French fries and donuts. A trans fat is any unsaturated fat with at least one double bond in the trans configuration. Trans fats are commonly produced by the partial hydrogenation of vegetable oils, an industrial process that converts a liquid oil into a semisolid state. Trans fats have been shown to have very detrimental effects on the lipid profile, as they both increase LDL-C and at increased doses, decrease HDL-C [39]. It has now become well established that trans fats are detrimental and should be avoided and minimized as much as possible [40]. Patients with hyperlipidemia and/or CHD should be instructed to avoid industrially produced trans fats as much as possible by avoiding foods that list trans fat on the nutrition label or have partially hydrogenated oils in the ingredient list.

Nuts and Cardiovascular Health

There is emerging evidence that many kinds of nuts have beneficial cardiovascular effects. As discussed earlier under the "Lowering LDL-C" section, almonds are one of the major foods used in the Portfolio diet studies to reduce cholesterol [15]. In general, about 30 g per day of almonds, which is about 20–25 almonds, is consistent with the Portfolio diet and can be recommended to patients for LDL lowering. This amount of almonds contains about 180–200 calories and can be incorporated as a healthy snack alternative.

In addition to effects on lipids, certain nuts have other desirable vascular effects. In two diet intervention studies, patients randomized to walnuts had improved endothelial function as measured by brachial artery flow mediated vasodilation. In both of these studies, patients in the intervention group were given 40–65 g of walnuts, which is about 8–13 walnuts per day [41, 42].

Since nuts are calorie-dense, they should be recommended with specific instruction, especially to overweight and obese patients. In general, we recommend unroasted, unsalted (plain) raw nuts since the beneficial effects of nuts are likely diluted or counterbalanced by roasting in oils, coating with sugars, or salting. Eating a small handful of nuts everyday is a healthy snack that improves cardiovascular health and can be used to replace less healthy snacks.

DASH Diet for Hypertension

Although the main focus of this chapter is on lifestyle approaches for the prevention and treatment of hyperlipidemia and CHD, we would be remiss if we did not mention dietary approaches to prevent and treat hypertension. The Dietary Approaches to Stop Hypertension (DASH) diet studies have shown that a diet rich in fruits and vegetables and low in sodium can reduce blood pressure [43, 44]. The DASH and DASH-sodium trials were both randomized studies of a diet emphasizing fruits, vegetables, low-fat dairy, and including whole grains, poultry, fish, and nuts; DASH diets limit red meats, sweets, and sugar-sweetened beverages. The DASH-sodium study showed a synergistic effect of the DASH diet with sodium restriction, and blood pressure lowering effect was most prominent among patients with hypertension.

The DASH diet should be a starting point in the prevention and treatment of all patients with prehypertension or hypertension. We have found the online printout published by the National Heart, Lung, and Blood Institute (NHLBI) to be a very helpful educational resource for patients. This document is free and available through the NHLBI website at http://www.nhlbi.nih.gov or by google searching for "dash diet" and following the link titled, "Your Guide to Lowering Your Blood Pressure with DASH." The full website address is included in the citations [45].

Weight Loss Diets

Observational studies on weight loss of interest include the National Weight Control Registry that has enrolled over 3,500 successful weight loss maintainers, defined as weight loss of 60 lbs sustained over 6 years [46]. The profile of these patients shows that they:

- Consume a low-calorie, low-fat diet (24% of calories from fat) which includes regular breakfasts.
- Expend large amount of energy in voluntary physical activity (2,800 kcal/week; about 1 h of exercise per day).
- They are physically active and spend few hours in watching TV.

There are several misconceptions about weight loss diets. First, weight loss is not easy to accomplish. Most patients drop out of the weight loss effort without obtaining the benefits they sought. In one important study where patients were randomized to the Atkins, Zone, Weight Watchers, and Pritikin type diets, only about 50% completed the 1-year study [47]. Moreover, when subjects were given different diets at a workplace, the investigators noted that a Mediterranean style or low carbohydrate seemed to offer advantages over the low-fat diet [48].

Second, there is no magic diet that works for everyone. A more definitive study was the Pounds Lost study in 2009 [49]. In this carefully designed clinical trial, investigators randomized subjects to one of the four dietary interventions: (1) low fat (20% of energy), average protein (15% of energy); (2) moderate fat (40%), average protein (15%); (3) low fat (20%), high protein (25%); and (4) moderate fat (40%), high protein (25%). They concluded that "reduced-calorie diets result in clinically meaningful weight loss" that was independent of the macronutrients they emphasized. Another recent randomized study comparing low-fat and low-carbohydrate diets found similar weight loss in both groups at 2 years [50]. A further paper noted that early adherence during the first 6 months of Pounds Lost study was crucial to achieving both short-term and long-term weight goals [51]. Thus, the importance of structured interventions such as self-monitoring and counseling that target improved nutrition, increased physical activity, and weight loss cannot be emphasized strongly enough.

To put this into practice, we believe that an effective clinic visit should include a motivational assessment integrated into the dietary and physical activity assessment. To optimize the time, we use the following approach employing forms that are filled out in advance and reviewed by the clinician (Table 6.2).

Table 6.2 Patient dietary history interview form

Questions	Patient answers
1. How would you define good health? Is it important to you? Why?	
2. What concerns you about your current lifestyle? Dietary concerns? What are the barriers to staying on a good dietary regimen? What has worked in the past? Exercise/physical activity concerns? What are the barriers to doing this? Any symptoms that occur with effort? Any special precautions?	
3. What is your diet like? Please review the 8 Fs: (a) Frequency? How many meals/day? Do you eat breakfast? (b) Fast foods? Yes/No and how often per week (c) Fruits and vegetables? 5 or more servings/day recommended; if not, why not? (d) Fruit juices and other sweetened drinks such as soda? What beverages do you drink in an average day? Many patients lose weight successfully by getting rid of the sweetened fruit juices and soft drinks they consume daily (e) Fish? How many times/week? How many are fatty fish? (good choices include salmon or trout) (f) Fried foods? How often? Important to avoid (g) Fats: Table fats? Butter, stick margarine, or soft spreads? Salad fats? Oil and vinegar dressing (our preferred) or creamy dressing? Nuts? Nuts are a good snack to cut down on sweets. Cooking fats: We recommend canola or olive oil (h) Fiber? We emphasize soluble fiber such as cooked oatmeal, or oat cereals as well as whole grains	
4. How motivated are you on a scale of 1 (not at all) to 10 (I am going to do it for sure) to succeed in both the short-term and longer-term lifestyle intervention?	

Please note the last question, which asks the patient to rate their willingness to change. If the response is 1–3, clearly the patient is not interested. This may not be the time to spend great efforts on teaching lifestyle change. We do offer resources to these patients if and when they feel more motivated to change and remind them that many patients often come back when they are ready and at that time can accomplish meaningful lifestyle change.

If the response is 4–10, we ask why it is not a 2 or 3? How do they know that they are truly interested in changing? This helps them clarify why they want to change. If the response is 8–10, we ask why are they so sure that this will work this time?

To help our patients' change, we rely on self-assessment, counseling sessions, and goal setting. First, we have asked them to keep a diet diary for 2 weeks and bring it to their visit with a dietitian. Second, we have asked our patients to get a pedometer and set a goal for daily steps. We make the initial goal about 1,000 steps more than what they average for the first week they wear the pedometer. Their eventual goal is 8–10,000 steps daily. We also recommend for those with a smart phone or computer, apps such as Lose It! [52] which tracks food intake and exercise calories. We also ask them to remember a sound byte from the visit "eat less, eat smart, move more daily."

Table 6.3 Dietary prescription to reduce cardiovascular risk

Food group	Practical comments and recommendations
Saturated fats (SFA)	Substitute high-fat animal products and full-fat dairy products with leaner or lower fat products; for cooking, use unsaturated plant oils such as olive oil or canola oil instead of saturated fats from animal products
Trans fatty acids (TFA)	Avoid stick margarines, donuts, fried foods, commercially baked products with trans fats, or foods that list partially hydrogenated oils in the ingredients
Fruits and vegetables	Five or more servings daily are suggested by the Dietary Alternatives to Stop Hypertension (DASH) diet and by many other recommendations for good health
	Here is a quick tip: the more colors the better! Eat meals with green, yellow, red, and as many other colored vegetables as you can get. Eat fruit with every meal and for a healthy snack to make sure you get enough fruit every day
Beans and legumes	Eat beans and legumes for a healthy and lean source of protein and fiber
Whole grains and cereal fiber	Eat whole wheat instead of white bread and flour; sweetened cereals diminish the beneficial effects of cereal fiber
Omega-3-fatty acids	1–2 servings per week of oily fish (salmon or trout are good choices; sardines have omega-3-fatty acids but watch out for the salt!)
Nuts	Nuts like almonds were used in the Portfolio diet to lower "bad" cholesterol; eat a handful a day; Walnuts improve artery function; raw (unroasted, unsalted) nuts are best
Alcohol	Moderate alcohol may be beneficial, although we do not know for sure. A "standard drink" is one half ounce of alcohol (contained in an average glass of wine, one average can of beer, or one and a half ounces of liquor). Moderate consumption is seven or less drinks per week for women and 14 or less drinks per week for men with no more than 2 drinks on any day
	If patients cannot limit alcohol intake, they have increased risks for heart disease (atrial fibrillation and cardiomyopathy), liver disease, accidents, and stroke. If you drink, do not drive or operate heavy machinery
Mediterranean-style diet	Eat more fruits, vegetables, nuts, and legumes. Olive oil is the preferred oil, but canola oil is recommended as a healthy oil as well
	Use a healthy oil and balsamic or red wine vinegar for salad dressing
	Moderate alcohol is acceptable
	Eat less fatty meats
	Eat less fatty dairy products like milk, cheese, and yogurt (use low-fat versions)
	Replace fatty meats with fish, poultry, or vegetable sources of protein such as beans and legumes
Sodium	Limit sodium (salt) intake; high sodium in your diet increases your risk for high blood pressure. Aim for less than 1,500 mg per day of sodium. Read nutrition labels on the foods you buy to get a sense for how much sodium you eat
Lifestyle change: diet and moderate activity and mild (7–8%) weight loss to prevent diabetes	Clinical trial evidence shows lifestyle change (diet and exercise) in overweight middle-aged men and women with impaired glucose tolerance (prediabetes) can reduce the rate of Type 2 diabetes by almost 60%
	Lose a few pounds by eating less and moving more to prevent diabetes!

Table 6.4 Exercise prescription

Exercise parameter	Practical recommendations
Frequency	Exercise at least 5 days per week; the key is regular exercise
Intensity	If you have not exercised regularly for a while, start easy and build up gradually. Always warm-up and cool-down. If you get symptoms such as lightheadedness, unexpected or severe shortness of breath, or chest heaviness, tightness, pressure (does not have to be pain) that occur with effort, let your doctor know right away and do not exercise again until you get medical clearance. Flexibility exercises such as stretching or yoga should be an important part of your regimen especially as you get older. Some patients may want to ask their doctor for an exercise prescription
Time	Aim to build up to 30–60 min per session; start with something you enjoy and can do easily and build up duration over time. Sometimes it may be more practical to break this up into two sessions per day. Work the sessions into your day by walking to the train, walking during lunch, walking when you get home at night, or walking after dinner. Always have an indoor option when weather makes outside exercise impossible (treadmill, stationery bicycle, or step aerobics)
Type	Choose from various types of aerobic exercise such as walking, swimming, bicycling, or running; weight lifting and resistance training are also useful, but should supplement aerobic exercise
Monitor your progress	Monitor your progress with a pedometer. Set a goal of 1,000 steps more per day than you do the first week you wear it and every 2–4 weeks increase that goal until you are getting in 8–10,000 steps per day

In summary, this chapter reviews up to date and concise information about macronutrients and diets that the clinician will hear about from his/her patients. For some, using diet approaches and regular exercise to keep LDL-C lower and avoid gaining weight will be very effective. For the growing number with weight gain, metabolic syndrome, and/or Type 2 diabetes, understanding the importance of motivation and structured interventions such as feedback and effective counseling should help control risk factors in the short-term and hopefully achieve meaningful metabolic change in the longer term. Readers can feel free to use our dietary and exercise prescriptions (Tables 6.3 and 6.4) as a starting point for recommendations and motivating change in patient behaviors.

References

1. Stamler J. Population-wide adverse dietary patterns: a pivotal cause of epidemic coronary heart disease/cardiovascular disease. J Am Diet Assoc. 2008;108:228–32.
2. Ford ES, Ajani UA, Croft JB, et al. Explaining the decrease in U.S. deaths from coronary disease, 1980–2000. N Engl J Med. 2007;356:2388–98.
3. McGill Jr HC, McMahan CA, Herderick EE, et al. Effects of coronary heart disease risk factors on atherosclerosis of selected regions of the aorta and right coronary artery. PDAY Research Group. Pathobiological Determinants of Atherosclerosis in Youth. Arterioscler Thromb Vasc Biol. 2000;20:836–45.

4. McMahan CA, Gidding SS, Viikari JS, et al. Association of Pathobiologic Determinants of Atherosclerosis in Youth risk score and 15-year change in risk score with carotid artery intima-media thickness in young adults (from the Cardiovascular Risk in Young Finns Study). Am J Cardiol. 2007;100:1124–9.
5. Pletcher MJ, Bibbins-Domingo K, Liu K, et al. Nonoptimal lipids commonly present in young adults and coronary calcium later in life: The CARDIA (Coronary Artery Risk Development in Young Adults) Study. Ann Intern Med. 2010;153:137–46.
6. Weiss R, Dziura J, Burgert TS, et al. Obesity and the metabolic syndrome in children and adolescents. N Engl J Med. 2004;350:2362–74.
7. American Heart Association Healthy Diet Goals. http://www.americanheart.org/presenter.jhtml?identifier=3071616. Accessed 31 May 2010.
8. Brown MS, Goldstein JL. Biomedicine. Lowering LDL–not only how low, but how long? Science. 2006;311:1721–3.
9. Cohen JC, Boerwinkle E, Mosley Jr TH, Hobbs HH. Sequence variations in PCSK9, low LDL, and protection against coronary heart disease. N Engl J Med. 2006;354:1264–72.
10. Jones P, Kafonek S, Laurora I, Hunninghake D. Comparative dose efficacy study of atorvastatin versus simvastatin, pravastatin, lovastatin, and fluvastatin in patients with hypercholesterolemia (the CURVES study). Am J Cardiol. 1998;81:582–7.
11. Alberti KG, Eckel RH, Grundy SM, et al. Harmonizing the metabolic syndrome: a joint interim statement of the International Diabetes Federation Task Force on Epidemiology and Prevention; National Heart, Lung, and Blood Institute; American Heart Association; World Heart Federation; International Atherosclerosis Society; and International Association for the Study of Obesity. Circulation. 2009;120:1640–5.
12. Mann JI. Diet and risk of coronary heart disease and type 2 diabetes. Lancet. 2002;360:783–9.
13. Sacks FM, Katan M. Randomized clinical trials on the effects of dietary fat and carbohydrate on plasma lipoproteins and cardiovascular disease. Am J Med. 2002;113(Suppl 9B):13S–24.
14. Jenkins DJ, Kendall CW, Faulkner DA, et al. Assessment of the longer-term effects of a dietary portfolio of cholesterol-lowering foods in hypercholesterolemia. Am J Clin Nutr. 2006;83:582–91.
15. Jenkins DJ, Kendall CW, Marchie A, et al. Effects of a dietary portfolio of cholesterol-lowering foods vs lovastatin on serum lipids and C-reactive protein. JAMA. 2003;290:502–10.
16. Ornish D, Brown SE, Scherwitz LW, et al. Can lifestyle changes reverse coronary heart disease? The Lifestyle Heart Trial. Lancet. 1990;336:129–33.
17. Barnard RJ, DiLauro SC, Inkeles SB. Effects of intensive diet and exercise intervention in patients taking cholesterol-lowering drugs. Am J Cardiol. 1997;79:1112–4.
18. Mensink RP, Zock PL, Kester AD, Katan MB. Effects of dietary fatty acids and carbohydrates on the ratio of serum total to HDL cholesterol and on serum lipids and apolipoproteins: a meta-analysis of 60 controlled trials. Am J Clin Nutr. 2003;77:1146–55.
19. Nicholls SJ, Lundman P, Harmer JA, et al. Consumption of saturated fat impairs the anti-inflammatory properties of high-density lipoproteins and endothelial function. J Am Coll Cardiol. 2006;48:715–20.
20. Welsh JA, Sharma A, Abramson JL, Vaccarino V, Gillespie C, Vos MB. Caloric sweetener consumption and dyslipidemia among US adults. JAMA. 2010;303:1490–7.
21. Ansell BJ, Navab M, Hama S, et al. Inflammatory/antiinflammatory properties of high-density lipoprotein distinguish patients from control subjects better than high-density lipoprotein cholesterol levels and are favorably affected by simvastatin treatment. Circulation. 2003;108:2751–6.
22. McLaughlin T, Carter S, Lamendola C, et al. Clinical efficacy of two hypocaloric diets that vary in overweight patients with type 2 diabetes: comparison of moderate fat versus carbohydrate reductions. Diabetes Care. 2007;30:1877–9.
23. Grundy SM, Vega GL, Tomassini JE, Tershakovec AM. Correlation of non-high-density lipoprotein cholesterol and low-density lipoprotein cholesterol with apolipoprotein B during simvastatin+fenofibrate therapy in patients with combined hyperlipidemia (a subanalysis of the SAFARI trial). Am J Cardiol. 2009;104:548–53.

24. Tuomilehto J, Lindstrom J, Eriksson JG, et al. Prevention of type 2 diabetes mellitus by changes in lifestyle among subjects with impaired glucose tolerance. N Engl J Med. 2001;344:1343–50.
25. Knowler WC, Barrett-Connor E, Fowler SE, et al. Reduction in the incidence of type 2 diabetes with lifestyle intervention or metformin. N Engl J Med. 2002;346:393–403.
26. Franz MJ. Is there a role for the glycemic index in coronary heart disease prevention or treatment? Curr Atheroscler Rep. 2008;10:497–502.
27. Vega-Lopez S, Ausman LM, Griffith JL, Lichtenstein AH. Interindividual variability and intra-individual reproducibility of glycemic index values for commercial white bread. Diabetes Care. 2007;30:1412–7.
28. Mozaffarian D, Micha R, Wallace S. Effects on coronary heart disease of increasing polyunsaturated fat in place of saturated fat: a systematic review and meta-analysis of randomized controlled trials. PLoS Med. 2010;7:e1000252.
29. Kris-Etherton PM, Harris WS, Appel LJ. Omega-3 fatty acids and cardiovascular disease: new recommendations from the American Heart Association. Arterioscler Thromb Vasc Biol. 2003;23:151–2.
30. Jacobson TA. Role of n-3 fatty acids in the treatment of hypertriglyceridemia and cardiovascular disease. Am J Clin Nutr. 2008;87:1981S–90S.
31. Burr ML, Fehily AM, Gilbert JF, et al. Effects of changes in fat, fish, and fibre intakes on death and myocardial reinfarction: diet and reinfarction trial (DART). Lancet. 1989;2:757–61.
32. Dietary supplementation with n-3 polyunsaturated fatty acids and vitamin E after myocardial infarction: results of the GISSI-Prevenzione trial. Gruppo Italiano per lo Studio della Sopravvivenza nell'Infarto miocardico. Lancet 1999;354:447–55.
33. de Lorgeril M, Renaud S, Mamelle N, et al. Mediterranean alpha-linolenic acid-rich diet in secondary prevention of coronary heart disease. Lancet. 1994;343:1454–9.
34. de Lorgeril M, Salen P, Martin JL, Monjaud I, Delaye J, Mamelle N. Mediterranean diet, traditional risk factors, and the rate of cardiovascular complications after myocardial infarction: final report of the Lyon Diet Heart Study. Circulation. 1999;99:779–85.
35. Kris-Etherton P, Eckel RH, Howard BV, St Jeor S, Bazzarre TL. AHA Science Advisory: Lyon Diet Heart Study. Benefits of a Mediterranean-style, National Cholesterol Education Program/American Heart Association Step I Dietary Pattern on Cardiovascular Disease. Circulation. 2001;103:1823–5.
36. Yokoyama M, Origasa H, Matsuzaki M, et al. Effects of eicosapentaenoic acid on major coronary events in hypercholesterolaemic patients (JELIS): a randomised open-label, blinded endpoint analysis. Lancet. 2007;369:1090–8.
37. Mente A, de Koning L, Shannon HS, Anand SS. A systematic review of the evidence supporting a causal link between dietary factors and coronary heart disease. Arch Intern Med. 2009;169:659–69.
38. Trichopoulou A, Bamia C, Trichopoulos D. Anatomy of health effects of Mediterranean diet: Greek EPIC prospective cohort study. BMJ. 2009;338:b2337.
39. Mensink RP, Katan MB. Effect of dietary trans fatty acids on high-density and low-density lipoprotein cholesterol levels in healthy subjects. N Engl J Med. 1990;323:439–45.
40. Mozaffarian D, Katan MB, Ascherio A, Stampfer MJ, Willett WC. Trans fatty acids and cardiovascular disease. N Engl J Med. 2006;354:1601–13.
41. Ros E, Nunez I, Perez-Heras A, et al. A walnut diet improves endothelial function in hypercholesterolemic subjects: a randomized crossover trial. Circulation. 2004;109:1609–14.
42. Cortes B, Nunez I, Cofan M, et al. Acute effects of high-fat meals enriched with walnuts or olive oil on postprandial endothelial function. J Am Coll Cardiol. 2006;48:1666–71.
43. Appel LJ, Moore TJ, Obarzanek E, et al. A clinical trial of the effects of dietary patterns on blood pressure. DASH Collaborative Research Group. N Engl J Med. 1997;336:1117–24.
44. Sacks FM, Svetkey LP, Vollmer WM, et al. Effects on blood pressure of reduced dietary sodium and the Dietary Approaches to Stop Hypertension (DASH) diet. DASH-Sodium Collaborative Research Group. N Engl J Med. 2001;344:3–10.
45. Your guide to lowering your blood pressure with DASH. http://www.nhlbi.nih.gov/health/public/heart/hbp/dash/new_dash.pdf. Accessed 2 Aug 2010.

46. Wing RR, Hill JO. Successful weight loss maintenance. Annu Rev Nutr. 2001;21:323–41.
47. Dansinger ML, Gleason JA, Griffith JL, Selker HP, Schaefer EJ. Comparison of the Atkins, Ornish, Weight Watchers, and Zone diets for weight loss and heart disease risk reduction: a randomized trial. JAMA. 2005;293:43–53.
48. Shai I, Schwarzfuchs D, Henkin Y, et al. Weight loss with a low-carbohydrate, Mediterranean, or low-fat diet. N Engl J Med. 2008;359:229–41.
49. Sacks FM, Bray GA, Carey VJ, et al. Comparison of weight-loss diets with different compositions of fat, protein, and carbohydrates. N Engl J Med. 2009;360:859–73.
50. Foster GD, Wyatt HR, Hill JO, et al. Weight and metabolic outcomes after 2 years on a low-carbohydrate versus low-fat diet: a randomized trial. Ann Intern Med. 2010;153:147–57.
51. Williamson DA, Anton SD, Han H, et al. Early behavioral adherence predicts short and long-term weight loss in the POUNDS LOST study. J Behav Med. 2010;33:305–14.
52. Lose it! weightloss app. http://itunes.apple.com/us/app/lose-it/id297368629?mt=8. Accessed 25 July 2010.

Chapter 7
Drug Therapy for Dyslipidemia

Matthew J. Sorrentino

Keywords Statins • Hepatotoxicity • Myopathy • Resins • Ezetimibe • Fibrates • Niacin

Coronary heart disease (CHD) remains the number one cause of death for men and women in the USA and is rapidly becoming a major cause of morbidity and mortality in developing nations as well. The recognition and treatment of coronary risk factors such as dyslipidemia, hypertension, smoking, obesity, and diabetes has made a substantial impact on reducing CHD events. The National Cholesterol Education Program guidelines recommend that low-density lipoprotein cholesterol (LDL-C) should be the primary target of therapy to reduce cardiovascular events. The HMG CoA reductase inhibitors or statins are effective in lowering LDL-C and have become some of the most prescribed medications in the world. Recent studies have extended the boundaries of treatment to different risk groups and have shown that this treatment strategy is beneficial across the cardiovascular risk spectrum.

Epidemiologic studies such as the Framingham Heart Study demonstrated that cholesterol levels are associated with survival [1]. The Multiple Risk Factor Intervention Trial documented an increased death rate at cholesterol levels above 200 mg/dl establishing the relationship between cholesterol levels and mortality [2]. A meta-analysis of over 40 cholesterol treatment trials indicated that a 10% reduction in serum cholesterol translates into a 15% reduction in CHD mortality and an 11% reduction in total mortality [3]. This relationship applies to most cholesterol reducing modalities including diet, pharmacological, and surgical approaches.

M.J. Sorrentino (✉)
Department of Medicine, Section of Cardiology,
University of Chicago Pritzker School of Medicine, Chicago, IL 60637, USA
e-mail: msorrent@medicine.bsd.uchicago.edu

M.J. Sorrentino (ed.), *Hyperlipidemia in Primary Care: A Practical Guide to Risk Reduction*, Current Clinical Practice, DOI 10.1007/978-1-60327-502-6_7,

Treatment Guidelines

The National Cholesterol Education Program (NCEP) Adult Treatment Panel III guidelines recommend that the LDL-C should be the primary target of therapy for at-risk individuals [4]. A summary of how to implement the NCEP guidelines is outlined in Table 7.1. All individuals aged 20 and above should have a fasting lipid panel as a screening evaluation. A patient's risk status can then be determined by evaluating for the presence of clinical atherosclerotic disease and for major cardiovascular risk factors. Individuals can be classified into three risk categories for a cardiac event:

- Low risk (<10% 10-year risk of a coronary event)
- Moderate risk (10–20% 10-year risk)
- High risk (>20% 10-year risk)

The high-risk category includes patients with established CHD as well as non-CHD patients who carry the same risk for major coronary events as CHD patients. This includes patients with diabetes mellitus and patients with other clinical forms of atherosclerosis (referred to as CHD risk-equivalent disease) such as symptomatic carotid artery disease, an abdominal aortic aneurysm, or peripheral arterial disease.

In 2004, the NCEP published a committee report reviewing trials published after the Adult Treatment Panel III guidelines and suggested further modification of the risk categories [5]. Low-risk patients, having at most only one additional risk factor to LDL-C, were left unchanged. Moderate-risk patients were divided into two groups. The patients in the first category have two or more risk factors but the Framingham risk calculation indicates less than 10% 10-year risk. The second category or moderately high-risk patients have two or more risk factors with a 10-year risk of 10–20%. High-risk individuals include patients with documented CHD or CHD risk-equivalent disease. Within this category, patients at *very high* risk can be identified. Factors that would classify a patient as very high risk are summarized in Table 7.2. LDL-C treatment goals are set based on the risk category. Risk calculators are available at http://www.nhlbi.nih.gov/guidelines/cholesterol.

Table 7.1 Summary of the implementation of the National Cholesterol Education Program Adult Treatment Panel III Guidelines (from [4])

1. Measure fasting lipoprotein levels
2. Identify clinical atherosclerosis
3. Determine the presence of major cardiovascular risk factors
4. If two or more risk factors present, calculate 10-year risk
5. Determine risk category and establish LDL goal
6. Initiate lifestyle modification in LDL above goal
7. Add drug therapy if LDL continues to exceed goal
8. Identify metabolic syndrome and treat if present despite lifestyle modification
9. Treat elevated triglycerides to non-HDL-C goal

Table 7.2 Factors that place a patient into the very high-risk category [5]

The presence of established coronary heart disease plus
1. Multiple risk factors (especially diabetes mellitus)
2. Severe and poorly controlled risk factors (especially continued cigarette smoking)
3. Multiple risk factors of the metabolic syndrome
(a) High triglycerides ≥ 200 mg/dl plus
(b) Low HDL-C (<40 mg/dl)
4. Patients with acute coronary syndromes

Table 7.3 LDL-C and non-HDL-C goals according to risk categories

Risk category	LDL-C goal (mg/dl)	Non-HDL-C goal (triglycerides ≥ 200 mg/dl) (mg/dl)
Very high risk	<70 Optional goal	<100 Optional goal
High risk (CHD or CHD risk equivalent, 10-year risk >20%)	<100	<130
Moderate high risk (≥2 risk factors, 10–20% 10-year risk)	<130 (<100 optional goal)	<160 (<130 optional goal)
Moderate risk (≥2 risk factors, <10% 10-year risk)	<130	<160
Low risk (0 or 1 risk factor)	<160	<190

Adapted from NCEP ATPIII guidelines [4] and the National Heart, Lung, and Blood Institute update [5]

Once a risk category is determined, an LDL-C goal is chosen based on the risk group (Table 7.3). Therapeutic lifestyle changes (TLCs) are begun (diet and exercise program) and the LDL-C re-evaluated after a 3- to 6-month trial. If the LDL-C goal is not reached, drug therapy is recommended. For patients at high risk, drug therapy may be implemented at the time of diagnosis.

Once the LDL-C is at goal, additional lipid parameters can be assessed and targeted for further risk reduction. Non HDL cholesterol (non HDL C) is the secondary target for patients with fasting triglycerides greater than 200 mg/dl. The non-HDL-C goals are 30 mg/dl higher than the LDL-C goal. Recently, the American Diabetes Association/American College of Cardiology Foundation recommended that apolipoprotein B_{100} (apo B) should be considered a third treatment goal for patients with cardiometabolic risk after LDL-C and non-HDL-C are at goal [6]. Patients with multiple cardiometabolic risk factors but no clinical cardiovascular disease or diabetes are considered high risk and the apo B target is less than 90 mg/dl. Patients with cardiometabolic risk factors and diabetes or clinical cardiovascular disease are at very high risk and have an apo B target of less than 80 mg/dl (Table 7.4).

Table 7.4 Treatment goals in patients with cardiometabolic risk and lipoprotein abnormalities [6]

	Goals		
	LDL-C (mg/dl)	Non-HDL-C (mg/dl)	Apolipoprotein B (mg/dl)
Highest risk patients:			
Known CVD or diabetes plus one additional risk factor	<70	<100	<80
High-risk patients:			
No diabetes or known clinical CVD but two or more risk factors or diabetes but no other CVD risk factors	<100	<130	<90

Other risk factors beyond dyslipoproteinemia include smoking, hypertension, and family history of CAD

Lipid Lowering with the Statin Drugs

The HMG CoA reductase inhibitors (statins) are the most commonly prescribed drugs for lowering LDL-C. There are currently seven statins in the US market (Table 7.5). They differ in terms of efficacy, half-life, and metabolism. All are effective LDL-C-lowering drugs. The statins work by inhibiting the enzyme that catalyzes the rate-limiting step in cholesterol synthesis. This leads to clearance of LDL-C particles from the circulation by the liver. In addition, statins minimally raise HDL-cholesterol (HDL-C) and lower triglyceride containing particles. They all reduce levels of hs-CRP and other inflammatory markers.

Two early primary prevention trials have shown that treatment with statins reduce cardiovascular events between 19 and 37%. Individuals with multiple risk factors have a greater absolute reduction in risk. The West of Scotland Coronary Prevention (WOSCOP) study used pravastatin in a high-risk cohort of middle-aged men with high cholesterol levels and showed that a 26% reduction in LDL-C resulted in a 31% relative reduction in risk of nonfatal myocardial infarction and death from CHD [7]. The Air Force/Texas Coronary Atherosclerosis Prevention Study (AFCAPS/TexCAPS) evaluated whether cholesterol lowering with statin therapy can benefit individuals with average cholesterol levels but low HDL-C levels. In this study, lovastatin reduced the risk of a first major cardiac event by 37% [8]. This study suggests that statin therapy to lower LDL-C can be an effective treatment to lower cardiovascular risk in individuals with average LDL-C levels and low HDL-C as their primary lipid abnormality. More recently, the JUPITER study evaluated older individuals with multiple risk factors, an LDL-C less than 130 mg/dl and an elevated hs-CRP, and showed that an LDL-C reduction of 50% with high-dose rosuvastatin significantly reduced the rates of a first major cardiovascular event and all-cause mortality [9].

The vulnerable patient with multiple risk factors is more likely to benefit from lipid-lowering therapy. A calculation of the number of patients needed to be treated (NNT) over a given period of time to prevent a cardiac event shows that this number decreases in higher-risk individuals (Table 7.6). Analysis of the WOSCOPS and AFCAPS/TexCAPS studies, for example, showed a lower NNT in subgroups of

Table 7.5 Statins

Statin (generic)	Brands available	Available doses (mg)	LDL-lowering efficacy (%)
Lovastatin	Generic lovastatin, Mevacor (Merck), Altocor (Andrx)	10, 20, 40	21–42
Pravastatin	Generic pravastatin, Pravachol (Bristol-Myers Squibb)	10, 20, 40, 80	22–37
Fluvastatin	Lescol, Lescol XL (Novartis)	20, 40, 80	22–36
Simvastatin	Generic simvastatin, Zocor (Merck)	10, 20, 40, 80	26–47
Atorvastatin	Lipitor (Pfizer)	10, 20, 40, 80	39–60
Rosuvastatin	Crestor (AstraZeneca)	5, 10, 20, 40	40–60
Pitavastatin	Livalo (Kowa)	1, 2, 4	32–43

Table 7.6 Number needed to treat by subgroup analysis (from [10])

Study	NNT overall	NNT smokers	NNT diabetics	NNT hypertensives
WOSCOPS	44	34	–	–
AFCAPS/TexCAPS	49	19	27	31

NNT number needed to treat, *WOSCOPS* West of Scotland Coronary Prevention Study, *AFCAPS/TexCAPS* Air Force/Texas Coronary Atherosclerosis Prevention Study

patients with additional risk factors [10]. Extrapolation of the JUPITER trial over a 5-year treatment period calculated that the number needed to treat to prevent the occurrence of one primary event with high-dose rosuvastatin is 25 [9].

Secondary prevention trials studied the use of statins in patients diagnosed with CHD to determine if these agents would reduce subsequent cardiac events. The Scandinavian Simvastatin Survival Study (4S) evaluated the effect of cholesterol lowering with simvastatin in 4,444 patients with angina or a previous myocardial infarction and reported a 30% reduction in risk of death compared with the placebo group [11]. This was the first major study to show a total mortality benefit with lipid-lowering therapy. Additional studies such as the Cholesterol and Recurrent Events (CARE) trial using pravastatin demonstrated similar results in individuals with lower average cholesterol levels than the 4S study [12].

The Medical Research Council Heart Protection Study extended these findings to CHD risk-equivalent patients. This large collaborative study of over 20,000 individuals treated patients with coronary disease, other atherosclerotic disease including carotid artery disease and peripheral arterial disease, or diabetes [13]. Patients were randomized to simvastatin 40 mg daily or placebo. The treatment group had a 24% reduction in major vascular events regardless of their disease category. This study proved influential to guideline recommendations. The Heart Protection Study included a large number of individuals who at randomization had LDL-C values below 100 mg/dl; below NCEP treatment guideline levels at the time. These patients received the same relative risk reduction as subjects with higher LDL-C levels suggesting that high-risk candidates will receive significant risk reduction by an

LDL-lowering strategy regardless of their presenting LDL levels. The American Diabetes Association (ADA), in response to the Heart Protection Study, recommended that for patients with diabetes over the age of 40 years and a total cholesterol ≥135 mg/dl, statin therapy may be appropriate regardless of baseline LDL levels [14].

Hypertension patients are at increased risk for cardiovascular events and tend to present with a clustering of risk factors. The Anglo-Scandinavian Cardiac Outcomes Trial (ASCOT) studied the benefits of cholesterol-lowering therapy in hypertensive patients without substantially elevated cholesterol levels [15]. Over 10,000 individuals with a total cholesterol level of less than 6.5 mmol/L (average 5.5 mmol/L or 213 mg/dl) were randomized to atorvastatin 10 mg or placebo. The study ended early after 3.3 years of follow-up because ongoing analysis showed a significant reduction in the primary end point in treated subjects. The ASCOT study population is an older high-risk group of individuals with an average of 3.7 risk factors in addition to hypertension per subject. This study suggests that individuals with multiple risk factors will benefit from an LDL-C-lowering strategy regardless of what primary cardiac risk factor led to the increased risk.

Recent studies have also looked at the highest risk level of the spectrum. Patients who suffer from an acute coronary syndrome are at substantially increased risk for future events both in the short and long term. Studies have explored more intensive strategies for lowering cholesterol in this group of patients. The Pravastatin or Atorvastatin Evaluation and Infection Therapy (PROVE IT) study compared standard lipid-lowering therapy (pravastatin 40 mg) with an intensive regimen (atorvastatin 80 mg) in over 4,000 patients hospitalized for an acute coronary syndrome [16]. The primary end point of death, myocardial infarction, unstable angina requiring hospitalization, revascularization, or stroke was reduced by 16% in the intensive treatment group (absolute risk reduction 2.2%) compared with the standard therapy group. In patients not previously receiving statin therapy, the intensive treatment group had an average reduction in LDL-C of 51% compared with only a 22% reduction in the standard treatment group. This suggests that patients with an acute coronary syndrome may benefit from more aggressive lipid lowering than has been achieved in the major secondary prevention trials to date. The Treating to New Targets (TNT) trial extended this finding to patients with chronic CHD [17]. Higher-dose statin (atorvastatin 80 mg) compared with a starting dose statin (atorvastatin 10 mg) achieved a further 22% relative risk reduction (2.2% absolute risk reduction) with a mean LDL-C of 77 mg/dl achieved in the high-dose group.

Statin Medications

Lovastatin

The statin medications are competitive inhibitors of 3-hydroxy-3-methylglutaryl coenzyme A (HMG CoA) reductase, a rate-limiting enzyme in the synthesis of cholesterol (Table 7.7). The first statin was found by investigators at Sankyo as a fungal

Table 7.7 Statins (from [18])

	Absorption (%)	Effect of food on systemic bioavailability (%)	Plasma protein binding (%)	Hepatic extraction (% of absorbed dose)	Renal excretion (%)	Plasma half-life (h)
Lovastatin	31	+50	>95	>69	30	3
Simvastatin	61–85	0	98	>79	13	
Pravastatin	34	−32	43 48	46	60	3
Fluvastatin	>90	−22	>99	>68	6	0.5–0.8
Atorvastatin			>98		<17	11–24
Rosuvastatin	50		88	60	16	19

compound from *Penicillium citrinum* (called mevastatin). Investigators at Merck isolated a similar compound (it differs by a single methyl group) from the common soil fungus *Aspergillus terreus* called lovastatin. Mevastatin was not further developed because of possible tumor formation in animal studies. Lovastatin was approved by the FDA in 1987 for cholesterol reduction.

Approximately 33% of lovastatin is absorbed following an oral dose [18]. The drug's mechanism of action is in the liver and it is taken up by hepatocytes by first-pass hepatic extraction. Lovastatin is a prodrug and is hydrolyzed within hepatocytes to the active agent. When taken with food, the systemic bioavailability of lovastatin increases by 50% which is why it was recommended that this drug be taken with the evening meal. Its elimination half-life is approximately 3 h. Lovastatin typically lowers LDL-C between 30 and 40%. It is available as a generic medication.

Simvastatin

Simvastatin is a synthetically derived statin and differs from lovastatin by the addition of a single methyl group. Simvastatin is also a prodrug that is enzymatically hydrolyzed in the liver to an open ring active form of the drug. The pharmacokinetics of simvastatin is similar to lovastatin [19]. About 30% of the oral dose is absorbed and the majority of the drug is extracted by the liver on first pass. Only a small amount of the drug reaches the systemic circulation. Simvastatin is mainly eliminated through biliary excretion. Simvastatin is about twice as potent as lovastatin and is also available as a generic medication.

Pravastatin

Pravastatin is produced by chemical modification of lovastatin. Pravastatin is administered as the sodium salt of the active compound and is rapidly absorbed. Food decreases systemic bioavailability of pravastatin but this does not seem to change its lipid lowering efficacy [20]. The elimination half-life of pravastatin is about 3 h, similar to lovastatin. Pravastatin's route of excretion is both biliary and renal with 47% of the drug eliminated through the kidney. Pravastatin is hydrophilic and the least bound to plasma proteins.

Fluvastatin

Fluvastatin is the first fully synthetic statin with a chemical structure that differs substantially from the fungal derivatives [18]. Fluvastatin is a racemic mixture with highly active and weakly active enantiomers. Fluvastatin is highly absorbed after an oral dose. Absorption is decreased when fluvastatin is given with a meal. Fluvastatin is highly protein bound which is thought to possibly minimize toxicity in peripheral tissues. Fluvastatin has the shortest elimination half-life of less than an hour. Fluvastatin is less efficacious than the other statins so is not useful when a significant reduction in LDL-C is required.

Atorvastatin

Atorvastatin is a potent HMG CoA reductase inhibitor that can lower LDL-C as much as 50–60%. The drug is rapidly absorbed and metabolized by first-pass mechanisms in the liver. The cytochrome P450 3A4 metabolism produces metabolites that are also potent lipid-lowering compounds. The half-life of atrovastatin is about 14 h but the duration of HMG CoA reductase inhibition can last 20–30 h secondary to the effects of the active metabolites. Food can change the rate of absorption of atrovastatin but this does not affect lipid lowering [21]. The drug is highly protein bound and is excreted mainly by biliary mechanism. It will remain a patent-protected medication until November 2011.

Rosuvastatin

Rosuvastatin was introduced to the market in 2003 and, like atorvastatin, is a very potent statin achieving LDL-C reductions in the 50–60% range. About 10% of the drug is metabolized by the cytochrome P450 2C9 enzyme into a weakly active metabolite [22]. The elimination half-life for rosuvastatin is about 19 h and it is eliminated largely by the gastrointestinal route. The plasma concentration can be increased as much as threefold in patients with severe renal impairment. Japanese and Chinese individuals may have a twofold increase in plasma concentrations when given the same dose as Caucasians.

Pitavastatin

Pitavastatin is the newest statin on the market. Pitavastatin is a lipophilic synthetic statin that comes in 1, 2, and 4 mg doses. It has been available in Japan since 2003. The full dose of pitavastatin lowers LDL-C by about 46%. Pitavastatin is minimally metabolized by the liver cytochrome enzymatic system which gives this drug the potential to have less drug interactions than the other statins [23].

Adverse Effects of Statins

The major adverse effects of statins are the potential for hepatotoxicity and myopathy. Hepatotoxicity occurs in about 1% of patients with standard doses of the statins. It is dose related and may increase in prevalence at increased doses. Hepatotoxicity is defined as an elevation in transaminases (ALT and AST) over three times the upper limits of normal. It is recommended to obtain baseline transaminases before starting a statin since a small subset of patients will present with elevated liver enzymes either due to fat deposition in the liver or other subclinical liver diseases. Enzymes should then be re-measured 6–8 weeks after starting a statin or after an increase in dose to monitor for toxicity. If the enzymes are elevated greater than three times the upper limit of normal, then the drug can be discontinued and the enzymes usually slowly return to normal. Statins should not be used in patients with advanced liver disease since the systemic exposure can be significantly increased in these patients.

Myopathy can be broken down into the categories of myalgias, myositis, and rhabdomyolysis. Rhabdomyolysis is a serious consequence of statin use and can lead to renal failure. This is a very rare adverse reaction with these agents and is more likely to occur if there is a drug–drug interaction causing systemic accumulation of the drug. Myopathy and myositis can cause muscle weakness, sometimes only noticeable with exercise, muscle soreness, and uncommon elevations in the creatine kinase (CK) enzyme. Statins should be discontinued if the CK elevates greater than ten times the upper limit of normal.

All statins are contraindicated during pregnancy and for nursing mothers since cholesterol is essential for fetal development and there is concern that statins may cause deficiencies of important compounds necessary for fetal growth.

Drug–Drug interactions

Toxicity may be increased in patients who are taking multiple medications that share a similar mechanism of metabolism in the liver. Table 7.8 lists a number of medications that have been shown to have an interaction with statins. In general,

Table 7.8 Selected drug interactions with statins

	Lovastatin	Simvastatin	Pravastatin	Fluvastatin	Atorvastatin	Rosuvastatin
Antifungal/macrolide antibiotics	Avoid or suspend use during therapy	Avoid or suspend use during therapy	Avoid	Caution when used together	↑ Risk of myopathy, 40% ↑ atorvastatin concentration with erythromycin	No clinically significant interactions with ketoconazole, erythromycin
Fibrates	20 mg Max dose	Contra indicated with gemfibrozil	Avoid	Avoid	↑ Risk of myopathy	10 mg Max dose with gemfibrozil
Niacin (>1 g daily)	20 mg Max dose	Use caution	Not recommended with lipid-lowering doses	No effect	↑ Risk of myopathy	–
Amiodarone	40 mg Max dose	10 mg Max dose	–	–	–	–
Verapamil	40 mg Max dose	10 mg Max dose	No effect with diltiazem	–	–	–
Warfarin	No effect on PT but recommend monitoring	Modest increase in INR	No effect on PT but recommend monitoring	No effect on PT but recommend monitoring	No effect on PT	Clinically significant ↑ in INR
Cyclosporin	20 mg Max dose	Contra indicated	10 mg Starting dose, 20 mg max dose	No effect on cyclosporin levels, fluvastatin levels ↑	↑ Risk of myopathy	5 mg Max dose
Digoxin	No effect on levels	Slight elevation in digoxin levels	No effect	11% Increase in digoxin	20% Increase in digoxin	No effect
Grapefruit Juice	Avoid >1 quart daily	Avoid >1 quart daily	No change[a]	–	↑ Atorvastatin levels have been reported[a]	–

Data extracted from Mevacor 2008, Zocor 2008, Pravachol 2007, Lescol 2008, Lipitor 2008, Crestor 2008 package inserts
[a]Data from ref. [24]

antifungal agents and certain macrolide antibiotics (erythromycin and clarithromycin but not azithromycin) can increase concentrations of statin medications (with the possible exception of rosuvastatin) and increase the risk of muscle toxicity. Statin therapy should be suspended during the course of antibiotic therapy to avoid toxicity in patients at high risk of developing toxicity. Fibrates and gemfibrozil in particular can lead to an increase risk of myopathy when used concomitantly with statins. Fenofibrate may be a safer choice. Rosuvastatin can significantly increase the INR in patients on warfarin therapy. All patients on a statin and warfarin should have close monitoring of the INR. Finally, large amounts (>1 quart daily) of grapefruit juice can delay metabolism of many medications and temporarily increase serum levels of the drugs. Lovastatin, simvastatin, and atorvastatin can have significant increases in bioavailability when taken with grapefruit juice. This could potentially lead to increased toxicity. Pravastatin is not affected because the drug uses a different metabolic pathway [24].

How to Choose a Statin

When choosing a statin, four general considerations should be taken into account; namely efficacy, toxicity, outcome data, and cost. Atorvastatin and Rosuvastatin are the most efficacious statins and can achieve a greater than 50% LDL-C lowering. As monotherapy, all the statins have about the same incidence of liver and muscle toxicity. They differ, however, in drug–drug interactions and certain drugs will need to be avoided or used at lower doses to avoid these interactions. When a number of medications can be chosen with similar efficacy and safety, it is recommended to choose the agent that has a convincing outcome study that applies to your patient. The dose used should be the same as used in the study to hopefully achieve the same risk reduction in your patient. Finally, cost is a major concern for patients to obtain medications and to ensure compliance. Three statins are currently available as low cost generics and may be preferable to the higher cost branded agents if they can achieve the same efficacy, safety, and outcome for your patient.

When to Use a Statin

Statins are first line pharmacological therapy for LDL-C lowering in at-risk individuals. Benefit has been seen in both primary and secondary prevention trials. For primary prevention, statins are typically used in patients that cannot achieve an LDL-C goal with a therapeutic lifestyle program alone. For secondary prevention, statins are typically recommended for all patients unless there is a contraindication to their use.

Intestinal Agents

Bile Acid Sequestrants (Resins)

The resins bind bile acids (not cholesterol) in the gastrointestinal tract preventing the return of the bile acids to the liver through the enterohepatic circulation. To produce more bile acids, the liver increases synthesis of cholesterol and up regulates LDL receptors increasing the clearance of LDL-C from the circulation. The resins can reduce LDL-C by 10–20% when used as monotherapy. Reduction in LDL-C reaches steady state after about 2 weeks of therapy.

Cholestyramine and colestipol were the first two available resins but their use was limited because of poor tolerability by many patients. Colesevelam (Welchol) is a more recently available resin that can be taken in tablet form improving its tolerability. The amount of colesevelam needed to reduce LDL-C is less than the earlier resins because each colesevelam molecule has multiple bile acid binding sites. Six to nine tablets are required daily, however, to achieve a similar 10–20% reduction in LDL-C [25].

The main adverse effects of the resins are gastrointestinal. As many as a third of patients will develop abdominal fullness and constipation although these symptoms are less with colesevelam [26]. Triglycerides can increase by about 10% because of increased liver synthesis of VLDL particles. The older bile acid sequestrants may inhibit the absorption of vitamin D and a number of medications including warfarin, digoxin, thiazide diuretics, thyroxine, and statins.

Outcome data with resins is limited. The only major trial is the Lipid Research Clinics Coronary Primary Prevention Trial which evaluated over 3,800 asymptomatic men with hypercholesterolemia and randomized the population to cholestyramine or placebo over an average of 7.4 years [27]. There was a 20.3% reduction in LDL-C in the treatment group that led to a 19% reduction in CHD death and nonfatal myocardial infarction.

There is increased interest in using resins as combination therapy with statins. An additional 20–25% reduction in LDL-C can be achieved with the addition of a resin to a statin. Colesevelam has also been shown to improve glycemic control in patients with type 2 diabetes mellitus with a mean reduction in hemoglobin A_{1c} between 0.5 and 1% compared with placebo [28]. Based on these data, colesevelam received FDA approval to improve glycemic control in patients with type 2 diabetes in January 2008.

When to Use Bile Acid Sequestrants

Statins remain the primary pharmacologic agent when the goal is to reduce LDL-C. Resins are reasonable alternatives when statins cannot be tolerated although LDL-C lowering will be limited to about 20%. Colesevelam is better tolerated than the earlier resins and concern remains about the increased noncardiac mortality seen with colestipol. Colesevelam is not currently available as a generic. Combination therapy with statins is an effective method for further reduction in LDL-C. It is recommended to begin with the highest tolerable statin dose to reduce LDL-C. If further LDL-C reduction is required, a resin can be added. This combination is used frequently in patients with familial hypercholesterolemia. There is emerging evidence to suggest that colesevelam may be useful as an additional agent for glycemic control in patients with type 2 diabetes mellitus.

Ezetimibe

Ezetimibe is a selective cholesterol absorption inhibitor that prevents the absorption of dietary and biliary cholesterol and other exogenous phytosterols through the intestinal wall. The selectivity of this compound does not affect absorption of triglycerides, bile acids, or fat soluble vitamins. The target of ezetimibe is the Niemann-Pick C1-Like 1 (NPC1L1) protein [29]. The binding of ezetimibe to this protein blocks cholesterol uptake in the brush border membrane of the enterocyte. Following absorption, ezetimibe is glucoronidated in the intestinal wall and undergoes enterohepatic recirculation. The drug is then returned to its primary site of action in the intestine where it remains active. This limits its systemic exposure.

Similar to the bile acid sequestrants, ezetimibe lowers LDL-C between 15 and 20% as monotherapy. When combined with maximal doses of statins in patients with familial hypercholesterolemia, up to an additional 20.7% reduction in LDL-C was achieved [30]. Outcome studies to determine if combination therapy with statins will achieve further risk reduction are ongoing. A surrogate marker study evaluating regression of atherosclerosis by carotid artery ultrasound with combination therapy compared with statin therapy alone failed to show any incremental benefit in carotid artery thickness but this study was too small to determine if there were any reductions in clinical events [31].

When to Use Ezetimibe

Ezetimibe can be used as monotherapy in patients who are intolerant of statins. As with the resins, only a 15–20% reduction in LDL-C would be expected. Ezetimibe can be added to the highest tolerable dose of a statin if further LDL-C reduction is required. Ezetimibe may be better tolerated than resins used in a similar manner. Long-term toxicity data need to be collected although ezetimibe appears to be very well tolerated.

Fibrates

The fibrates are a class of medications that are weak agonists of the peroxisome proliferator-activated receptor α (PPAR-α). The PPARs are nuclear transcription factors that modulate gene expression with effects on lipid and glucose metabolism. The PPAR-α agonists lower triglyceride levels and mildly raise HDL-C. They may lower LDL-C although if there is a substantial decrease in triglyceride levels, LDL-C may increase slightly in some patients. This increase in LDL-C may be due to an increase in particle size and thus cholesterol content of the LDL particles and not an increase in absolute number of LDL particles. These less dense LDL particles may be less atherogenic than small, dense LDL. Gemfibrozil and fenofibrate are the two most widely used fibrates in the USA and are available as generic medications. Table 7.9 summarizes the fibrate drugs that are available.

The fibrates were available before the statins for lipid lowering but concerns were raised early about possible noncardiac toxicity. The World Health Organization's Cooperative Primary Prevention Trial using clofibrate showed an excess risk of gall bladder disease, cancer, and all-cause mortality [32]. Clofibrate is not widely available and rarely prescribed. Gemfibrozil was studied in the primary prevention Helsinki Heart Study which showed a 34% reduction in the incidence of cardiac events although no decrease in total mortality in part because of excess noncardiac deaths [33].

The Veterans Affairs High-Density Lipoprotein Cholesterol Intervention Trial (VA-HIT) is a secondary prevention trial that compared 1,200 mg of gemfibrozil with placebo in over 2,500 men with CHD and low HDL-C levels (40 mg/dl or less) [34]. HDL-C levels were increased by 6%, triglycerides lowered 31%, and no change was observed in LDL-C levels with gemfibrozil therapy. There was a 24% reduction in the combined end point of death from coronary disease, nonfatal myocardial infarction, and stroke. Patients with metabolic syndrome or diabetes (high triglycerides and low HDL-C) seemed to derive the most benefit from therapy with gemfibrozil [35].

Table 7.9 Fibrates

Fibrate (generic)	Brands available	Doses available (mg)
Gemfibrozil	Generic and Lopid (Parke-Davis)	600
Fenofibrate	Generic and generic micronized fenofibrate Multiple brands in Tricor (Abbott), Lofibra (Teva), Triglide (SkyePharma), TriLipix delayed release tablets (Abbott), Antara (Oscient), and others	Micronized – 67, 134, 200 Tricor – 45, 145 Lofibra – 54, 160 Triglide – 50, 160 TriLipix – 45, 135 Antara – 43, 130
Bezafibrate (not in USA)	Generic and Bezalip (Roche), Bezalip SR	200, 400
Clofibrate (not widely available)	Generic and Atromid-S (Wyeth)	500

Fenofibrate was studied in diabetic patients in the Fenofibrate Intervention and Event Lowering in Diabetes (FIELD) study [36]. Prior cardiovascular disease was present in 22% of the patients, and statins and other lipid-lowering agents were allowed during the study. The primary composite end point of CHD death or nonfatal myocardial infarction was not significantly different between the fenofibrate and the placebo group, but the secondary end point of total cardiovascular disease events was significantly lower in the fenofibrate group. Patients in the placebo group were more likely treated with other lipid-lowering agents (17% vs. 8%) that may have influenced the results of the study. The Action to Control Cardiovascular Risk in Diabetes (ACCORD) study evaluated the combination of simvastatin plus fenofibrate in comparison to simvastatin alone and failed to show any further cardiovascular risk reduction raising the question about the benefit of this combination in diabetic patients [37].

Gemfibrozil

Gemfibrozil has been the most studied of the fibrates in both primary and secondary prevention trials. It is completely absorbed after an oral dose. The rate and extent of absorption is increased if the drug is given before a meal. It is metabolized in the liver by the cytochrome 3A4 system. Its half-life is 1.5 h. Greater than 70% of the drug is excreted through the kidney. It should not be used in patients with advanced liver or kidney disease. Gemfibrozil is usually dosed as a 600 mg tablet 30 min before the morning and the evening meals. It should not be used with repaglinide since the combination can lead to severe hypoglycemia. Caution should be taken when combined with statins or high-dose niacin because of the increase risk of myopathy. It is a pregnancy C category medication.

Fenofibrate

Fenofibrate is a PPARα agonist like gemfibrozil that can reduce very low-density lipoproteins and triglycerides. It is a prodrug metabolized to the active compound fenofibric acid. Fenofibrate has a 20 h half-life. It is a pregnancy category C. It is available by a number of manufacturers including as a generic medication (Table 7.9). There are multiple doses available as well as a micronized fenofibrate (particles <400 nm) which has improved bioavailability due to its smaller size. There is a potential for myopathy and rhabdomyolysis with fenofibrate, although no events occurred in the FIELD trial including in patients on combination with a statin [36]. Fenofibrate doses should be lowered in patients with advanced renal failure. Fenofibrate may increase serum levels of statins so it is recommended to give the two medications at different times of the day.

When to Use Fibrates

Fibrates are generally recommended to treat hypertriglyceridemia. Fibrates may be an alternative therapy to statins in patients who cannot tolerate statins. Patients with a low HDL-C or a mixed hyperlipidemia as typically seen in diabetic patients may achieve the greatest benefit from fibrates. Fibrates may be used with caution with statins because an increased risk of muscle toxicity may occur especially with gemfibrozil. Outcome studies combining statins and fibrates have not shown further clinical benefit.

Niacin

Niacin therapy has the greatest potential to raise HDL-C levels. Niacin is available as a short acting supplement or as a prolonged release preparation to attempt to avoid cutaneous side effects such as flushing. Brands available in the USA include Niaspan (Kos) and Slo-Niacin (Upsher-Smith). High doses of niacin can raise HDL-C greater than any other currently available therapy. There have been few outcome studies, however, that document cardiovascular risk reduction with niacin. The Coronary Drug Project conducted between 1966 and 1975 evaluated the long-term efficacy of 3 g of niacin daily in a group of men who had a previous myocardial infarction [38]. After 6 years, the patients taking niacin had a lower incidence of nonfatal myocardial infarction. After 15 years of follow-up, the patients assigned to niacin had an 11% lower mortality than the placebo group even though these subjects had stopped the therapy 9 years earlier [39]. No further studies with niacin monotherapy have been performed that clearly show risk reduction.

Niacin is difficult to take and nearly 50% of individuals cannot tolerate the drug because of side effects. Niacin is used in lower doses in combination with statins with the hope that a combined effect of lowering LDL-C with the statin and raising HDL-C with niacin will translate into further risk reduction. Outcome studies will need to be done to determine if this strategy will achieve further risk reduction. The HDL-Atherosclerosis Treatment Study (HATS) enrolled 160 men and women with clinical coronary disease and low HDL-C, and observed the effects of simvastatin plus niacin compared with placebo or antioxidant vitamins on angiographic coronary artery disease [40]. Measurable benefits were observed with the combination therapy but since there was no statin group alone it is unclear what role the niacin played in the results of this study.

When to Use Niacin

Niacin can be used as monotherapy to lower LDL-C or raise HDL-C. Statins are drugs of first choice in reducing LDL-C but niacin can be an alternative strategy if statins are not tolerated. Niacin can be considered a first choice agent in individuals with isolated low HDL-C although there is no outcome data to support its use. Niacin has most appeal as an add-on agent to statins to achieve further LDL-C lowering or to get non-HDL-C to goal. Combination extended-release niacin and statin products are available (Advicor = extended release niacin + lovastatin, Simcor = extended release niacin + simvastatin, both manufactured by Abbott).

Conclusions

Pharmacological therapy designed to lower cholesterol levels has become an important development in the treatment of CHD and for individuals at increased cardiovascular risk. Treatment strategies to lower LDL-C and raise HDL-C have been shown to reduce cardiovascular risk regardless of the risk factors present. The reduction in cardiac events in this country has been attributed in part to aggressive treatment of hyperlipidemia. Unfortunately, heart disease remains the number one cause of death worldwide despite these important breakthroughs. Identifying patients at risk is the important first step in achieving further success in reducing the ravages of heart disease.

References

1. Anderson KM, Castelli WP, Levy D. Cholesterol and mortality. 30 years of follow-up from the Framingham study. JAMA. 1987;257(16):2176–80.
2. Neaton JD, Blackburn H, Jacobs D, et al. Serum cholesterol level and mortality findings for men screened in the Multiple Risk Factor Intervention Trial. Multiple Risk Factor Intervention Trial Research Group. Arch Intern Med. 1992;152(7):1490–500.
3. Gould AL, Rossouw JE, Santanello NC, Heyse JF, Furberg CD. Cholesterol reduction yields clinical benefit: impact of statin trials. Circulation. 1998;97(10):946–52.
4. Third Report of the National Cholesterol Education Program (NCEP) Expert Panel on Detection, Evaluation, and Treatment of High Blood Cholesterol in Adults (Adult Treatment Panel III) final report. Circulation 2002;106(25):3143–21.
5. Grundy SM, Cleeman JI, Merz CN, et al. Implications of recent clinical trials for the National Cholesterol Education Program Adult Treatment Panel III guidelines. Circulation. 2004;110(2): 227–39.
6. Brunzell JD, Davidson M, Furberg CD, et al. Lipoprotein management in patients with cardiometabolic risk: consensus statement from the American Diabetes Association and the American College of Cardiology Foundation. Diabetes Care. 2008;31(4):811–22.
7. Shepherd J, Cobbe SM, Ford I, et al. Prevention of coronary heart disease with pravastatin in men with hypercholesterolemia. West of Scotland Coronary Prevention Study Group. N Engl J Med. 1995;333(20):1301–7.
8. Downs JR, Clearfield M, Weis S, et al. Primary prevention of acute coronary events with lovastatin in men and women with average cholesterol levels: results of AFCAPS/TexCAPS. Air Force/Texas Coronary Atherosclerosis Prevention Study. JAMA. 1998;279(20):1615–22.
9. Ridker PM, Danielson E, Fonseca FA, et al. Rosuvastatin to prevent vascular events in men and women with elevated C-reactive protein. N Engl J Med. 2008;359(21):2195–207.
10. Kumana CR, Cheung BM, Lauder IJ. Gauging the impact of statins using number needed to treat. JAMA. 1999;282(20):1899–901.

11. Randomised trial of cholesterol lowering in 4444 patients with coronary heart disease: the Scandinavian Simvastatin Survival Study (4 S). Lancet 1994;344(8934):1383–9.
12. Sacks FM, Pfeffer MA, Moye LA, et al. The effect of pravastatin on coronary events after myocardial infarction in patients with average cholesterol levels. Cholesterol and Recurrent Events Trial investigators. N Engl J Med. 1996;335(14):1001–9.
13. Heart Protection Study Collaborative Group. MRC/BHF Heart Protection Study of cholesterol lowering with simvastatin in 20,536 high-risk individuals: a randomised placebo-controlled trial. Lancet 2002;360(9326):7–22.
14. Haffner SM. Dyslipidemia management in adults with diabetes. Diabetes Care. 2004;27 Suppl 1:S68–71.
15. Sever PS, Dahlof B, Poulter NR, et al. Prevention of coronary and stroke events with atorvastatin in hypertensive patients who have average or lower-than-average cholesterol concentrations, in the Anglo-Scandinavian Cardiac Outcomes Trial–Lipid Lowering Arm (ASCOT-LLA): a multicentre randomised controlled trial. Lancet. 2003;361(9364):1149–58.
16. Cannon CP, Braunwald E, McCabe CH, et al. Intensive versus moderate lipid lowering with statins after acute coronary syndromes. N Engl J Med. 2004;350(15):1495–504.
17. LaRosa JC, Grundy SM, Waters DD, et al. Intensive lipid lowering with atorvastatin in patients with stable coronary disease. N Engl J Med. 2005;352(14):1425–35.
18. Blum CB. Comparison of properties of four inhibitors of 3-hydroxy-3-methylglutaryl-coenzyme A reductase. Am J Cardiol. 1994;73(14):3D–11.
19. Jones PH. Lovastatin and simvastatin prevention studies. Am J Cardiol. 1990;66(8):39B–43.
20. Haria M, McTavish D. Pravastatin. A reappraisal of its pharmacological properties and clinical effectiveness in the management of coronary heart disease. Drugs. 1997;53(2):299–336.
21. Radulovic LL, Cilla DD, Posvar EL, Sedman AJ, Whitfield LR. Effect of food on the bioavailability of atorvastatin, an HMG-CoA reductase inhibitor. J Clin Pharmacol. 1995;35(10):990–4.
22. Cheng JW. Rosuvastatin in the management of hyperlipidemia. Clin Ther. 2004;26(9):1368–87.
23. Watson KE. Pitavastatin: the newest HMG-CoA reductase inhibitor. Rev Cardiovasc Med. 2010;11(1):26–32.
24. Lilja JJ, Kivisto KT, Neuvonen PJ. Grapefruit juice increases serum concentrations of atorvastatin and has no effect on pravastatin. Clin Pharmacol Ther. 1999;66(2):118–27.
25. Insull Jr W, Toth P, Mullican W, et al. Effectiveness of colesevelam hydrochloride in decreasing LDL cholesterol in patients with primary hypercholesterolemia: a 24-week randomized controlled trial. Mayo Clin Proc. 2001;76(10):971–82.
26. Knopp RH. Drug treatment of lipid disorders. N Engl J Med. 1999;341(7):498–511.
27. The Lipid Research Clinics Coronary Primary Prevention Trial results. I. Reduction in incidence of coronary heart disease. JAMA 1984;251(3):351–64.
28. Bays HE, Goldberg RB, Truitt KE, Jones MR. Colesevelam hydrochloride therapy in patients with type 2 diabetes mellitus treated with metformin: glucose and lipid effects. Arch Intern Med. 2008;168(18):1975–83.
29. Garcia-Calvo M, Lisnock J, Bull HG, et al. The target of ezetimibe is Niemann-Pick C1-Like 1 (NPC1L1). Proc Natl Acad Sci USA. 2005;102(23):8132–7.
30. Gagne C, Gaudet D, Bruckert E. Efficacy and safety of ezetimibe coadministered with atorvastatin or simvastatin in patients with homozygous familial hypercholesterolemia. Circulation. 2002;105(21):2469–75.
31. Kastelein JJ, Akdim F, Stroes ES, et al. Simvastatin with or without ezetimibe in familial hypercholesterolemia. N Engl J Med. 2008;358(14):1431–43.
32. WHO cooperative trial on primary prevention of ischaemic heart disease with clofibrate to lower serum cholesterol: final mortality follow-up. Report of the Committee of Principal Investigators. Lancet 1984;2(8403):600–4.
33. Frick MH, Elo O, Haapa K, et al. Helsinki Heart Study: primary-prevention trial with gemfibrozil in middle-aged men with dyslipidemia. Safety of treatment, changes in risk factors, and incidence of coronary heart disease. N Engl J Med. 1987;317(20):1237–45.
34. Rubins HB, Robins SJ, Collins D, et al. Gemfibrozil for the secondary prevention of coronary heart disease in men with low levels of high-density lipoprotein cholesterol. Veterans Affairs

High-Density Lipoprotein Cholesterol Intervention Trial Study Group. N Engl J Med. 1999;341(6):410–8.
35. Rubins HB, Robins SJ, Collins D, et al. Diabetes, plasma insulin, and cardiovascular disease: subgroup analysis from the Department of Veterans Affairs high-density lipoprotein intervention trial (VA-HIT). Arch Intern Med. 2002;162(22):2597–604.
36. Keech A, Simes RJ, Barter P, et al. Effects of long-term fenofibrate therapy on cardiovascular events in 9795 people with type 2 diabetes mellitus (the FIELD study): randomised controlled trial. Lancet. 2005;366(9500):1849–61.
37. Ginsberg HN, Elam MB, Lovato LC, et al. Effects of combination lipid therapy in type 2 diabetes mellitus. N Engl J Med. 2010;362(17):1563–74.
38. Clofibrate and niacin in coronary heart disease. JAMA 1975;231(4):360–81.
39. Canner PL, Berge KG, Wenger NK, et al. Fifteen year mortality in Coronary Drug Project patients: long-term benefit with niacin. J Am Coll Cardiol. 1986;8(6):1245–55.
40. Brown BG, Zhao XQ, Chait A, et al. Simvastatin and niacin, antioxidant vitamins, or the combination for the prevention of coronary disease. N Engl J Med. 2001;345(22):1583–92.

Chapter 8
Hypertriglyceridemia

Sonal Chandra and Matthew J. Sorrentino

Keywords Hypertriglyceridemia • Chylomicrons • Atherogenic dyslipidemia • Omega-3-fish oils • Fibrates

Case Report

A 57-year-old pharmacist with a history of hypertension and recent increase in weight gain came in for an annual physical checkup. The pharmacist had gained 22 pounds over the past year since the death of his wife. The patient had been eating indiscriminately and drinking heavily for the past 6 months. A fasting lipid panel revealed total cholesterol of 248 mg/dl, triglycerides 423 mg/dl, and high-density lipoprotein (HDL) cholesterol 44 mg/dl. The low-density lipoprotein (LDL) cholesterol was not calculated. He asked about therapies to help reduce the triglycerides.

Introduction

Triglyceride Metabolism

Triglycerides (TGs) are utilized as storage molecules of metabolic energy and fatty acids for the synthesis of membrane lipids. TG levels are determined by dietary sources as well as de novo synthesis [1]. TGs are major lipids in chylomicrons and very low-density lipoprotein (VLDL) particles. These particles are closely related to

M.J. Sorrentino (✉)
Department of Medicine, Section of Cardiology,
University of Chicago Pritzker School of Medicine, Chicago, IL 60637, USA
e-mail: msorrent@medicine.bsd.uchicago.edu

M.J. Sorrentino (ed.), *Hyperlipidemia in Primary Care: A Practical Guide to Risk Reduction*, Current Clinical Practice, DOI 10.1007/978-1-60327-502-6_8,

the metabolism of other lipoproteins, including HDL particles. During its passage through the intestinal system, ingested fat is lipolyzed, dissolved into micelles, hydrolyzed by pancreatic lipase, and absorbed as fatty acids into the small intestine. After fatty acids are converted into TG, they make their way into the systemic circulation in the form of apolipoprotein B-48 containing chylomicrons [2–4]. De novo synthesis takes place in the liver in response to a carbohydrate-rich diet from excess fatty acids stored in cellular reserves [5]. The apolipoprotein B-100 containing nascent VLDL particles in the liver is initially deficient in TG until converted into highly lipidated TG-rich VLDL versions [6].

While in circulation, TGs are subject to enzymatic activity of lipoprotein lipase (LPL) with Apolipoprotein C-II (apoC-II) acting as an important co-factor. Deficiency in apoC-II can cause severe hypertriglyceridemia [7]. A decrease in the TG content of the lipoprotein particle leads to the formation of lipid-poor apolipoprotein A-I enriched pre-β HDL particles, mediated in part by phospholipid transfer protein (PLTP) [8]. Conversely, cholesterol ester transfer protein (CETP) and PLTP activity will increase in the presence of an increased pool of TG-rich lipoprotein particles, thereby, contributing to decreased HDL-cholesterol (HDL-C) levels and increased concentration of atherogenic small, dense LDL seen in hypertriglyceridemia [9, 10]. Importantly, almost all LDL is derived from VLDL. A number of different proteins such as apolipoprotein C-III, apolipoprotein A-V, and angiopoietin-like proteins 3 and 4 may act as potential inhibitors for the action of LPL, thereby, contributing to dyslipidemic states.

Defining Hypertriglyceridemia

The National Cholesterol Education Program–Adult Treatment Panel III (NCEP-ATP III) defines acceptable serum levels of TG as below 150 mg/dl [11]. The American Heart Association cardiovascular risk assessment for fasting TG levels are as follows. Borderline values range from 150 to 199 mg/dl; high values from 200 to 499 mg/dl, and levels above 500 mg/dl are considered to be in the very high range (Table 8.1).

Primary vs. Acquired Hypertriglyceridemia

Hypertriglyceridemia usually refers to elevations in VLDL-cholesterol (VLDL-C) and chylomicrons and causes could be familial or genetic (primary) vs. acquired (secondary).

Table 8.1 Classification of triglycerides

<150 mg/dl	Normal
150–199 mg/dl	Borderline risk
200–400 mg/dl	High risk
>500 mg/dl	Extreme high risk

Table 8.2 Clinical classification of primary hypertriglyceridemias (from refs. [13, 14])

1. Chylomicronemia (type I hyperlipoproteinemia)
   Caused by lipoprotein lipase (LPL) deficiency or apolipoprotein c-II deficiency
   Autosomal recessive
   Fasting chylomicronemia
   Triglycerides between 1,000 and 4,500 mg/dl
   Heterozygotes have normal fasting triglycerides, increased after fatty meal
   Recurrent pancreatitis
2. Type V hyperlipoproteinemia
   Fasting chylomicronemia, elevated VLDL
   Hypertriglyceridemia can be aggravated by factors increasing VLDL production, i.e., alcohol intake, estrogens, rapid weight gain, poorly controlled diabetes
   Triglycerides 500–3,000 mg/dl
   Pancreatitis, neurologic symptoms, xanthomas, heart disease
3. Hepatic lipase deficiency
4. Remnant hyperlipidemia (type III hyperlipoproteinemia and familial dysbetalipoproteinemia)
   Binding defect of apolipoprotein E
   Chylomicrons and VLDL accumulate
   Xanthomas, atherosclerotic disease
5. Familial hypertriglyceridemia
   Autosomal dominant, overproduction of VLDL
   Isolated hypertriglyceridemia, present also in family members
   Triglycerides 200–500 mg/dl
   Associated with the metabolic syndrome
6. Familial combined hyperlipidemia
   VLDL elevation, LDL elevation, or both
   Family history of premature atherosclerosis

Primary or familial TG disorders include genetic conditions that are known to significantly elevate plasma triglyceride levels such as primary chylomicronemia, familial hypertriglyceridemia, familial combined hyperlipoproteinemia, and familial dysbetalipoproteinemia [12]. These disorders are characterized by deficiencies in LPL or its cofactors, insufficient removal mechanisms of TG-rich lipoproteins with resultant increase in chylomicrons, VLDL-C, LDL-cholesterol (LDL-C), or combination of remnants. Table 8.2 provides a clinical classification of the primary hypertriglyceridemias. Genetic abnormalities contributing to high TG levels such as LPL deficiency and apoC-II deficiency in homozygous individuals are readily diagnosed because of marked fasting chylomicronemia. Chylomicrons are normally not present in the plasma when fasting. Identification of heterozygotes can be challenging as they may have normal fasting TG levels. However, there may be a propensity for abnormal postprandial TG levels. Type V hyperlipidemia results in both elevated levels of VLDL particles and chylomicrons [13]. The major risk in these patients is the development of life-threatening pancreatitis. Other overt clinical features in patients with chylomicronemia syndromes include eruptive xanthomas, hepatosplenomegaly, lipemia retinalis, abdominal pain with or without pancreatitis, peripheral neuropathy, dyspnea, memory loss, and dementia. Remainder of the clinical syndromes

Table 8.3 Acquired causes of hypertriglyceridemia (from ref. [15])

Metabolic influences
Diabetes mellitus
Obesity
Hyperuricemia
Glycogen storage disease type I
Hormonal influences
Insulin
Estrogen
Thyroid hormone
Nutritional influences
Alcohol
High carbohydrate intake
Disease states
Renal disease: nephrotic syndrome, renal failure
Paraproteinemias
Drugs
Diuretics, beta-blockers, steroids (estrogen replacement therapy)

listed in Table 8.2 is poorly characterized and may not be distinguishable from acquired causes of hypertriglyceridemia except for the presence of a strong family history. For example, in familial disorder of type III hyperlipoproteinemia or dysbetalipoproteinemia, the patients usually are homozygous for apolipoprotein E2; but its manifestation requires an additional trigger such as diabetes, obesity, hypothyroidism, or renal disease [14–16]. Clinically, these patients present with tuberoeruptive xanthomas and xanthomas in palm creases (xanthoma palmaris striata), and with features of coronary and peripheral arterial disease [17].

A wide range of factors can trigger lipogenesis and therefore, raise the levels of TG in the circulation (Table 8.3) [18]. Secondary etiologies of hypertriglyceridemia include hypothyroidism, kidney abnormalities (e.g., nephrotic syndrome or chronic kidney failure), diabetes mellitus, heavy alcohol consumption, carbohydrate-rich diets, and obesity. These disorders could be second hits on a genetically predisposed substrate. Gender and age contribute to variability in TG levels. In men and postmenopausal women, it appears that estrogen deficiency is responsible for higher postprandial TG levels compared with premenopausal women. Conversely, hormone replacement therapy has also demonstrated an increase in TG-VLDL levels, especially in those with preexisting or familial disease [19, 20].

Whether it is fasting or postprandial states, women demonstrate lower plasma TG levels compared with men [21, 22]. Decreased levels are a result of increased muscular TG uptake and storage in addition to higher clearance. There is also an impact of age on plasma TG increase irrespective of total body fat content, regional fat distribution, and behavioral variables [23, 24]. Hypertriglyceridemia (TG>150 mg/dl) is one of the diagnostic criteria of metabolic syndrome. Several drugs have the potential to increase TG levels (e.g., steroids, retinoids, oral estrogens, protease inhibitors, bile acid sequestrants, chlorthalidone, tamoxifen, or beta-blockers).

Hypertriglyceridemia is often observed in patients with metabolic syndrome, type 2 diabetes, or familial combined hyperlipidemia [25, 26]. The hallmark of these clinical phenotypes is the presence of insulin resistance resulting in abnormal regulation of lipid homeostasis [27]. This eventually leads to abnormalities in lipid handling in those organs that are particularly sensitive to insulin regulation such as adipose tissue, liver, and skeletal muscle [28]. It has since long been recognized that fatty acids are important ligands for several nuclear receptors that control lipid metabolism [28]. Abnormal signaling, as observed in the insulin resistant state, contributes to the upregulation in hepatic lipoprotein leading to increased production of VLDL particles. In addition, hyperglycemia impairs removal of TG-rich particles. Accumulation of chylomicrons and VLDL along with TG leads to high levels of potentially atherogenic particles and low levels of HDL-C [29]. With abnormal glucose and attendant fatty acid homeostasis, despite TG levels remaining within the so-called normal range, abnormalities in HDL and LDL become apparent. A fluctuating glucose profile leads to higher TG levels compared with diabetics with consistent control. Despite not very high levels of TG among the diabetics (30–40% of diabetics have triglyceride values over 200 mg/dl and only 10% are over 400 mg/dl), there is growing evidence that postprandial hyperlipidemia is prolonged in diabetics exposing the arteries to atherogenic particles for a longer period of time [30].

TG levels are frequently elevated in patients with chronic kidney disease as a result of increased concentration and/or impaired clearance of VLDL influenced by low LPL levels [31]. Animal studies indicate an association between hypoalbuminemia and reduced endothelial-bound LPL [32]. In addition to low lipase levels contributing to higher VLDL levels in nephrotic syndrome, reduced binding of VLDL to LPL as a result of dysfunctional HDL particles has also been demonstrated, thereby, contributing to an increase in the atherogenic burden [33]. Insulin resistance, a factor in renal insufficiency, promotes lipogenesis (VLDL particles) as well.

Obesity and nutritional factors also contribute to hypertriglyceridemia. Insulin resistance with hyperinsulinemia is common in the truncally obese patient and may promote VLDL production. Long-term alcohol consumption can raise TG levels and an alcohol binge in a susceptible individual can lead to a precipitous rise in levels leading to acute pancreatitis. High carbohydrate diets (>60% of total energy) consisting of simple sugars particularly have an impact on TG levels [34]. Specifically, consumption of simple sugars, such as the increasingly prevalent fructose found in soft drinks and processed foods, has greater glyceridemic effects with consequent elevation in plasma TG compared with complex carbohydrates or carbohydrate meals rich in fiber [35, 36]. Paradoxically, an emphasis on dietary fat reduction has resulted in more carbohydrate-rich diets with worsening obesity trends in this country resulting in higher levels of serum TG [37].

Drugs can further exacerbate borderline or high TG levels. Diuretics and beta-blockers have known to cause a modest rise in TG levels. Postmenopausal estrogen replacement therapy may raise TG levels as much as 25% from the baseline level. Long-term glucocorticoid use may increase TG as well. These elevations are worse in those with genetic susceptibilities.

Triglycerides and Cardiovascular Risk Assessment

The role of TG as a risk factor for coronary heart disease has been controversial and it is unclear whether high levels of TG are an independent risk factor for coronary artery disease (CAD), and importantly, whether it should be a target for therapy. When controlling for other lipoproteins, many studies have not found TG as an independent risk factor for the development of coronary heart disease. Emerging evidence does suggest however that abnormal TG levels, in setting of other lipoprotein abnormalities, may have a synergistic effect on cardiovascular risk.

Initial studies to evaluate an association between TG and incidence of coronary events were case-controlled studies. Prospective studies have demonstrated an association between TG levels and CAD with relative risks ranging between 1.2 and 1.6 [38]. When the studies were controlled for other lipoproteins, especially HDL-C, TG became less significant as an independent risk factor for CAD.

A number of intriguing observations can be derived from these epidemiologic studies. Triglyceride levels were not independently associated with coronary mortality in the Lipid Research Clinics Follow-up Study in the entire cohort, but rather in younger individuals and in subjects with lower HDL-C and LDL-C levels [39]. The Prospective Cardiovascular Munster Study (PROCAM) evaluated 4,559 male participants over a 6-year period [40]. Although TG levels were not found to be an independent predictor of risk, the study was able to identify a very high-risk group of individuals with LDL-C to HDL-C ratio of greater than 5.0. When the triglyceride levels were greater that 200 mg/dl in this subgroup, the number of coronary disease events over a 6-year period is more than doubled compared with the group with TG value less than 200 mg/dl. The Helsinki Heart Study found a similar increase in relative risk for cardiac events in individuals with a high LDL to HDL ratio (>5) and TG greater than 200 mg/dl compared with those with lower TG levels or alternatively lower LDL/HDL ratio with high TG [38]. These studies indicate that high-risk subgroups consist of those individuals with low HDL-C or a high LDL:HDL ratio in association with elevated TG levels. Many diabetic patients fit this pattern.

Some meta-analyses do suggest cardiovascular risk from TG, albeit as an attenuated predictor after adjustment for other risk factors. This still potentially implicates a direct atherogenic effect from TG particles [41]. A meta-analysis of 17 population-based prospective studies demonstrated that increased plasma TG levels were associated with greater cardiovascular risk in both men and women, after adjustment for HDL-C and other risk factors [42]. Similarly, another meta-analysis found the risk to be significant in individuals with TG levels in the top third of the population after adjusting for established coronary risk factors, including HDL-C when compared with those in the bottom third [43]. In line with these results are the data derived from a study of patients with CAD, TG levels were significantly associated with secondary cardiovascular events independent of HDL-C and LDL-C (hazard ratio of 1.50) [44].

Recently, there is emphasis being placed on elevated nonfasting TG levels indicative of remnant lipoproteins with high atherogenecity potential. Interestingly, the Women's Health Study after adjusting for levels of total and HDL-C, and measures of insulin resistance (diabetes, BMI, and C-reactive protein), failed to demonstrate a significant association between TG levels and the risk of cardiovascular events [41, 45]. In contrast, nonfasting TG levels were associated with an increase in cardiovascular events, independent of traditional risk factors and levels of other lipids, and markers of insulin resistance [45]. Similarly, in the Copenhagen City Heart Study, nonfasting TG levels were associated with increased risk of myocardial infarction, ischemic heart disease, and death after adjustment for age, total cholesterol, BMI, hypertension, diabetes, smoking, alcohol consumption, physical inactivity, lipid-lowering therapy, postmenopausal status, and hormone therapy in women [46]. The levels of nonfasting TG were highly correlated with those of remnant lipoprotein cholesterol. Recently, data obtained from a prospective study of 26,330 healthy women followed over an 11-year period revealed that the association with cardiovascular disease was stronger for nonfasting TG compared with fasting measurements of TG [47].

A number of studies have investigated if triglycerides are a risk factor in women. The Framingham Heart Study showed that women who have high triglyceride levels and a low HDL-C have a significantly higher risk of coronary disease and that this pattern of high triglyceride–low HDL-C is an independent risk factor for heart disease [48]. Secondary analysis of the Multiple Risk Factor Intervention Trial, The Lipid Research Clinics Coronary Primary Prevention Trial, and The Lipid Research Clinics Prevalence and Mortality Follow-Up Study showed that TG levels in men do not predict cardiovascular risk, but may remain a possibility for women [49].

Studies demonstrating TG as an independent or as a synergistic risk factor for cardiovascular event has borne mixed results. The Copenhagen Male Study evaluated 2,906 men over an 8-year period who were initially free of heart disease [50]. The incidence of heart disease increased from the lowest to the highest tercile of triglyceride levels. After adjusting for HDL-C, risk of cardiovascular disease remained persistent with increasing TG values within each level of HDL-C including the highest HDL-C category. Combined effects of HDL, TG, and total cholesterol on the incidence of atherosclerotic disease were examined prospectively in the Japanese-American men from the Honolulu Heart Program [51]. Risk of atherosclerotic disease appeared to be elevated in subjects with low HDL-C and high TG levels independent of other cardiovascular risk factors. The Scandinavian Simvastatin Survival Study similarly demonstrated an increased risk with increase in TG levels [52]. In addition, the Bezafibrate Infarction Prevention Study showed a small increase in mortality from elevated TG levels in men and women with established coronary heart disease, especially in the subgroup of patients with elevated LDL-C [53]. This is suggestive of hypertriglyceridemia as a synergistic risk factor in the presence of other abnormal lipid parameters. In a study of asymptomatic men, initially free from ischemic heart disease, an increase in fatal acute myocardial infarction events were noted in those with high TG/HDL ratio, indicating that TG is a significant amplifier of cardiovascular disease in the presence of high LDL-C and low HDL-C [54].

Table 8.4 Characteristics of the metabolic syndrome

Postprandial hypertriglyceridemia
Low HDL-C
Small, dense easily oxidized LDL-C
Insulin resistance
Hyperinsulinemia
Glucose intolerance or diabetes mellitus
Hypertension
Central obesity
Procoagulant state

Elevated TG levels are a marker for insulin resistant conditions such as metabolic syndrome and diabetes mellitus. Individuals with insulin resistance are susceptible to atherosclerotic disease. The abnormalities listed in Table 8.4 frequently coexist in the same individual. Physical inactivity, central obesity, high carbohydrate and saturated fat intake, aging, and genetic factors probably contribute to the syndrome. The triad of hypertriglyceridemia, elevated small, dense LDL-C particles, and low HDL-C is common in this syndrome and in diabetes mellitus and is referred to as atherogenic dyslipidemia. Because these conditions are defined by the presence of cardiovascular risk factors, it is difficult to prove whether TG independently predicts risk in these patients.

Aside from increasing cardiovascular disease rates, high TG levels also correlate with a greater risk of stroke. Nine hundred and forty one patients were followed for 8 years to detect transient ischemic attack (TIA) or ischemic stroke. Besides cholesterol levels, other contributing factors, such as smoking, complete medical history, and age, were taken into consideration [55]. High TG constituted an independent risk factor for ischemic stroke/TIA across subgroups of age, sex, patient characteristics, and cholesterol fractions. Patients with serum TG levels over 200 mg/dl had three times greater risk of suffering from a TIA.

Hypertriglyceridemia may predict the presence of small, dense LDL particles. LDL particles occur in a wide range of particle sizes. Two distinct families of LDL particles have been identified [12]. Pattern A is characterized by large, buoyant LDL particles with lower apolipoprotein B-100 (apoB) levels and pattern B consists of small, dense LDL particles with higher apoB levels. TG levels below 95 mg/dl are highly associated with pattern A, whereas levels greater than 160 mg/dl predict pattern B over 50% of the time, and those greater than 200 mg/dl predict pattern B nearly 80% of the time. The prospective Quebec Cardiovascular Study showed that the presence of small, dense LDL particles is associated with an increased risk of developing coronary heart disease [56]. Small, dense LDL particles are also thought to be more susceptible to oxidation, increasing their atherogenicity. Since elevated plasma TG level is strongly associated with low HDL-C levels, it may be difficult to tease out their individual atherogenic potential or contribution [57]. Therefore, non-HDL-C may be a better prognosticator along with TG since it includes all the atherogenic particles, including LDL, small dense LDL, and VLDL remnants [58].

Treatment of Hypertriglyceridemia

A classification of triglyceride levels is presented in Table 8.1. Triglyceride levels under 150 mg/dl are considered to be in the normal range. Because the incidence of pattern B small, dense LDL-C particles begins to increase above TG levels of 100 mg/dl [59], some experts would suggest a lower cutoff for the normal value in the at-risk individuals. Levels between 150 and 199 mg/dl are considered to be in the borderline risk range. Lifestyle modifications to lower the TG levels are recommended below 499 mg/dl; values above this connote higher risk. Most experts recommend a lifestyle modification program, but if TG remain above 500 mg/dl despite good adherence, then pharmacologic therapy is recommended. Triglyceride values above 1,000 mg/dl put an individual at high risk of developing acute pancreatitis. Pharmacologic therapy in combination with a lifestyle program is recommended. If a history of previous pancreatitis is present, then medication should be started immediately.

Lifestyle Modification

Prevention of cardiovascular events begins with a therapeutic lifestyle program. Table 8.5 provides an overview of lifestyle modifications to lower triglyceride levels. Treatment of high TG should begin with a lifestyle modification program that includes diet and exercise. Lifestyle changes demonstrated to be effective in modifying cardiovascular risk factors and reducing cardiovascular events include reduction in the intake of saturated fat and cholesterol, refined carbohydrates, and higher intake of fiber-rich diet (30–40 g/day). An adequate diet and exercise program decreases TG in over 50% of those who are adherent to it. This is especially true in patients with acquired hypertriglyceridemia; a lifestyle modification program alone will be adequate to return TG levels to the normal range. Compared with saturated fats, monounsaturated and polyunsaturated fats common in the Mediterranean diet have

Table 8.5 Lifestyle modification to lower triglycerides

Diet
Low sugar, low carbohydrate diet (diabetic diet)
Limit fat intake
Limit alcohol – in patients with very high triglycerides, alcohol should be eliminated
Dietary fish and fish oil supplementation may help lower triglycerides
Try to obtain and maintain an ideal body weight
Exercise
Regular consistent exercise program
Exercise may help raise HDL-C but vigorous exercise is usually needed
Smoking cessation
May help raise HDL-C

demonstrated beneficial effects in lowering atherogenic lipid profiles, specifically by reducing TG and small, dense LDL particles while maintaining appropriate HDL levels [60]. Although fruits and vegetables are rich in carbohydrates, studies have shown that they do not exert any effects on TG levels [61, 62]. The recommended level of dietary fat is 25–35% of caloric intake, within this range complex carbohydrates and a high-fiber diet are advised to facilitate TG lowering and to increase the levels of HDL and larger, more buoyant LDL particles. Carbohydrates need to be limited especially in diabetics and individuals with very high TG levels.

Red yeast rice may have cholesterol-lowering ability due to hydroxymethylglutaryl–coenzyme A reductase inhibitor activity. Its use has demonstrated modest reductions in TG levels [63]. Omega-3-fatty acids in the form of marine fish or fish oils can help lower TG levels. In patients with very high TG levels, fish oil capsules in higher doses can be used. Alcohol should be limited or completely eliminated in individuals with very high TG levels; patients at risk for pancreatitis need to be warned about the potential dangers of an alcohol or carbohydrate binge. A sudden rise in TG levels in circulation can cause acute life-threatening pancreatitis.

An exercise regimen can be very beneficial in lowering triglycerides and help raise HDL-C [64, 65]. Aerobic exercise at moderate to high intensity, 5–7 days/week, for at least 30 min/day is recommended for lifestyle maintenance with gradual increase to ≥60 min/day by people who need to achieve weight loss. Adherence to an appropriate exercise and dietary regimen would obviate the need for medication therapy in some people. For significant increases in HDL-C, more vigorous exercise may be needed. Large reduction in serum TG concentration after exercise training is achievable in previously inactive people with higher baseline concentrations, although those with initially low TG concentrations have smaller reductions after exercise training [66, 67].

Pharmacologic Therapy

When dietary therapy and exercise cannot achieve normalization of triglyceride levels, pharmacologic therapy should be considered. Omega-3-fatty acids, niacin, fibric acid derivatives, and statin drugs have all been used in patients with elevated triglyceride levels.

Omega-3-Fatty Acids

Omega-3-fatty acids include alpha-linolenic acid, found in plant sources such as flaxseed, nuts, and soy and in plant-based oils such as canola and soybean oils, and eicosapentaenoic (EPA) and docosahexaenoic (DHA) acids which are found primarily in cold-water fish, including salmon, mackerel, lake trout, tuna, and herring and fish oils.

A meta-analysis analyzing randomized controlled trials of omega-3 diets or supplementation and their effects on cardiovascular end points reported average TG reductions of 20% with no significant effect on LDL-C or HDL-C [68]. An omega-3 intervention irrespective of its form was associated with a significant reduction in cardiovascular mortality compared with control groups (relative risk 0.08, 95% CI 0.7–0.9). TG levels were decreased by 30% after treatment with omega-3-fatty acids in diabetic patients without adversely affecting hemoglobin A1c levels, but with some borderline worsening of blood glucose levels [69]. High doses (>6 g/day) can inhibit the synthesis of VLDL-TG and apoB, thus reducing levels of TG, and even though higher doses (15 g/day) could yield a 50% reduction in TG levels, they contribute to an overall increase in cholesterol levels [70, 71]. Cardiovascular protection conferred by omega-3 is inferred to be from reduced plaque growth, decreased platelet aggregation, reduced blood pressure by inhibition of eicosanoid-derived vasoconstriction factors and improved endothelial function, reduced occurrence of arrhythmias, and improved lipid profiles [72, 73].

Omega-3-fatty acids have been observed to lower VLDL and TGs by 15–40%, usually at doses of 3–4 g/day for EPA and DHA. However, current guidelines recommend omega-3 intake of 1 g/day for CAD patients or two fish servings per week consisting of a variety of fish and shellfish with low mercury content. This therapy results in smaller, less dense, presumably less atherogenic, VLDL and LDL particles [74]. In patients with TG levels >500 mg/dl, omega-3-fatty acids at doses of 3 g/day have been shown to decrease hypertriglyceridemia by 30%. ATP III recommends that omega-3-fatty acids be used as an adjunct to pharmacological therapy for lowering TG. The most practical way to achieve this quantity of omega-3-fatty acids is through the use of fish oil supplements.

Niacin

Niacin is a water-soluble B vitamin and when given in large amounts it can be used to lower cholesterol levels. The dose required to lower cholesterol levels is usually greater than 1,500 mg/day. The mechanism of action of niacin is still unclear, but is postulated that niacin inhibits lipolysis of TG, and thus decreases the production of VLDL particles, which in turn reduces production of LDL and triglycerides. The degree of cholesterol reduction is dose related and high doses of niacin are required for substantial reduction in triglycerides and LDL-C. In addition, high doses of niacin can significantly increase HDL-C and at the 2–3 g range may be the most potent HDL-raising agent. Niacin decreases LDL-C by about 5–25%, increases HDL-C by 15–35%, and decreases TG by 20–50% [11]. Unfortunately, doses in this range can produce intolerable side effects of flushing, itching, and heartburn making compliance a problem. In addition, there is a small incidence of liver toxicity especially with the long-acting preparations. Hyperglycemia may worsen in diabetic patients treated with niacin, however, there is no evidence of clinically relevant deterioration in glycemic control at recommended doses (≤2 g/day) [75].

The only major trial evaluating the efficacy of niacin is the Coronary Drug Project consisting of men with a prior myocardial infarction being treated with 3.0 g of niacin daily. There was no mortality benefit noted during the 6 years of the trial although nonfatal myocardial infarction decreased by 27% in the niacin group compared with placebo. At 15 years of follow-up (9 years after termination of the study), however, there was an unexpected 11% lower mortality in the niacin vs. the placebo group [76]. There was a 10% reduction in cholesterol levels and a 25% reduction in triglycerides in the niacin group, however, no significant correlation between the change in serum triglyceride levels and mortality was demonstrated. Not unexpectedly, nearly 30% of niacin-treated patients were poorly compliant with the treatment regimen due to drug intolerance. Currently, no other drugs are capable of a greater increase in HDL-C. Patients with high TG–low HDL are the most suitable candidates for this drug.

Fibric Acid Derivatives

Fibric acid derivatives are well known for their efficacy in treating hypertriglyceridemia. The mechanism of action of fibric acid derivatives is still unclear, although it is postulated that it triggers peroxisome proliferator activated receptors (PPARs), which regulate gene transcription and influence blood lipid levels [77]. Fibric acid derivatives have been demonstrated to decrease LDL by approximately 5–20%, increase HDL by 10–20%, and decrease TG by 20–50% [11]. The Cooperative Trial using clofibrate and the Helsinki Heart Study using gemfibrozil were primary prevention trials that showed a decrease in the incidence of nonfatal myocardial infarction but an unexpected increase in noncardiac deaths in the treated groups [25, 26]. In the Helsinki Heart Study, the subgroup of individuals with high TG and low HDL-C along with diabetic patients received the greatest benefit. In subjects with metabolic syndrome and hypertriglyceridemia, fenofibrate treatment (160 mg/day) reduced fasting and postprandial TG by about 45%, mainly due to reduction in large VLDL particles. Fibrate therapy has also resulted in reductions in non-HDL-C, apoB levels, and small LDL particles [78].

A secondary prevention trial demonstrating benefit from the treatment with fibrates is the Veterans Affairs High-Density Lipoprotein Cholesterol Intervention (VA-HIT) trial [79]. Over 2,500 men with coronary disease, an HDL-C ≤40 mg/dl, and an LDL-C ≤140 mg/dl were treated with gemfibrozil or placebo. Gemfibrozil treatment increased HDL by 6% and decreased triglycerides by 31%. LDL-C remained unchanged, but a nested case-controlled analysis demonstrated a decrease in concentration and an increase in particle size. There was a 22% relative risk reduction in major cardiac event in the treated group. Recent emerging results are suggesting that individuals with a pattern of low HDL, high triglycerides, and low LDL-C can benefit from therapy with a fibrate and statin. However, there are real concerns about an enhanced risk of myopathy with fibrate–statin combination therapy, especially, with gemfibrozil.

In the Fenofibrate Intervention and Event Lowering in Diabetes (FIELD) study, patients with type 2 diabetes were allocated to fenofibrate resulting in an initially promising, but nonsustained reductions in LDL-C, TG, and apoB with mild increase in HDL-C [80]. However, the use of statins in the control group and a deficiency in mixed hyperlipidemia (atherogenic mixed dyslipidemia) in the study group may have potentially confounded the results. Some of the side effects of fibrate therapy are myopathy, gallstones, dyspepsia, and heptopathy, therefore necessitating liver function testing at baseline, 3 months after initiation, and in regular intervals thereafter.

Statins

The statin drugs have a proven record in lowering cardiovascular risk without increasing the risk of noncardiac complications. These drugs are potent LDL-C-lowering agents, but are known to increase HDL-C and lower apoB in high-risk patients with elevated TG (<500 mg/dl), including those with metabolic syndrome or diabetes. Reductions of 40–50% in non-HDL-C, apoB, TG, and other TG-rich atherogenic lipoproteins have been reported with atorvastatin or rosuvastatin [81–84]. The benefit seen with the statin drugs has been attributed to the LDL-lowering effects of these agents. These studies suggest that a strategy of further lowering LDL-C in individuals with a low HDL-C, high triglycerides, and average LDL-C may achieve significant reduction in cardiac risk.

Combination Therapy

The ACCORD study (lipid arm) compared patients with fenofibrate and simvastatin to simvastatin therapy alone with a follow-up duration of 4.3 years. While there was no significant benefit on the primary end point (composite of nonfatal MI, nonfatal stroke, and CVD death) or any of the prespecified secondary end points [85], a beneficial trend was evident in patients with both high TG (≥204 mg/dl) and low HDL-C (<34 mg/dl) levels. This was supported by subgroup and post hoc analyses of the FIELD study. In terms of side effects, the group on combined therapy (fenofibrate and simvastatin) did not show a statistically significant increase in myositis or rhabdomyolysis. While combination medications can be safe most of the time, there is an increased incidence of liver toxicity that has to be monitored carefully. Statins should be used with caution when combined with niacin and fibrate (potentially an increased risk for myopathy).

Summary

High triglyceride levels are associated with a number of risk factors that substantially increase the risk of coronary heart disease. The metabolic syndrome is a constellation of signs and symptoms that has been linked to a high incidence of heart disease. Treatment begins with an aggressive lifestyle modification program. Dietary restriction of alcohol and carbohydrates can significantly lower triglyceride levels in many individuals. Those patients at high risk for cardiac disease should be considered for pharmacologic therapy. The lipid profile can tailor therapy for lipid reduction. Patients with borderline or high TG levels should undergo treatment for coexisting conditions and adopt lifestyle modifications aimed at lowering TG levels. Patients with coronary disease should be treated with a strategy to further lower LDL-C since this has demonstrated the greatest risk reduction. In patients with low LDL-C, low HDL-C, and high triglycerides, fibric acid derivatives are a reasonable option as demonstrated in the VA-HIT trial results. Isolated hypertriglyceridemia can be challenging to treat. Patients with TG levels greater than 1,000 mg/dl should be placed on drug therapy in addition to aggressive dietary change. The fibric acid derivatives are the drugs of first choice for this group of patients.

Our case: The pharmacist was advised to undergo a strict lifestyle modification. It appears that he was mostly eating processed, packaged food available at his drugstore. He was encouraged to reduce his carbohydrate and fat intake (especially refined carbohydrates), increase his fiber intake, and begin a 5 days/week exercise regimen. On follow-up, 6 months later, the patient had lost 20 lbs after adhering to a diet and exercise program and his new lipid profile demonstrated the following: triglycerides 130 mg/dl, HDL 47 mg/dl, and LDL 110 mg/dl.

References

1. Yen CL, Stone SJ, Koliwad S, Harris C, Farese Jr RV. Thematic review series: glycerolipids. DGAT enzymes and triacylglycerol biosynthesis. J Lipid Res. 2008;49:2283–301.
2. Mu H, Hoy CE. The digestion of dietary triacylglycerols. Prog Lipid Res. 2004;43:105–33.
3. Twickler T, Dallinga-Thie GM, Chapman MJ, Cohn JS. Remnant lipoproteins and atherosclerosis. Curr Atheroscler Rep. 2005;7:140–7.
4. Williams KJ. Molecular processes that handle – and mishandle – dietary lipids. J Clin Invest. 2008;118:3247–59.
5. Adiels M, Olofsson SO, Taskinen MR, Boren J. Overproduction of very low-density lipoproteins is the hallmark of the dyslipidemia in the metabolic syndrome. Arterioscler Thromb Vasc Biol. 2008;28:1225–36.
6. Olofsson SO, Stillemark-Billton P, Asp L. Intracellular assembly of VLDL: two major steps in separate cell compartments. Trends Cardiovasc Med. 2000;10:338–45.
7. Santamarina-Fojo S. The familial chylomicronemia syndrome. Endocrinol Metab Clin North Am. 1998;27:551–67. viii.
8. Kontush A, Chapman MJ. Functionally defective high-density lipoprotein: a new therapeutic target at the crossroads of dyslipidemia, inflammation, and atherosclerosis. Pharmacol Rev. 2006;58:342–74.
9. Dallinga-Thie GM, Dullaart RP, van Tol A. Concerted actions of cholesteryl ester transfer protein and phospholipid transfer protein in type 2 diabetes: effects of apolipoproteins. Curr Opin Lipidol. 2007;18:251–7.
10. Harchaoui KE, Visser ME, Kastelein JJ, Stroes ES, Dallinga-Thie GM. Triglycerides and cardiovascular risk. Curr Cardiol Rev. 2009;5:216–22.
11. Executive Summary of the Third Report of the National Cholesterol Education Program (NCEP) Expert Panel on Detection, Evaluation, and Treatment of High Blood Cholesterol in Adults (Adult Treatment Panel III). JAMA 2001;285:2486–97.
12. Assmann G, Brewer Jr HB. Genetic (primary) forms of hypertriglyceridemia. Am J Cardiol. 1991;68:13A–6A.
13. Greenberg BH, Blackwelder WC, Levy RI. Primary type V hyperlipoproteinemia. A descriptive study in 32 families. Ann Intern Med. 1977;87:526–34.

14. Brewer Jr HB, Zech LA, Gregg RE, Schwartz D, Schaefer EJ. NIH conference. Type III hyperlipoproteinemia: diagnosis, molecular defects, pathology, and treatment. Ann Intern Med. 1983;98:623–40.
15. Kushwaha RS, Hazzard WR, Wahl PW, Hoover JJ. Type III hyperlipoproteinemia: diagnosis in whole plasma by apolipoprotein-E immunoassay. Ann Intern Med. 1977;87:509–16.
16. Henneman P, van der Sman-de Beer F, Moghaddam PH, et al. The expression of type III hyperlipoproteinemia: involvement of lipolysis genes. Eur J Hum Genet. 2009;17:620–8.
17. Jialal I, Amess W, Kaur M. Management of hypertriglyceridemia in the diabetic patient. Curr Diab Rep. 2010;10:316–20.
18. Mancini M, Steiner G, Betteridge DJ, Pometta D. Acquired (secondary) forms of hypertriglyceridemia. Am J Cardiol. 1991;68:17A–21A.
19. Walsh BW, Schiff I, Rosner B, Greenberg L, Ravnikar V, Sacks FM. Effects of postmenopausal estrogen replacement on the concentrations and metabolism of plasma lipoproteins. N Engl J Med. 1991;325:1196–204.
20. Glueck CJ, Lang J, Hamer T, Tracy T. Severe hypertriglyceridemia and pancreatitis when estrogen replacement therapy is given to hypertriglyceridemic women. J Lab Clin Med. 1994;123:59–64.
21. Freedman DS, Jacobsen SJ, Barboriak JJ, et al. Body fat distribution and male/female differences in lipids and lipoproteins. Circulation. 1990;81:1498–506.
22. Cullen P, Schulte H, Assmann G. The Munster Heart Study (PROCAM): total mortality in middle-aged men is increased at low total and LDL cholesterol concentrations in smokers but not in nonsmokers. Circulation. 1997;96:2128–36.
23. Bonora E, Targher G, Branzi P, et al. Cardiovascular risk profile in 38-year and 18-year-old men. Contribution of body fat content and regional fat distribution. Int J Obes Relat Metab Disord. 1996;20:28–36.
24. Greenfield MS, Kraemer F, Tobey T, Reaven G. Effect of age on plasma triglyceride concentrations in man. Metabolism. 1980;29:1095–9.
25. WHO cooperative trial on primary prevention of ischaemic heart disease with clofibrate to lower serum cholesterol: final mortality follow-up. Report of the Committee of Principal Investigators. Lancet 1984;2:600–4.
26. Frick MH, Elo O, Haapa K, et al. Helsinki Heart Study: primary-prevention trial with gemfibrozil in middle-aged men with dyslipidemia. Safety of treatment, changes in risk factors, and incidence of coronary heart disease. N Engl J Med. 1987;317:1237–45.
27. Grundy SM. Small LDL, atherogenic dyslipidemia, and the metabolic syndrome. Circulation. 1997;95:1–4.
28. Downs JR, Clearfield M, Weis S, et al. Primary prevention of acute coronary events with lovastatin in men and women with average cholesterol levels: results of AFCAPS/TexCAPS. Air Force/Texas Coronary Atherosclerosis Prevention Study. JAMA. 1998;279:1615–22.
29. Mazzone T, Chait A, Plutzky J. Cardiovascular disease risk in type 2 diabetes mellitus: insights from mechanistic studies. Lancet. 2008;371:1800–9.
30. Kreisberg RA. Diabetic dyslipidemia. Am J Cardiol. 1998;82:67U–73U. discussion 85U–6U.
31. Sorrentino MJ. Early intervention strategies to lower cardiovascular risk in early nephropathy: focus on dyslipidemia. Cardiol Clin. 2010;28:529–39.
32. Shearer GC, Stevenson FT, Atkinson DN, Jones H, Staprans I, Kaysen GA. Hypoalbuminemia and proteinuria contribute separately to reduced lipoprotein catabolism in the nephrotic syndrome. Kidney Int. 2001;59:179–89.
33. Vaziri ND. Dyslipidemia of chronic renal failure: the nature, mechanisms, and potential consequences. Am J Physiol Renal Physiol. 2006;290:F262–72.
34. Parks EJ, Hellerstein MK. Carbohydrate-induced hypertriacylglycerolemia: historical perspective and review of biological mechanisms. Am J Clin Nutr. 2000;71:412–33.
35. Teff KL, Elliott SS, Tschop M, et al. Dietary fructose reduces circulating insulin and leptin, attenuates postprandial suppression of ghrelin, and increases triglycerides in women. J Clin Endocrinol Metab. 2004;89:2963–72.

36. Teff KL, Grudziak J, Townsend RR, et al. Endocrine and metabolic effects of consuming fructose- and glucose-sweetened beverages with meals in obese men and women: influence of insulin resistance on plasma triglyceride responses. J Clin Endocrinol Metab. 2009;94:1562–9.
37. Parks EJ. Changes in fat synthesis influenced by dietary macronutrient content. Proc Nutr Soc. 2002;61:281–6.
38. Manninen V, Tenkanen L, Koskinen P, et al. Joint effects of serum triglyceride and LDL cholesterol and HDL cholesterol concentrations on coronary heart disease risk in the Helsinki Heart Study. Implications for treatment. Circulation. 1992;85:37–45.
39. Criqui MH, Heiss G, Cohn R, et al. Plasma triglyceride level and mortality from coronary heart disease. N Engl J Med. 1993;328:1220–5.
40. Assmann G, Schulte H. Relation of high-density lipoprotein cholesterol and triglycerides to incidence of atherosclerotic coronary artery disease (the PROCAM experience). Prospective Cardiovascular Munster study. Am J Cardiol. 1992;70:733–7.
41. Bitzur R, Cohen H, Kamari Y, Shaish A, Harats D. Triglycerides and HDL cholesterol: stars or second leads in diabetes? Diabetes Care. 2009;32 Suppl 2:S373–7.
42. Hokanson JE, Austin MA. Plasma triglyceride level is a risk factor for cardiovascular disease independent of high-density lipoprotein cholesterol level: a meta-analysis of population-based prospective studies. J Cardiovasc Risk. 1996;3:213–9.
43. Sarwar N, Danesh J, Eiriksdottir G, et al. Triglycerides and the risk of coronary heart disease: 10,158 incident cases among 262,525 participants in 29 Western prospective studies. Circulation. 2007;115:450–8.
44. von Eynatten M, Hamann A, Twardella D, Nawroth PP, Brenner H, Rothenbacher D. Atherogenic dyslipidaemia but not total- and high-molecular weight adiponectin are associated with the prognostic outcome in patients with coronary heart disease. Eur Heart J. 2008;29:1307–15.
45. Bansal S, Buring JE, Rifai N, Mora S, Sacks FM, Ridker PM. Fasting compared with nonfasting triglycerides and risk of cardiovascular events in women. JAMA. 2007;298:309–16.
46. Nordestgaard BG, Benn M, Schnohr P, Tybjaerg-Hansen A. Nonfasting triglycerides and risk of myocardial infarction, ischemic heart disease, and death in men and women. JAMA. 2007;298:299–308.
47. Mora S, Rifai N, Buring JE, Ridker PM. Fasting compared with nonfasting lipids and apolipoproteins for predicting incident cardiovascular events. Circulation. 2008;118:993–1001.
48. Castelli WP. Epidemiology of triglycerides: a view from Framingham. Am J Cardiol. 1992;70:3H–9H.
49. Avins AL, Neuhaus JM. Do triglycerides provide meaningful information about heart disease risk? Arch Intern Med. 2000;160:1937–44.
50. Jeppesen J, Hein HO, Suadicani P, Gyntelberg F. Triglyceride concentration and ischemic heart disease: an eight-year follow-up in the Copenhagen Male Study. Circulation. 1998;97:1029–36.
51. Burchfiel CM, Laws A, Benfante R, et al. Combined effects of HDL cholesterol, triglyceride, and total cholesterol concentrations on 18-year risk of atherosclerotic disease. Circulation. 1995;92:1430–6.
52. Pedersen TR, Olsson AG, Faergeman O, et al. Lipoprotein changes and reduction in the incidence of major coronary heart disease events in the Scandinavian Simvastatin Survival Study (4S). Circulation. 1998;97:1453–60.
53. Haim M, Benderly M, Brunner D, et al. Elevated serum triglyceride levels and long-term mortality in patients with coronary heart disease: the Bezafibrate Infarction Prevention (BIP) Registry. Circulation. 1999;100:475–82.
54. Jeppesen J, Hein HO, Suadicani P, Gyntelberg F. High triglycerides/low high-density lipoprotein cholesterol, ischemic electrocardiogram changes, and risk of ischemic heart disease. Am Heart J. 2003;145:103–8.
55. Tanne D, Koren-Morag N, Graff E, Goldbourt U. Blood lipids and first-ever ischemic stroke/transient ischemic attack in the Bezafibrate Infarction Prevention (BIP) Registry: high triglycerides constitute an independent risk factor. Circulation. 2001;104:2892–7.

56. St-Pierre AC, Cantin B, Dagenais GR, et al. Low-density lipoprotein subfractions and the long-term risk of ischemic heart disease in men: 13-year follow-up data from the Quebec Cardiovascular Study. Arterioscler Thromb Vasc Biol. 2005;25:553–9.
57. Ginsberg HN, Bonds DE, Lovato LC, et al. Evolution of the lipid trial protocol of the Action to Control Cardiovascular Risk in Diabetes (ACCORD) trial. Am J Cardiol. 2007;99:56i–67i.
58. Kastelein JJ, van der Steeg WA, Holme I, et al. Lipids, apolipoproteins, and their ratios in relation to cardiovascular events with statin treatment. Circulation. 2008;117:3002–9.
59. Austin MA, King MC, Vranizan KM, Krauss RM. Atherogenic lipoprotein phenotype. A proposed genetic marker for coronary heart disease risk. Circulation. 1990;82:495–506.
60. Grundy SM. Hypertriglyceridemia, insulin resistance, and the metabolic syndrome. Am J Cardiol. 1999;83:25F–9F.
61. Zino S, Skeaff M, Williams S, Mann J. Randomised controlled trial of effect of fruit and vegetable consumption on plasma concentrations of lipids and antioxidants. BMJ. 1997;314:1787–91.
62. Mittendorfer B, Sidossis LS. Mechanism for the increase in plasma triacylglycerol concentrations after consumption of short-term, high-carbohydrate diets. Am J Clin Nutr. 2001;73:892–9.
63. Lin CC, Li TC, Lai MM. Efficacy and safety of *Monascus purpureus* Went rice in subjects with hyperlipidemia. Eur J Endocrinol. 2005;153:679–86.
64. Grandjean PW, Crouse SF, O'Brien BC, Rohack JJ, Brown JA. The effects of menopausal status and exercise training on serum lipids and the activities of intravascular enzymes related to lipid transport. Metabolism. 1998;47:377–83.
65. Kokkinos PF, Holland JC, Narayan P, Colleran JA, Dotson CO, Papademetriou V. Miles run per week and high-density lipoprotein cholesterol levels in healthy, middle-aged men. A dose-response relationship. Arch Intern Med. 1995;155:415–20.
66. Thompson PD, Yurgalevitch SM, Flynn MM, et al. Effect of prolonged exercise training without weight loss on high-density lipoprotein metabolism in overweight men. Metabolism. 1997;46:217–23.
67. Wood PD, Haskell WL, Blair SN, et al. Increased exercise level and plasma lipoprotein concentrations: a one-year, randomized, controlled study in sedentary, middle-aged men. Metabolism. 1983;32:31–9.
68. Bucher HC, Hengstler P, Schindler C, Meier G. N-3 polyunsaturated fatty acids in coronary heart disease: a meta-analysis of randomized controlled trials. Am J Med. 2002;112:298–304.
69. Luo J, Rizkalla SW, Vidal H, et al. Moderate intake of n-3 fatty acids for 2 months has no detrimental effect on glucose metabolism and could ameliorate the lipid profile in type 2 diabetic men. Results of a controlled study. Diabetes Care. 1998;21:717–24.
70. Harris WS, Connor WE, Illingworth DR, Rothrock DW, Foster DM. Effects of fish oil on VLDL triglyceride kinetics in humans. J Lipid Res. 1990;31:1549–58.
71. Nestel PJ, Connor WE, Reardon MF, Connor S, Wong S, Boston R. Suppression by diets rich in fish oil of very low density lipoprotein production in man. J Clin Invest. 1984;74:82–9.
72. De Caterina R, Madonna R, Massaro M. Effects of omega-3 fatty acids on cytokines and adhesion molecules. Curr Atheroscler Rep. 2004;6:485–91.
73. Massaro M, Scoditti E, Carluccio MA, Campana MC, De Caterina R. Omega-3 fatty acids, inflammation and angiogenesis: basic mechanisms behind the cardioprotective effects of fish and fish oils. Cell Mol Biol (Noisy-le-grand). 2010;56:59–82.
74. Lichtenstein AH, Appel LJ, Brands M, et al. Diet and lifestyle recommendations revision 2006: a scientific statement from the American Heart Association Nutrition Committee. Circulation. 2006;114:82–96.
75. Crouse 3rd JR. New developments in the use of niacin for treatment of hyperlipidemia: new considerations in the use of an old drug. Coron Artery Dis. 1996;7:321–6.
76. Canner PL, Berge KG, Wenger NK, et al. Fifteen year mortality in Coronary Drug Project patients: long-term benefit with niacin. J Am Coll Cardiol. 1986;8:1245–55.

77. Kersten S, Desvergne B, Wahli W. Roles of PPARs in health and disease. Nature. 2000;405:421–4.
78. Rosenson RS, Wolff DA, Huskin AL, Helenowski IB, Rademaker AW. Fenofibrate therapy ameliorates fasting and postprandial lipoproteinemia, oxidative stress, and the inflammatory response in subjects with hypertriglyceridemia and the metabolic syndrome. Diabetes Care. 2007;30:1945–51.
79. Rubins HB, Robins SJ, Collins D, et al. Gemfibrozil for the secondary prevention of coronary heart disease in men with low levels of high-density lipoprotein cholesterol. Veterans Affairs High-Density Lipoprotein Cholesterol Intervention Trial Study Group. N Engl J Med. 1999;341:410–8.
80. Keech A, Simes RJ, Barter P, et al. Effects of long-term fenofibrate therapy on cardiovascular events in 9795 people with type 2 diabetes mellitus (the FIELD study): randomised controlled trial. Lancet. 2005;366:1849–61.
81. Ballantyne CM, Bertolami M, Hernandez Garcia HR, et al. Achieving LDL-C, non-HDL-C, and apolipoprotein B target levels in high-risk patients: Measuring Effective Reductions in Cholesterol Using Rosuvastatin therapY (MERCURY) II. Am Heart J. 2006;151:975.e1–9.
82. Stalenhoef AF, Ballantyne CM, Sarti C, et al. A comparative study with rosuvastatin in subjects with metabolic syndrome: results of the COMETS study. Eur Heart J. 2005;26:2664–72.
83. Bakker-Arkema RG, Davidson MH, Goldstein RJ, et al. Efficacy and safety of a new HMG-CoA reductase inhibitor, atorvastatin, in patients with hypertriglyceridemia. JAMA. 1996;275:128–33.
84. Hunninghake DB, Stein EA, Bays HE, et al. Rosuvastatin improves the atherogenic and atheroprotective lipid profiles in patients with hypertriglyceridemia. Coron Artery Dis. 2004;15:115–23.
85. Ginsberg HN, Elam MB, Lovato LC, et al. Effects of combination lipid therapy in type 2 diabetes mellitus. N Engl J Med. 2010;362:1563–74.

Chapter 9
Isolated Low HDL

Robert S. Rosenson

Keywords High-density lipoprotein • Lipoprotein subclasses • Cardiovascular risk • Hypoalphalipoproteinemia

Case Report

A 24-year-old male graduate student was referred for evaluation and management of low high-density lipoprotein cholesterol (HDL-C). His father had a myocardial infarction at an age of 49 years and a second myocardial infarction 1 month after the first event. His father has a low HDL-C level that was been consistently less than 35 mg/dL. The paternal grandfather had four myocardial infarctions with the first event occurring in his late 40-year range.

The past medical and surgical history is noncontributory. He does not take any medications. He eats what is convenient and nearly always neglects breakfast. At lunch, he consumes sandwiches on wheat bread with turkey, and for dinner he eats a salad with a main course that includes poultry or beef. He consumes 2–4 cans of beer weekly. His exercise is sporadic, and at a maximum he jogs 1.5–2 miles in 15–20 min one or two times weekly.

He is 5 ft 8 in. and he weighs 188 lbs. His body mass index is 29.31 kg/m^2. His blood pressure is 104/70 mmHg and pulse is 70 per minute and regular. The physical examination was normal with no xanthelasmas, corneal arcus, evidence of cataract formation, or cardiac murmers.

The lipid profile obtained by his primary care physician revealed a total cholesterol of 196 mg/dL, low-density lipoprotein cholesterol (LDL-C) of 136 mg/dL,

R.S. Rosenson (✉)
Mount Sinai School of Medicine, New York, NY 10029-6324, USA
e-mail: robert.rosenson@mssm.edu

M.J. Sorrentino (ed.), *Hyperlipidemia in Primary Care: A Practical Guide to Risk Reduction*, Current Clinical Practice, DOI 10.1007/978-1-60327-502-6_9,

triglycerides of 138 mg/dL, and HDL-C of 22 mg/dL (Table 9.1) Fasting blood glucose was 84 mg/dL and serum creatinine was 0.8 mg/dL. TSH was normal.

Assessment

Primary Hypoalphalipoproteinemia

The HDL-C levels are below the tenth percentile (less than tenth percentile) for a man at this age (Table 9.2). He does not have elevated levels of triglycerides that would characterize the phenotype hypertriglyceridemia with hypoalphalipoproteinemia or elevated LDL-C levels that would suggest familial combined hyperlipidemia. In the interim, the patient has been counseled on a low-fat, low-cholesterol, and hypocaloric diet. He has been asked to increase his exercise to a minimum of three times per week with a goal of exercising 3 h weekly.

At 3-month follow-up, he has made minimal changes in his lifestyle. He has reduced his visits to fast food restaurants from every week to every other week. He has recently purchased a bicycle and plans to use it for transportation. Despite these efforts, he reports a recent 8 pound weight gain that occurred around his final examinations. A fasting NMR lipoprofile was obtained (Table 9.1). The apolipoprotein B concentration was elevated at 114 mg/dL.

He returns to clinic after 6 months from the initial visit and he has reported for the past 3 months he has rode his bicycle to work on a daily basis. Further, he has modified his diet by making sandwiches at home and taking them to work and this has reduced his intake of fast foods and restaurant dining. At this visit, his weight is 202 lbs. The lipoprotein profile is illustrated in Table 9.1.

He now manifests hypertriglyceridemia with hypoalphalipoproteinemia. With continued weight gain, the fasting triglycerides have increased (≥200 mg/dL). The LDL particle concentration is elevated despite the near-optimal LDL-C level. This case highlights HDL–LDL interactions that are commonly seen in patients with low HDL-C levels. At this time, it remains unresolved whether lowering excess LDL particles or increasing reduced HDL particles will produce optimal cardiovascular event reduction. As discussed later, combined therapy directed at lowering excess LDL particles and increasing reduced HDL particles has been accompanied by reduced atherosclerosis progression and cardiovascular event reduction.

Treatment Plan

He was placed on simvastatin 40 mg nightly and extended-release niacin 500 mg with food. After 4 weeks, he was asked to increase the niacin dosage to 1,000 mg daily.

Table 9.1 Fasting lipid and lipoprotein subclasses

	Lipids				Lipoproteins					
	LDL-C (mg/dL)	HDL-C (mg/dL)	Triglycerides (mg/dL)	Total cholesterol (mg/dL)	LDL-P (nmol/L)	Small LDL-P (nmol/L)	Large HDL-P (μmol/L)	Large VLDL-P (nmol/L)	LDL-P size (nm)	Weight (lbs)
Referral visit	136	33	138	196	–	–	–	–	–	185
Initial visit	112	32	260	196	1,915	1,804	2.4	5.9	19.3	188
3-Month	129	31	220	204	1,910	1,746	3.6	2.3	19.3	196
6-Month	137	30	243	216	2,186	2,106	2.1	4.3	19.1	202

LDL-P: <1,000 nmol/L optimal, 1,000–1,299 nmol/L near or above optimal, 1,300–1,599 nmol/L borderline-high, 1,600–2,000 nmol/L high, >2,000 nmol/L very high; small LDL-P: <600 nmol/L low, 600–849 nmol/L moderate, 850–1,200 nmol/L borderline-high, >1,200 nmol/L high; large HDL-P: >9.0 μmol/L low risk, 4.0–9.0 μmol/L intermediate, <4.0 μmol/L high risk; large VLDL-P: <0.5 nmol/L low risk, 0.5–5.0 nmol/L intermediate, >5.0 nmol/L high risk; LDL-P size: large (pattern A) 23.0–20.6 nm, small (pattern B) 20.5–18.0 nm

Table 9.2 Percentile range for lipid levels

	Age	HDL-C (90th percentile)	Total cholesterol (90th percentile)	LDL-C (90th percentile)	Triglycerides (90th percentile)
White men	20–34	34	236	165	199
	35–44	30	258	176	241
	45–54	31	268	187	228
	55–64	31	274	194	280
	65–74	31	270	185	256
	≥75	32	257	186	219
White women	20–34	38	229	155	164
	35–44	37	242	155	209
	45–54	38	279	182	212
	55–64	37	291	189	213
	65–74	37	290	192	253
	≥75	39	287	197	248
Non-Hispanic white men		30	260	179	248
Non-Hispanic white women		37	271	176	228
Mexican-American men		33	257	172	266
Mexican-American women		37	258	166	240
Non-Hispanic black men		35	252	186	171
Non-Hispanic black women		40	262	174	162

Reference values in the USA for the 10th percentile for HDL-C and the 19th percentile for total and LDL-C and triglycerides. Values are shown according to age for white men and women, and mean values are given for different groups. (Units are mg/dL.) Data from: National Health and Nutrition Examination Survey (NHANES) III

Plasma HDL-C Level: An Inverse Risk Predictor for Cardiovascular Disease

Low HDL-C can confer additional risk for cardiovascular disease (CVD) irrespective of total cholesterol levels [1]. Epidemiologic studies have demonstrated that the level of HDL-C is an independent risk factor for coronary heart disease (CHD) with a continuous, inverse relationship to CHD [2, 3]. In a 12-year follow-up of the Framingham study, individuals with high HDL-C (80th percentile) were at 50% lower risk of CHD than those with low HDL-C (20th percentile) [4]. Similarly, Prospective Cardiovascular Münster (PROCAM) study participants with HDL-C≥35 mg/dL were found to have four times less risk of CHD at 6-year follow-up than patients with HDL-C<35 mg/dL [3]. An independent reduction in CHD risk of 2–3% has been estimated for every 1-mg/dL increase in HDL-C [5, 6].

Among Framingham participants, low HDL-C was significantly associated with increased incidence of myocardial infarction (MI). This association persisted even in subjects with the lowest concentrations of total cholesterol (≤192 mg/dL in men and ≤211 mg/dL in women) [7]. In a 21-year study of 8,000 men, low HDL-C (<35 mg/dL) was also shown to carry an excess risk of CHD death regardless of total cholesterol level [8].

Importantly, baseline HDL-C level has been shown in several statin trials to predict CVD risk [9]. For example, in the Cholesterol and Recurrent Events (CARE) trial, which enrolled 4,159 patients with CHD and average cholesterol levels, the proportion of pravastatin-treated patients who experienced a cardiovascular (CV) event was significantly higher among those with pretreatment HDL-C levels ≤37 mg/dL compared with those with pretreatment HDL-C levels >37 mg/dL (23% vs. 19%, respectively) [10]. Importantly, baseline HDL-C level has been shown in several statin trials to predict CVD risk [9]. In the Treating to New Targets (TNT) trial, 9,770 stable CHD patients are included with mean LDL-C levels <70 mg/dL. Low HDL-C levels in that subgroup remained a significant predictor of major cardiovascular events [11]. The cardiovascular event rate was 40% lower for patients in the highest quintile (>55 mg/dL) vs. the lowest quintile (<38 mg/dL) of HDL-C.

Low HDL-C Levels: A Marker of Atherogenic Dyslipoproteinemia?

Low HDL-C is common among several patient populations with an increased risk of CVD, such as individuals with type 2 diabetes or metabolic syndrome [12, 13]. In these individuals, low HDL-C is frequently found in association with elevated triglycerides and a preponderance of small, dense LDL particles [14]. This lipid profile is termed the atherogenic dyslipidemia. Furthermore, evidence suggests that the CHD risk associated with low HDL-C may, in part, reflect a previously unrecognized shift in LDL size from large LDL to small LDL particles. Data from the Framingham Offspring study showed that in individuals with low HDL-C (<40 mg/dL), there was a substantial increase in the level of small LDL particles [14] (Fig. 9.1).

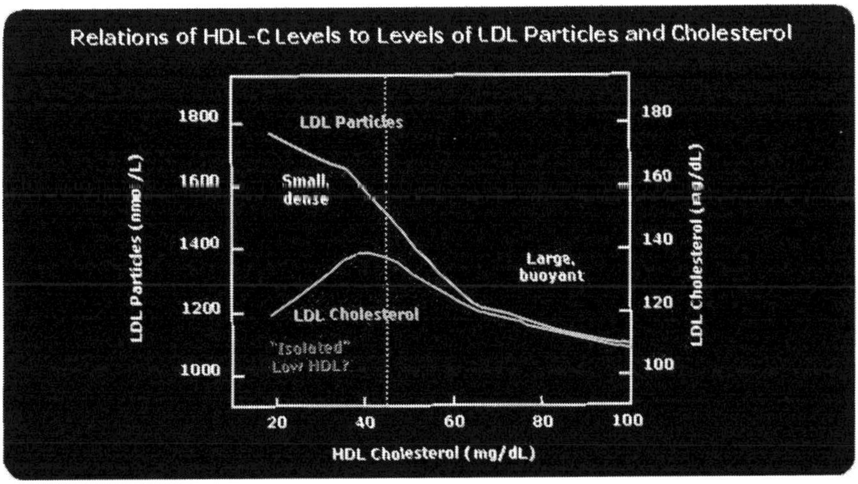

Fig. 9.1 Framingham offspring study: clinical implications of the disconnect between LDL-C and LDL particles in patients with low HDL-C [14]

Further, the dyslipidemic profile in patients with type 2 diabetes or metabolic syndrome may be characterized by the formation of small, dense HDL with altered physicochemical properties, such as abnormal composition (triglyceride-rich) and dysfunctional antiatherogenic activity (diminished antioxidative activity) [15]. Thus, while HDL-C level is a strong, independent, and inverse predictor of CVD, other factors that are closely associated with low HDL-C levels may also contribute to CVD risk.

HDL-C and Existing Guideline Recommendations

The NCEP guidelines recognize elevated LDL-C as the primary target for lipid modification [6]. Recommended targets reflect clear evidence from clinical trials that large reductions in LDL-C are associated with significant decreases in CV events. Nonetheless, the guidelines do recognize the importance of low HDL-C as a CHD risk factor and state that:

- In addition to intensive LDL-C lowering, risk assessment should cover high triglyceride and low HDL-C levels (low HDL-C being defined as <40 mg/dL).
- Low HDL-C modifies the goal for LDL-C lowering and should be used as a risk factor to estimate the 10-year CHD risk.
- HDL-C is a secondary therapeutic target in patients with isolated low HDL-C (where triglycerides are ≥200 mg/dL) or as a component of the metabolic syndrome.

However, NCEP guidelines do not stipulate a target level for HDL-C [6]. This is likely due to the absence of pharmacotherapies that can robustly raise HDL-C and a consequent lack of direct evidence from clinical outcomes trials. In contrast, other influential guidelines do suggest target levels for HDL-C. The American Diabetes Association recommends an optimal target of 40 mg/dL for men and 50 mg/dL for women with type 2 diabetes [2]. Similarly, an HDL-C target of ≥40 mg/dL is recommended by the Expert Group on HDL-C as a goal for patients with CVD and those without clinical CVD at high risk (e.g., patients with type 2 diabetes or metabolic syndrome) [16]. As has been the case with LDL-C targets, HDL-C targets will undoubtedly be reassessed as more trial data emerges. A treatment algorithm for low HDL disorders is outlined in Fig. 9.2.

What Are the Current Therapeutic Options for Raising HDL-C Levels?

It is important to consider secondary disorders that affect HDL metabolism as treating those conditions that may have clinically meaningful impact on HDL-C levels. Low HDL-C can occur as a consequence of acute infections or other inflammatory

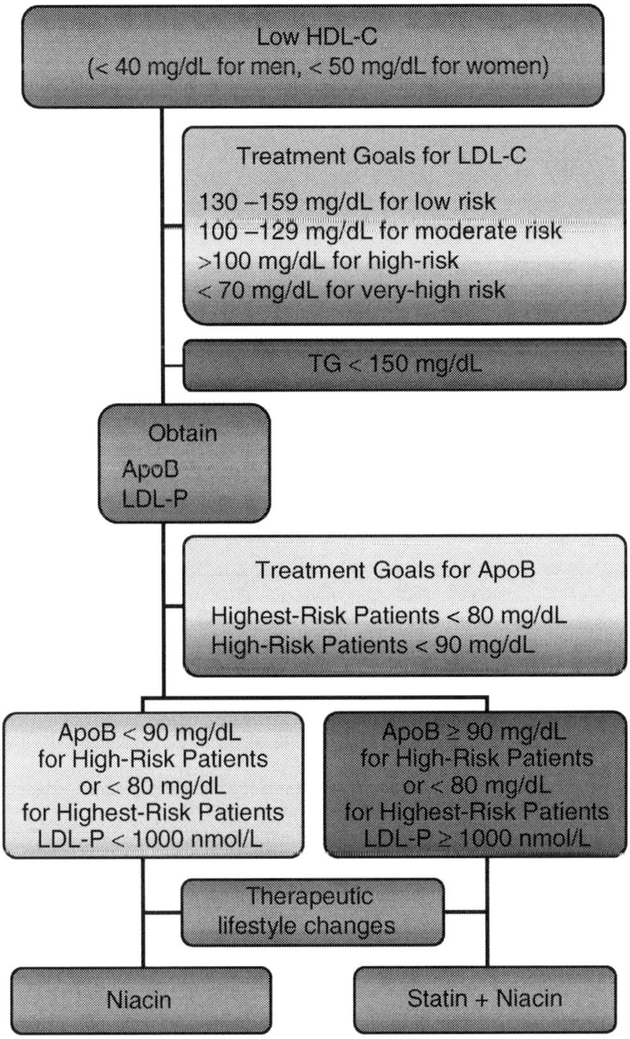

Fig. 9.2 Treatment algorithm for low HDL-C disorders. *HDL-C* high-density lipoprotein cholesterol, *LDL-C* low-density lipoprotein cholesterol, *TG* triglycerides, *ApoB* apolipoprotein B, *LDL-P* low-density lipoprotein particles

conditions or by artificially low HDL-C measures in patients with gammopathies. Low serum HDL-C concentration can be induced by pharmacological therapies such as beta blockers, benzodiazepines, and anabolic steroids.

Therapeutic lifestyle changes are the cornerstone for HDL-C raising strategies. Exercise, weight loss (in overweight subjects), smoking cessation, and substitution of monounsaturated for saturated fatty acids all can raise HDL-C (Table 9.3). Besides therapeutic lifestyle changes, including exercise, smoking cessation, and improvements in diet [17], a number of pharmacologic interventions are available for improving the HDL-C profile.

Table 9.3 Efficacy of lifestyle strategies for increasing HDL-C [9]

Strategy	Increase in HDL-C (%)
Weight reduction	5–20
Physical activity	5–30
Smoking cessation	5
Moderate alcohol consumption	8
Mediterranean-style diet vs. 30% fat diet[a]	2

[a]Compared with an average American diet

Table 9.4 Summary data of nicotinic acid (niacin) effects on HDL-C [20]

HDL-C	No. of subjects	Net change (mg/dL)	Percent change
ER-Niacin[a]	248	+9.2	+21.9
IR-Niacin[b]	814	+9.2	+22.5
SR-Niacin[c]	536	+6.0	+12.7
Pooled	2,490	+6.7	+15.7

[a]Extended release
[b]Immediate release
[c]Slow release

Niacin

Niacin (nicotinic acid) is the most effective HDL-C-raising drug currently available, and it also favorably affects LDL-C, LDL particle size, and triglyceride levels. While several mechanisms have been proposed for this activity, it is the binding of niacin to the G-protein-coupled receptor HM74 and the subsequent suppression of triacylglycerol lipolysis in adipose tissue that is the most well understood [18].

An extended-release form of niacin 3,000 mg has been shown to increase HDL-C by 30% in patients with primary hyperlipidemia [19], although a meta-analysis of randomized trials using various niacin preparations indicates the increase of HDL between 7 and 23% (Table 9.4) [20]. Regarding the effect of niacin on CVD end points, the most robust data come from the Coronary Drug Project. At 15-year follow-up, this study showed that niacin 3,000 mg daily significantly reduced all-cause mortality by 11% ($p<0.001$) vs. placebo in 8,341 men with previous MI [21].

Niacin is, however, associated with tolerability problems – side effects include skin flushing and pruritus can occur in up to 80% of patients, and liver toxicity and disruption of glucose control [20]. The extended-release formulation has improved tolerance, producing significantly less flushing than immediate-release of niacin [22].

Fibrates

Fibrates (peroxisome proliferator-activated receptor-alpha agonists) stimulate the formation of HDL in the serum by increasing the expression of proteins involved in HDL metabolism (e.g., apolipoproteins A-I and A-II, ABCA1, and SR-B1) [23]. Fibrates can increase HDL-C by up to 20%, as well as substantially reduce triglyceride levels (Table 9.5) [20]. Beneficial changes in the size and distribution of HDL and LDL subclasses are also produced [24].

Table 9.5 Summary data of fibrate effects on HDL-C [20]

HDL-C	No. of subjects	Net change (mg/dL)	Percent change
Bezafibrate	5,161	+4.3	+11.0
Ciprofibrate	91	+3.9	+10.0
Clofibrate	278	−0.1	−0.2
Fenofibrate	1,457	+4.5	+10.2
Gemfibrozil	7,461	+4.4	+10.7
Pooled	14,448	+4.1	+10.0

The benefits of fibrates in patients with low HDL-C (<40 mg/dL) are best demonstrated by the VA-HIT trial. In 2,531 patients with a history of CHD, average LDL-C, and low HDL-C, gemfibrozil 1,200 mg daily raised HDL-C by 6% after 1 year and, over 5 years, resulting in significant reductions in the primary end point of CHD death or nonfatal MI (22% reduction; $p=0.006$) [25]. Subsequent analysis revealed a weak correlation between increased HDL-C and CHD event reduction, whereas changes in LDL-C or triglyceride levels were unrelated to residual risk [26]. More meaningful insights into residual CHD risk were provided by HDL and LDL lipoprotein measurements [27]. On therapy, high levels of HDL particles were associated with a 0.71 (per standard deviation change) reduced risk of CHD events and high levels of LDL particles were associated with a 1.28 (per standard deviation change) increased risk of CHD events. This analysis provides strong support for HDL–LDL interactions commonly seen in patients with low HDL-C levels and disorders of insulin resistance. In the BIP study, which included 3,090 patients with prior MI or stable angina and low HDL-C levels [28], bezafibrate 400 mg daily increased HDL-C by 18% and reduced triglycerides by 21%, but produced no significant reduction in the primary end point (nonfatal or fatal MI, or sudden death). However, there was a reduction in this end point over 6 years in individuals with high triglycerides (≥200 mg/dL) (39.5%; $p=0.02$) [28]. In the Helsinki Heart study of 4,081 men with no CHD, gemfibrozil 1,200 mg/day produced a significant 34% reduction in the incidence of CHD events, which was strongly associated with elevated HDL-C [29]. More recently, the FIELD study assessed the effect of fenofibrate on CHD event rates in 9,795 diabetic patients [30]. Surprisingly, fenofibrate 200 mg daily did not significantly reduce the risk of the primary outcome of coronary events compared with placebo (risk reduction, 11%; $p=0.16$). Possible explanations for this finding include selection of diabetic patients in whom 63% had normal lipid levels, the small increase in HDL-C in the treatment group (1.2% relative to baseline), and/or the greater use of statins in the placebo group [31]. Total CV events, a secondary outcome measure, were significantly reduced (risk reduction, 11%; $p=0.035$).

Statins

In addition to their significant impact on LDL-C, statins produce small increases in HDL-C (5–15%) [9]. The underlying mechanism is not well understood, but may involve a reduction in CETP activity. Although the effect of these small changes in

HDL-C on reducing CHD risk is difficult to determine, given the larger simultaneous decreases in LDL-C, evidence suggests that the reduction in morbidity seen in at least some statin trials can be partly attributed to changes in HDL-C. For example, among patients with CHD and hypercholesterolemia who participated in the 4S trial [32], while decreases in major coronary events with simvastatin 20–40 mg/day were mostly due to reductions in LDL-C, increases in HDL-C also contributed to clinical outcome, with a 0.8% reduction in major coronary events for every 1% increase in HDL-C, independent of LDL-C [33]. Furthermore, statins may be especially beneficial in individuals with low HDL-C at baseline. In the AFCAPS/TexCAPS study, lovastatin 20–40 mg/day increased HDL-C by 6% after 1 year in patients with an average risk for CHD. Individuals whose baseline HDL-C was <40 mg/dL experienced a threefold reduction (45–15%) in risk for first-time, CHD-related events after 5.2 years compared with those with HDL-C ≥40 mg/dL [34]. In AFCAPS/TexCAPS study, CVD risk was linearly related to apoB levels [34]. More recently, a post hoc analysis of four prospective studies that used intravascular ultrasound (IVUS) to determine changes in atherosclerotic progression in 1,455 statin-treated patients with angiographic coronary disease showed that a ≥5% reduction in atheroma volume was observed in those patients in whom a 7% increase in HDL-C was accompanied by a reduction in LDL-C to <87.5 mg/dL [35]. Despite these observations, no significant difference was found with regard to clinical events.

Combination of Lipid Altering Therapies

Combining therapies may be the most effective strategy for reducing CV risk in patients with multiple lipid disorders. Niacin may be a particularly effective adjunct to other lipid therapies. In HATS, a study of 160 patients with CHD, the effects of combination therapy on coronary stenosis was measured by quantitative coronary angiography and CV events [36]. Treatment with simvastatin plus niacin produced significant changes in LDL-C and HDL-C levels compared with baseline measurements after 3 years (–42% and +26%, respectively; $p<0.001$). Although there was regression of coronary stenosis with combination therapy, as well as a reduction in CV events (24% with placebo vs. 3% with simvastatin/niacin; $p=0.04$ vs. placebo), these results should not be over-interpreted due to the placebo-controlled nature of this study. ARBITER 2 also evaluated the benefits of extended-release niacin (1,000 mg daily) in 167 patients with known CHD and low HDL-C on a background of statin treatment. After 1 year of treatment, HDL-C levels were elevated by 21% and atherosclerotic progression was reduced in the niacin/statin group compared with placebo [37]. AIM-HIGH (NCT00120289) is an ongoing randomized, double-blind clinical trial designed to determine whether extended-release niacin plus simvastatin is more effective than simvastatin alone in reducing the first major CV event in 3,300 patients with two components of the atherogenic dyslipidemia (HDL-C ≤ 40 mg/dL and triglycerides ≥ 150 mg/dL).

Statin–fibrate combinations are also effective at modifying adverse lipid profiles and may reduce CV risk more than monotherapy. Rosuvastatin/Fenofibric

(5, 10 or 20 mg) and (135 mg) resulted in a higher proportion of patients achieving optimal levels of HDL-C, TG, non-HDL-C, and apoB than corresponding dose of rosuvastatin monotherapies administered to 120 patients with type 2 diabetes raised HDL-C by 22% and lowered LDL-C by 46% ($p<0.0001$), which was significantly better than individual monotherapies [38]. Despite the impact on the overall lipid profile, convincing data on the effect of this combined treatment on CV outcomes is lacking. The results from the Action to Control Cardiovascular Risk in Diabetes (ACCORD) study with the combination of simvastatin plus fenofibrate in comparison to simvastatin alone showed no reduction in the primary end point with combination therapy [39].

Thiazolidinediones are a class of drugs used primarily to lower blood sugar levels by improving insulin resistance. These agents can increase HDL-C levels, but may also change the distribution of small LDL particles to larger cholesterol-enriched LDL particles, thus modestly increasing LDL-C levels [40]. Studies suggest that different agents in this drug class have divergent lipid effects. For example, in a study of 100 patients with type 2 diabetes previously receiving troglitazone, switching to pioglitazone was associated with a decrease in triglyceride levels, while changing to rosiglitazone was associated with an increase [41]. Although levels of HDL-C increased in both groups, pioglitazone improved HDL-C to a greater extent than rosiglitazone in patients with HDL-C <35 mg/dL at baseline.

Summary

Low HDL-C currently represents one of the strongest independent predictors of CHD risk. Targeting HDL-C is a promising strategy for combating CVD, and one that may help address the residual CVD risk in statin treated patients. In particular, pharmacologic elevation of HDL-C may also be associated with additional beneficial effects, such as a reduction in overall LDL particle number. This results from the redistribution of highly atherogenic, cholesterol-depleted small, dense LDL to larger, less atherogenic, cholesterol-enriched LDL particles that improves LDL particle–LDL receptor interaction and facilitates LDL clearance. However, there remains a lack of trial data confirming the clinical benefit of independently raising HDL-C to protective levels, particularly in patients with isolated low HDL-C levels.

References

1. Rosenson RS. Low HDL-c: a secondary target of dyslipidemia therapy. Am J Med. 2005;118(10):1067–77.
2. Gordon T, Castelli WP, Hjortland MC, Kannel WB, Dawber TR. High density lipoprotein as a protective factor against coronary heart disease. The Framingham Study. Am J Med. 1977;62:707–14.
3. Assmann G, Schulte H, von Eckardstein A, Huang Y. High-density lipoprotein cholesterol as a predictor of coronary heart disease risk. The PROCAM experience and pathophysiological implications for reverse cholesterol transport. Atherosclerosis. 1996;124:S11–20.

4. Castelli WP, Garrison RJ, Wilson PW, Abbott RD, Kalousdin S, Kannel WB. Incidence of coronary heart disease and lipoprotein cholesterol levels. The Framingham Study. JAMA. 1986;256:2835–8.
5. Gordon DJ, Probstfield JL, Garrison RJ, Neaton JD, Castelli WP, Knoke JD, et al. High-density lipoprotein cholesterol and cardiovascular disease. Four prospective American studies. Circulation. 1989;79:8–15.
6. Executive summary of the third report of the National Cholesterol Education Program (NCEP) expert panel on detection, evaluation, and treatment of high blood cholesterol in adults (Adult Treatment Panel III). JAMA 2001;285:2486–97.
7. Abbott RD, Wilson PW, Kannel WB, Castelli WP. High density lipoprotein cholesterol, total cholesterol screening, and myocardial infarction. The Framingham Study. Arteriosclerosis. 1988;8:207–11.
8. Goldbourt U, Yaari S, Medalie JH. Isolated low HDL cholesterol as a risk factor for coronary heart disease mortality. A 21-year follow-up of 8000 men. Arterioscler Thromb Vasc Biol. 1997;17:107–13.
9. Rosenson RS. Low high-density lipoprotein cholesterol and cardiovascular disease: Risk reduction with statin therapy. Am Heart J. 2006;151:556–63.
10. Sacks FM, Pfeffer MA, Moye LA, Rouleau JL, Rutherford JD, Cole TG, et al. The effect of pravastatin on coronary events after myocardial infarction in patients with average cholesterol levels. Cholesterol and Recurrent Events Trial investigators. N Engl J Med. 1996;335:1001–9.
11. Barter P, Gotto AM, LaRosa JC, Maroni J, Szarek M, Grundy SM, et al. HDL cholesterol, very low levels of LDL cholesterol, and cardiovascular events. N Engl J Med. 2007;357:1301–10.
12. Isomaa B, Almgren P, Tuomi T, Forsen B, Lahti K, Nissen M, et al. Cardiovascular morbidity and mortality associated with the metabolic syndrome. Diabetes Care. 2001;24:683–9.
13. American Diabetes A. Standards of medical care in diabetes–2007. Diabetes Care 2007;30:S4–41.
14. Otvos JD, Jeyarajah EJ, Cromwell WC. Measurement issues related to lipoprotein heterogeneity. Am J Cardiol. 2002;90:22i–9.
15. Nobecourt E, Jacqueminet S, Hansel B, Chantepie S, Grimaldi A, Chapman MJ, et al. Defective antioxidative activity of small dense hdl3 particles in type 2 diabetes: relationship to elevated oxidative stress and hyperglycaemia. Diabetologia. 2005;25:199–211.
16. Sacks FM. Cholesterol EGoH. The role of high-density lipoprotein (HDL) cholesterol in the prevention and treatment of coronary heart disease: expert group recommendations. Am J Cardiol. 2002;90:139–43.
17. Ashen MD, Blumenthal RS. Low HDL cholesterol levels. N Engl J Med. 2005;353:1252–60.
18. Karpe F, Frayn KN. The nicotinic acid receptor – a new mechanism for an old drug. Lancet. 2004;363:1892–4.
19. Goldberg A, Alagona P, Capuzzi DM, Guyton J, Morgan JM, Rodgers J, et al. Multiple-dose efficacy and safety of an extended-release form of niacin in the management of hyperlipidemia. Am J Cardiol. 2000;85:1100–5.
20. Birjmohun RS, Hutten BA, Kastelein JJP, Stroes ESG. Efficacy and safety of high-density lipoprotein cholesterol-increasing compounds: a meta-analysis of randomized controlled trials. J Am Coll Cardiol. 2005;45:185–97.
21. Canner PL, Berge KG, Wenger NK, Stamler J, Friedman L, Prineas RJ, et al. Fifteen year mortality in coronary drug project patients: long-term benefit with niacin. J Am Coll Cardiol. 1986;8:1245–55.
22. Chapman MJ, Assmann G, Fruchart J-C, Shepherd J, Sirtori C. Raising high-density lipoprotein cholesterol with reduction of cardiovascular risk: the role of nicotinic acid – a position paper developed by the European Consensus Panel on HDL-c*. Curr Med Res Opin. 2004;20:1253–68.
23. Fruchart JC, Staels B, Duriez P. The role of fibric acids in atherosclerosis. Curr Atheroscler Rep. 2001;3:83–92.
24. Rosenson RS, Wolff DA, Huskin AL, Helenowski IB, Rademaker AW. Fenofibrate therapy ameliorates fasting and postprandial lipoproteinemia, oxidative stress, and the inflammatory response in subjects with hypertriglyceridemia and the metabolic syndrome. Diabetes Care. 2007;30:1945–51.

25. Rubins HB, Robins SJ, Collins D, Fye CL, Anderson JW, Elam MB, et al. Gemfibrozil for the secondary prevention of coronary heart disease in men with low levels of high-density lipoprotein cholesterol. Veterans Affairs High-Density Lipoprotein Cholesterol Intervention Trial Study Group. N Engl J Med. 1999;341:410–8.
26. Robins SJ, Collins D, Wittes JT, Papademetriou V, Deedwania PC, Schaefer EJ, et al. Relation of gemfibrozil treatment and lipid levels with major coronary events: VA-HIT: a randomized controlled trial. JAMA. 2001;285:1585–91.
27. Otvos JD, Collins D, Freedman DS, Shalaurova I, Schaefer EJ, McNamara JR, et al. Low-density lipoprotein and high-density lipoprotein particle subclasses predict coronary events and are favorably changed by gemfibrozil therapy in the Veterans Affairs High-Density Lipoprotein Intervention Trial. Circulation. 2006;113:1556–63.
28. Secondary prevention by raising HDL cholesterol and reducing triglycerides in patients with coronary artery disease: The bezafibrate infarction prevention (BIP) study. Circulation 2000; 102:21–7.
29. Frick MH, Manninen V, Huttunen JK, Heinonen OP, Tenkanen L, Mänttäri M. HDL-cholesterol as a risk factor in coronary heart disease. An update of the Helsinki Heart Study. Drugs. 1990; 40:7–12.
30. Keech A, Simes RJ, Barter P, Best J, Scott R, Taskinen MR, et al. Effects of long-term fenofibrate therapy on cardiovascular events in 9795 people with type 2 diabetes mellitus (the field study): randomised controlled trial. Lancet. 2005;366:1849–61.
31. Rosenson RS. Field of confusion: future prospects for fibrate therapy in cardiovascular disease. Curr Atheroscler Rep. 2006;8:219–22.
32. Randomised trial of cholesterol lowering in 4444 patients with coronary heart disease: The Scandinavian Simvastatin Survival Study (4S). Lancet 1994;344:1383–9.
33. Pedersen TR, Olsson AG, Færgeman O, Kjekshus J, Wedel H, Berg K, et al. Lipoprotein changes and reduction in the incidence of major coronary heart disease events in the Scandinavian Simvastatin Survival Study (4 S). Circulation. 1998;97:1453–60.
34. Gotto Jr AM, Whitney E, Stein EA, Shapiro DR, Clearfield M, Weis S, et al. Relation between baseline and on-treatment lipid parameters and first acute major coronary events in the Air Force/Texas Coronary Atherosclerosis Prevention Study (AFCAPS/TexCAPS). Circulation. 2000;101:477–84.
35. Nicholls SJ, Tuzcu EM, Sipahi I, Grasso AW, Schoenhagen P, Hu T, et al. Statins, high-density lipoprotein cholesterol, and regression of coronary atherosclerosis. JAMA. 2007;297:499–508.
36. Brown BG, Zhao X-Q, Chait A, Fisher LD, Cheung MC, Morse JS, et al. Simvastatin and niacin, antioxidant vitamins, or the combination for the prevention of coronary disease. N Engl J Med. 2001;345:1583–92.
37. Taylor AJ, Sullenberger LE, Lee HJ, Lee JK, Grace KA. Arterial Biology for the Investigation of the Treatment Effects of Reducing Cholesterol (ARBITER) 2: a double-blind, placebo-controlled study of extended-release niacin on atherosclerosis progression in secondary prevention patients treated with statins. Circulation. 2004;110:3512–7.
38. Rosenson RS, Carlson DM, Kelly MT, Setze CM, Hirshbery B, Stolzenbach, Williams LA. Achievement of lipid targets with the combination of rosuvastatin and fenofibrate acid in patients with type 2 diabetes mellitus cardiovasc Drugs Ther 2011;25:47–57.
39. Ginsberg HN, Elam MB, Lovato LC, et al. Effects of combination lipid therapy in type 2 diabetes mellitus. N Engl J Med. 2010;362:1562–74.
40. Freed MI, Ratner R, Marcovina SM, Kreider MM, Biswas N, Cohen BR, et al. Effects of rosiglitazone alone and in combination with atorvastatin on the metabolic abnormalities in type 2 diabetes mellitus. Am J Cardiol. 2002;90:947–52.
41. Gegick CG, Altheimer MD. Thiazolidinediones: comparison of long-term effects on glycemic control and cardiovascular risk factors. Curr Med Res Opin. 2004;20:919–30.

Chapter 10
Lipoprotein(a)

Matthew J. Sorrentino

Keywords Lipoprotein(a) • Apolipoprotein(a) • Atherothrombosis • Plasminogen

Case Report

The patient is a 44-year-old Caucasian male who developed chest discomfort while playing ice hockey. He was seen at his local emergency department where an EKG showed evidence for an acute inferior wall myocardial infarction. Cardiac catheterization documented an occluded right coronary artery which was opened with a percutaneous intervention. In addition, he had a significant coronary stenosis in his left anterior descending and circumflex arteries that eventually led to a three-vessel coronary bypass surgery. His past medical history was otherwise unremarkable. He has a family history of coronary artery disease in his father also at a younger age.

His baseline lipid panel drawn a few months prior to the myocardial infarction revealed a total cholesterol of 177 mg/dl, high-density lipoprotein cholesterol (HDL-C) 39 mg/dl, triglycerides 159 mg/dl, and a calculated low-density lipoprotein cholesterol (LDL-C) 106 mg/dl. He was initially treated with a starting dose of atorvastatin with little change in his calculated LDL-C. Further lipid testing was done and he was found to have an elevated lipoprotein(a) of 89 mg/dl. The statin was continued and niacin added and eventually titrated to a dose of 1,500 mg daily. Current lipid panel on this combination is a total cholesterol of 160 mg/dl, HDL-C 46 mg/dl, triglycerides 145 mg/dl, and calculated LDL-C 85 mg/dl. His current Lp(a) is measured as 68 mg/dl.

M.J. Sorrentino (✉)
Department of Medicine, Section of Cardiology,
University of Chicago Pritzker School of Medicine, Chicago, IL 60637, USA
e-mail: msorrent@medicine.bsd.uchicago.edu

M.J. Sorrentino (ed.), *Hyperlipidemia in Primary Care: A Practical Guide to Risk Reduction*, Current Clinical Practice, DOI 10.1007/978-1-60327-502-6_10,

What is Lipoprotein(a)?

Lipoprotein(a) or Lp(a) refers to a family of particles that can be considered variants of LDL. The protein moiety of Lp(a) is similar in part to the protein moiety of LDL since it contains a single copy of apolipoprotein B_{100} (apoB). Linked to the apoB protein by disulfide bonds is a unique glycoprotein called apolipoprotein(a) or apo(a). Apo(a) is structurally similar to plasminogen which may lead to inhibition of fibrinolysis and an increased tendency for thrombus formation.

Lp(a) levels can vary over 1,000-fold in the human population from undetectable levels to an Lp(a) cholesterol of greater than 100 mg/dl. Genetic factors largely determine the level of Lp(a) so there is very little change in Lp(a) concentration in an individual during lifetime or due to environmental factors [1].

Lp(a) and Atherothrombosis

Lp(a) may have a number of roles in atherothrombosis. Since it is similar to LDL, Lp(a) may be proatherogenic. Lp(a) has been found in atherosclerotic plaques with higher concentrations found in culprit lesions of patients with unstable angina [2]. Lp(a) can undergo oxidative modification and be taken up by macrophages forming foam cells and, therefore, Lp(a) may add to the atherosclerotic potential of LDL. Lp(a) may be proinflammatory and stimulate the release of inflammatory cytokines, chemotactic factors, and the proliferation of smooth muscle cells in atherosclerotic plaques [3].

The apo(a) moiety of Lp(a) has homology with plasminogen and can bind to the plasminogen receptor. This may give the particle a prothrombotic potential. Studies have suggested that Lp(a) may interfere with plasmin generation, enhance platelet aggregation, increase the expression of plasminogen activator inhibitor 2, and inactivate the inhibitor of tissue factor [4]. Via these mechanisms, Lp(a) may represent a link between the atherosclerotic process and thrombotic complications.

There is emerging evidence that Lp(a) may undergo lipolytic and proteolytic modifications in addition to oxidative changes that may modify its function and toxicity. Phospholipase A-2 (PLA_2) can hydrolyse Lp(a) phospholipids (similar to LDL) enhancing binding in the subendothelium potentially making it more atherogenic [5]. In addition, elastase and metalloproteinase enzymes may modify apo(a) [4]. This enzymatic modification may convert large-size apo(a) molecules into a smaller size apo(a) similar to the small apo(a) isoforms that are thought to have the highest atherothrombotic potential.

Prevalence of Lp(a) in Different Populations

Lp(a) levels may vary significantly between different categories of patients and ethnic populations. Lp(a) levels tend to be higher in women than in men [6]. Patients with chronic kidney disease have elevated Lp(a) levels [7]. In addition,

Lp(a) levels may predict cardiovascular events in patients on dialysis [8]. Lp(a) may in part contribute to the high cardiovascular event rate in patients with chronic kidney disease.

African American individuals tend to have Lp(a) levels that are two to three times higher than Caucasians [9], although this increase may not correlate with an increased cardiovascular risk. Unlike in Caucasians, there is no correlation between Lp(a) levels and coronary artery calcium in blacks [10, 11]. In addition, there was no increased coronary heart disease risk in black patients with elevated Lp(a) levels in the Atherosclerosis Risk in Communities (ARIC) study [12].

Lp(a) levels have also been shown to be higher in individuals from the Indian subcontinent compared to Europeans [13]. Asian Indians have a mean Lp(a) level of 20 mg/dl and 30–40% of Asian Indians have levels greater than the 20–30 mg/dl level considered the upper limit of normal [14]. South Asians have a high risk of coronary artery disease in part due to a high prevalence of diabetes and mixed hyperlipidemia. The genetic predisposition for high levels of Lp(a) may significantly add to this risk. The combination of mixed hyperlipidemia and a high Lp(a) may magnify cardiovascular risk in this population. In one study, 42% of Asian Indians were found to have a clustering of high Lp(a) and a low HDL-C [15].

Lp(a) as a Cardiovascular Risk Factor

Soon after Lp(a) was identified, studies suggested an independent and continuous association between Lp(a) levels and the risk of coronary events. Some conflicting findings in these initial studies likely occurred because of variability in the measurement of Lp(a). A meta-analysis of studies published before 2000 with at least 1-year follow-up showed that individuals in the top tercile of Lp(a) values had about a 60% increased risk of coronary heart disease compared to those in the bottom third [16]. An updated meta-analysis including an additional 14 studies yielded an adjusted odds ratio of 1.45 for coronary heart disease events for individuals in the top third of Lp(a) distribution compared with those in the bottom third [17]. More recent assays have been developed that measure Lp(a) independent of apo(a) isoform size. In the Women's Health study using the updated assay, women with Lp(a) levels in the 90th percentile had increased cardiovascular risk particularly in women with high LDL-C levels as well [18]. Lp(a) is likely an independent risk factor in patients with established coronary heart disease as well. In a meta-analysis of nine studies in patients with known vascular disease, there was an independent association between Lp(a) levels and coronary risk although Lp(a) may be less predictive of risk in patients with established disease compared to those without [16].

Lp(a) levels have correlated with risk in noncardiac vascular beds as well. Elevations in Lp(a) is also an independent predictor of stroke in older adults [19]. Lp(a) levels have been found to be higher in patients with peripheral arterial disease (PAD) in some studies but has not been found to be a risk factor for the development of PAD in other surveys [20, 21]. Studies have also suggested that high levels of

Lp(a) are associated with venous thromboembolism [22] suggesting that the prothrombotic potential of Lp(a) may be an important aspect of this particle.

High Lp(a) levels in Asian Indians may be associated with a higher coronary heart disease [23] and ischemic stroke risk [24] as well. A high Lp(a) may be an especially important risk factor for coronary heart disease in younger individuals [25]. A small study of 50 consecutive north Indian male patients with a myocardial infarction at an age less than 45 years showed a higher Lp(a) and lower HDL-C in the patients and their first-degree relatives compared with controls [26].

Measurement of Lp(a)

Lp(a) shows a marked heterogeneity in density and size in large part due to different isoforms of apo(a) that can vary between 300 and 800 kDa due to differences in the number of kringle repeats of the molecule [27]. The size variation of apo(a) leads to poor correlation of Lp(a) values obtained by different measurement methods. More recently, a specific monoclonal antibody technique was developed to allow measurement of Lp(a) levels that are not influenced by the size heterogeneity of apo(a) [28]. Use of this method showed that immunochemical methods can give highly variable results that can lead to misclassification of CHD risk. Most laboratories report Lp(a) cholesterol levels. Lp(a), like LDL particles, can exist as multiple subclasses from smaller denser particles to larger more buoyant particles. The cholesterol content of the particles may be dependent in part by the size of the apo(a) molecule. Lp(a) cholesterol values will not be an accurate measurement of the number of particles that are present. Table 10.1 gives the recommended ranges for interpreting Lp(a) values and cardiovascular risk.

When to Measure Lp(a)

A number of epidemiologic studies have shown an association between high Lp(a) levels and cardiovascular disease (CVD) risk [16]. In addition, there is evidence to support high Lp(a) levels as a thrombotic risk factor as well [29]. Knowledge of Lp(a) values may help to determine CVD risk especially in certain subpopulations where Lp(a) may be a genetic trait. Therefore, it is reasonable to consider measuring

Table 10.1 Lipoprotein(a) values and cardiovascular risk

	Lp(a) cholesterol value (mg/dl)
Desirable	<14
Borderline risk	14–30
High risk	31–50
Very high risk	>50

Lp(a) in high-risk populations. This would include Caucasians and South Asians with a family history of CVD. It is not likely useful to measure Lp(a) in African American populations until we have more information about apo(a) isoforms that may be linked to CVD. In addition, occasionally a patient may be treated with an LDL-lowering therapy and not achieve the expected reduction in LDL-C. Since the Friedewald LDL-C includes Lp(a), this individual may have a high Lp(a) making up a large portion of the calculated LDL-C. An increased Lp(a) may also account for a large discrepancy between a calculated LDL-C and some direct LDL assays that are able to separate out the Lp(a). Measurement of Lp(a) would be useful in these groups. Many of the advanced lipid testing commercial products (VAP, Berkeley) include Lp(a) as a part of the lipid testing.

Levels of Lp(a) remain highly stable within individuals over many years [17]. In addition, the association of Lp(a) with coronary risk is independent of other cardiovascular risk factors. Therefore, most of the effect of Lp(a) on risk can be assessed by a single measurement and there is little reason for repeat measurements in an individual patient.

Treatment of High Lp(a)

At this point in time, there are no effective ways to lower Lp(a) levels and no studies that indicate that treatment directed at Lp(a) translates into reduced cardiovascular risk. It is not known what concentration of Lp(a) is considered a safe level. Lp(a) levels do not change with diet or exercise [30]. Alcohol consumption may lower Lp(a) levels somewhat although it is not known if this translates into reduced cardiovascular risk [31].

Lp(a) levels are relatively resistant to lowering by pharmacological agents. It is unclear if statins have a significant clinical effect on Lp(a) since studies have shown that statins may reduce [32], keep Lp(a) levels the same [33], or even increase levels especially in patients presenting with an acute coronary syndrome [34]. Only niacin and estrogen have been shown to modestly lower Lp(a) levels. Niacin may decrease Lp(a) levels up to 40% in patients with a mixed hyperlipidemia when used in maximum doses [35], although some studies have only shown a modest decline in Lp(a) levels using niacin either alone or in combination with a statin [36]. Hormone replacement therapy (HRT) in postmenopausal women can decrease Lp(a) levels, although HRT does not appear to reduce the incidence of cardiac events [37].

Currently, the best approach to treating a patient with high Lp(a) levels would be to modify all the correctable risk factors targeting LDL-C and non-HDL-C cholesterol as recommended by the NCEP guidelines. A combination of a statin plus niacin is commonly used in high-risk individuals with an elevated Lp(a) but there are no outcome studies verifying that this approach will further lower cardiovascular risk.

The patient in the case report was treated with a statin and niacin up to the dose that he was able to tolerate without side effects. His LDL-C level without the added Lp(a) cholesterol is 17 mg/dl [LDL-C minus the Lp(a)]. It is not likely that the

LDL-C can be driven down any further. The addition of niacin appears to have lowered the Lp(a) somewhat although it remains at the high-risk level. Since this patient is high risk, it is reasonable to continue combination therapy with the statin and niacin in conjunction with his lifestyle program even though we do not have an outcome study to guide us to the optimal therapy.

References

1. Koschinsky ML. Lipoprotein(a) and atherosclerosis: new perspectives on the mechanism of action of an enigmatic lipoprotein. Curr Atheroscler Rep. 2005;7(5):389–95.
2. Dangas G, Mehran R, Harpel PC, et al. Lipoprotein(a) and inflammation in human coronary atheroma: association with the severity of clinical presentation. J Am Coll Cardiol. 1998;32(7):2035–42.
3. Tziomalos K, Athyros VG, Wierzbicki AS, Mikhailidis DP. Lipoprotein a: where are we now? Curr Opin Cardiol. 2009;24(4):351–7.
4. Scanu AM. Lipoprotein(a) and the atherothrombotic process: mechanistic insights and clinical implications. Curr Atheroscler Rep. 2003;5(2):106–13.
5. Hoover-Plow J, Khaitan A, Fless GM. Phospholipase A2 modification enhances lipoprotein(a) binding to the subendothelial matrix. Thromb Haemost. 1998;79(3):640–8.
6. Ganotakis ES, Gazi IF, Papadakis JA, Jagroop IA, Nair DR, Mikhailidis DP. The relationship between circulating fibrinogen and lipoprotein (a) levels in patients with primary dyslipidemia. Clin Appl Thromb Hemost. 2007;13(1):35–42.
7. Sechi LA, Zingaro L, De CS, et al. Increased serum lipoprotein(a) levels in patients with early renal failure. Ann Intern Med. 1998;129(6):457–61.
8. Longenecker JC, Klag MJ, Marcovina SM, et al. High lipoprotein(a) levels and small apolipoprotein(a) size prospectively predict cardiovascular events in dialysis patients. J Am Soc Nephrol. 2005;16(6):1794–802.
9. Sorrentino MJ, Vielhauer C, Eisenbart JD, Fless GM, Scanu AM, Feldman T. Plasma lipoprotein (a) protein concentration and coronary artery disease in black patients compared with white patients. Am J Med. 1992;93(6):658–62.
10. Chironi G, Simon A, Denarie N, et al. Determinants of progression of coronary artery calcifications in asymptomatic men at high cardiovascular risk. Angiology. 2002;53(6):677–83.
11. Guerra R, Yu Z, Marcovina S, Peshock R, Cohen JC, Hobbs HH. Lipoprotein(a) and apolipoprotein(a) isoforms: no association with coronary artery calcification in the Dallas Heart Study. Circulation. 2005;111(12):1471–9.
12. Sharrett AR, Ballantyne CM, Coady SA, et al. Coronary heart disease prediction from lipoprotein cholesterol levels, triglycerides, lipoprotein(a), apolipoproteins A-I and B, and HDL density subfractions: The Atherosclerosis Risk in Communities (ARIC) Study. Circulation. 2001;104(10):1108–13.
13. Bhatnagar D, Anand IS, Durrington PN, et al. Coronary risk factors in people from the Indian subcontinent living in west London and their siblings in India. Lancet. 1995;345(8947):405–9.
14. Enas EA, Chacko V, Pazhoor SG, Chennikkara H, Devarapalli HP. Dyslipidemia in South Asian patients. Curr Atheroscler Rep. 2007;9(5):367–74.
15. Superko HR, Enas EA, Kotha P, Bhat NK, Garrett B. High-density lipoprotein subclass distribution in individuals of Asian Indian descent: the National Asian Indian Heart Disease Project. Prev Cardiol. 2005;8(2):81–6.
16. Danesh J, Collins R, Peto R. Lipoprotein(a) and coronary heart disease. Meta-analysis of prospective studies. Circulation. 2000;102(10):1082–5.
17. Bennet A, Di AE, Erqou S, et al. Lipoprotein(a) levels and risk of future coronary heart disease: large-scale prospective data. Arch Intern Med. 2008;168(6):598–608.

18. Suk DJ, Rifai N, Buring JE, Ridker PM. Lipoprotein(a), measured with an assay independent of apolipoprotein(a) isoform size, and risk of future cardiovascular events among initially healthy women. JAMA. 2006;296(11):1363–70.
19. Ariyo AA, Thach C, Tracy R. Lp(a) lipoprotein, vascular disease, and mortality in the elderly. N Engl J Med. 2003;349(22):2108–15.
20. Dieplinger B, Lingenhel A, Baumgartner N, et al. Increased serum lipoprotein(a) concentrations and low molecular weight phenotypes of apolipoprotein(a) are associated with symptomatic peripheral arterial disease. Clin Chem. 2007;53(7):1298–305.
21. Ridker PM, Stampfer MJ, Rifai N. Novel risk factors for systemic atherosclerosis: a comparison of C-reactive protein, fibrinogen, homocysteine, lipoprotein(a), and standard cholesterol screening as predictors of peripheral arterial disease. JAMA. 2001;285(19):2481–5.
22. Sofi F, Marcucci R, Abbate R, Gensini GF, Prisco D. Lipoprotein (a) and venous thromboembolism in adults: a meta-analysis. Am J Med. 2007;120(8):728–33.
23. Geethanjali FS, Jose VJ, Kanagasabapathy AS. Lipoprotein (a) phenotypes in south Indian patients with coronary artery disease. Indian Heart J. 2002;54(1):50–3.
24. Sharobeem KM, Patel JV, Ritch AE, Lip GY, Gill PS, Hughes EA. Elevated lipoprotein (a) and apolipoprotein B to AI ratio in South Asian patients with ischaemic stroke. Int J Clin Pract. 2007;61(11):1824–8.
25. Gambhir JK, Kaur H, Gambhir DS, Prabhu KM. Lipoprotein(a) as an independent risk factor for coronary artery disease in patients below 40 years of age. Indian Heart J. 2000;52(4):411–5.
26. Isser HS, Puri VK, Narain VS, Saran RK, Dwivedi SK, Singh S. Lipoprotein (a) and lipid levels in young patients with myocardial infarction and their first-degree relatives. Indian Heart J. 2001;53(4):463–6.
27. Scanu AM. Lp(a) lipoprotein–coping with heterogeneity. N Engl J Med. 2003;349(22):2089–90.
28. Marcovina SM, Albers JJ, Scanu AM, et al. Use of a reference material proposed by the International Federation of Clinical Chemistry and Laboratory Medicine to evaluate analytical methods for the determination of plasma lipoprotein(a). Clin Chem. 2000;46(12):1956–67.
29. Marcovina SM, Koschinsky ML. Evaluation of lipoprotein(a) as a prothrombotic factor: progress from bench to bedside. Curr Opin Lipidol. 2003;14(4):361–6.
30. Byrne DJ, Jagroop IA, Montgomery HE, et al. Lipoprotein (a) does not participate in the early acute phase response to training or extreme physical activity and is unlikely to enhance any associated immediate cardiovascular risk. J Clin Pathol. 2002;55(4):280–5.
31. Paassilta M, Kervinen K, Rantala AO, et al. Social alcohol consumption and low Lp(a) lipoprotein concentrations in middle aged Finnish men: population based study. BMJ. 1998;316(7131):594–5.
32. Gonbert S, Malinsky S, Sposito AC, et al. Atorvastatin lowers lipoprotein(a) but not apolipoprotein(a) fragment levels in hypercholesterolemic subjects at high cardiovascular risk. Atherosclerosis. 2002;164(2):305–11.
33. Goudevenos JA, Bairaktari ET, Chatzidimou KG, Milionis HJ, Mikhailidis DP, Elisaf MS. The effect of atorvastatin on serum lipids, lipoprotein(a) and plasma fibrinogen levels in primary dyslipidaemia – a pilot study involving serial sampling. Curr Med Res Opin. 2001;16(4):269–75.
34. Tsimikas S, Witztum JL, Miller ER, et al. High-dose atorvastatin reduces total plasma levels of oxidized phospholipids and immune complexes present on apolipoprotein B-100 in patients with acute coronary syndromes in the MIRACL trial. Circulation. 2004;110(11):1406–12.
35. Scanu AM, Bamba R. Niacin and lipoprotein(a): facts, uncertainties, and clinical considerations. Am J Cardiol. 2008;101(8A):44B–7B.
36. McKenney JM, Jones PH, Bays HE, et al. Comparative effects on lipid levels of combination therapy with a statin and extended-release niacin or ezetimibe versus a statin alone (the COMPELL study). Atherosclerosis. 2007;192(2):432–7.
37. Shlipak MG, Simon JA, Vittinghoff E, et al. Estrogen and progestin, lipoprotein(a), and the risk of recurrent coronary heart disease events after menopause. JAMA. 2000;283(14):1845–52.

Chapter 11
HIV with Dyslipidemia

Tochi Okwuosa

Keywords Human immunodeficiency virus • Antiretroviral therapy • Dyslipidemia • Lipodystrophy

Case Report

A 58 year old man who had been diagnosed with human immunodeficiency virus (HIV) disease and had been on antiretroviral therapy (ART) for about a year presents to his primary care physician for his yearly follow-up. He currently denies any complaints and states he had been following up closely with his infectious disease doctor who has been monitoring his CD4 counts and viral load for every 3–4 months. His medical history includes type 2 diabetes mellitus and HIV [no acquired immunodeficiency syndrome (AIDS)]. His ART regimen includes tenofovir/emtricitabine and lopinavir/ritonavir. He is also being treated with glyburide 20 mg daily for his diabetes.

On physical examination, his blood pressure is 140/78, weight 220 lbs, BMI 34 kg/m^2, and waist circumference 45 inches. The rest of his physical exam is unremarkable.

Fasting laboratory data reveal normal electrolytes and creatinine, hemoglobin A1c is 6.5%, total cholesterol 292 mg/dL, triglycerides 680 mg/dL, and high-density lipoprotein cholesterol (HDL-C) 28 mg/dL. Low-density lipoprotein cholesterol (LDL-C) could not be calculated due to the severely elevated triglyceride level. About a year ago, prior to initiation of ART, his lipid profile had been optimal.

- What are the considerations for treating dyslipidemia in this patient?
- Did ART contribute to his dyslipidemia?

T. Okwuosa (✉)
Division of Cardiology, Wayne State University School of Medicine, Detroit, MI 48201
e-mail: tokwuosa@med.wayne.edu

M.J. Sorrentino (ed.), *Hyperlipidemia in Primary Care: A Practical Guide to Risk Reduction*, Current Clinical Practice, DOI 10.1007/978-1-60327-502-6_11,

- What is his estimated 10-year risk of cardiovascular events and what role does HIV disease and ART play in this assessment and its management?
- Should his goal for lipid therapy be different from that of the general population without HIV disease?
- What drug–drug interactions are expected given his ART regimen, and how can they be avoided?
- Should his antiretroviral regimen be changed if his lipid profile continues to worsen despite optimal medical therapy?

Introduction

Cardiovascular disease (CVD) is the leading cause of death in the USA [1] and is a significant cause of morbidity and mortality in the patient population with HIV [2]. This risk of CVD increases as life expectancy in the HIV population increases with the advent and continued introduction of more effective ART [3–5]. As these HIV-infected patients live longer, they experience complications of illnesses, including CVD, not directly related to HIV infection [6]. The rationale for this increase in CVD risk in HIV patients is related to an increase in prevalence of Framingham cardiovascular (CV) risk factors [2, 7], especially dyslipidemia, insulin resistance, and hypertension; as well as direct effects of the virus on the heart and vasculature (e.g., inflammation and endothelial function) [2, 4]. Therapies for HIV infection also appear to be important contributors to the increase in CVD risk seen in this population [7] by their effects on traditional CVD risk factors including dyslipidemia; as well as direct effects on the vasculature and other inflammatory, immune, and viral factors related to HIV infection [4, 8].

In general, the higher the CVD risk, the more intense the risk-reducing interventions to prevent myocardial infarction (MI), stroke, or cardiovascular death. The relative effects of traditional risk factors on coronary heart disease (CHD) outcomes appear similar in both HIV-infected and -uninfected patients [9]. In the HIV patient, however, one must also take into account the co-morbidities (e.g., substance abuse, malignancy, liver disease, and other HIV complications) and multiple drug therapies in use, in addition to the CVD risk factors; while deciding the intensity of these interventions. Efforts to modify CV risk factors in this population should therefore focus on prevention and/or improvement of modifiable risks, e.g., smoking, hypertension, dyslipidemia, and glucose intolerance. An understanding of the interactions of these modifiable risks with the HIV disease process and its drug therapy is consequently necessary in order to make the best decisions for risk factor modification. This is unfortunately limited by certain factors. First, changes in preferred HIV drugs with time, as well as changes in drug therapy with each individual patient, make it difficult to study the effects of drug therapy on CV or any other risk for that matter [2]. Second, a lot of the studies are retrospective with short durations of follow-up [5]. Finally, HIV patients are more prone to alcohol abuse, drug abuse, and especially tobacco abuse; all contributing to impairment of CV function. Most of the HIV studies, however, do not match the HIV-uninfected control group, or make adjustments in analysis, for these confounding factors [2, 10, 11]. All of these factors limit the findings in most CVD in HIV studies, making it difficult to make associations and extrapolate findings to the general HIV population.

Factors Contributing to CVD Risk in HIV Patients

There is certainly increased risk of CVD in the HIV population [12–15], particularly among women [14], with variations across studies likely reflecting differences in populations studied as well as differences in definitions of end points in these studies [2]. HIV patients have higher rates of hospital admissions for CVD (particularly, acute MI) when compared to uninfected controls.

Traditional CV Risk Factors

The traditional risk factors including hypertension, diabetes mellitus (DM), and dyslipidemia affect CVD risk in HIV patients the same way and amount as in the general population [16]. However, there is a higher prevalence of these conventional CV risk factors in HIV patients compared with controls [14], a factor which could explain the increased risk of CVD observed in this population. In addition, studies controlling for HIV factors have demonstrated a significant effect of traditional risk factors on increased CVD risk suggesting that the traditional risk factors have a role to play in the increase in CVD risk observed in the HIV population [2]. Strong predictors of CVD risk in HIV patients include age, smoking, hypertension, and DM [4, 14]. Rates of tobacco use are consistently higher in the HIV population than that in age-matched controls [10, 11, 17]. HIV patients also have higher rates of dyslipidemia [18] and diet high in saturated fat [19] than the general population. Unfortunately, determination of role of treatment or disease-related dyslipidemia in CVD risk is limited by the absence of pre-HIV or pretreatment values [18].

HIV Disease Process

HIV directly infects myocytes causing inflammation with chronic virus-induced release of cytotoxic cytokines, leading to progressive tissue damage [20]. In the vasculature, HIV is associated with endothelial dysfunction [21] which is related to clinical manifestations of atherosclerosis [22]. It improves with ART, but does not return to baseline in the short term [21]. The mechanism of this endothelial dysfunction is likely related to lipid disorders with HIV infection [23], systemic inflammation with cytokine dysregulation, direct HIV effects on the endothelium and vascular smooth muscles [24], and/or viral protein-related endothelial activation [25]. Inflammation is certainly a likely player since inflammatory markers, e.g., interferon-α, are elevated in HIV patients [26]; and salicylates significantly improve endothelial dysfunction in HIV patients [27]. C-reactive protein (CRP) levels are elevated in AIDS [26].

Antiretroviral Therapy

ART has been positively correlated with increased CHD in multiple studies summarized by Currier et al. [2]. The Data Collection on Adverse Events of Anti-HIV Drugs (DAD) cohort study found a 26% relative increase in MI rates with longer exposure to ART (particularly, protease inhibitors), but did not find an association between MI incidence and markers of HIV disease including AIDS, CD4 lymphocyte counts, or HIV RNA [28]. This risk of MI was significantly reduced (from 16% per year to 10% per year) when lipid levels were adjusted for, suggesting that ART therapy contributed to CHD risk in this population of HIV patients. Interestingly, intermittent interruptions of ART therapy based on CD4 cell counts, as in the Strategic Management of Antiretroviral Therapy (SMART) study [29], led to an increase in CVD event rates. This finding could be related to increased total cholesterol to HDL-C ratio or inflammatory reaction within the vessel wall from unsuppressed HIV infection during intermittent therapy [2] and suggest a better risk profile with sustained therapy to suppress the virus.

Some studies have supported increased incidence of MI with the use of protease inhibitors (PIs) [30, 31], others have found no association between MI incidence and PI use [32], yet others have associated increased CV events with HIV seropositivity [12] and lower CD4 cell counts [33]; while some have correlated CVD event rates with nucleoside reverse transcriptase inhibitor (NRTI) use [33]. In addition, ART (particularly the PI – indinavir – now rarely used) has been associated with endothelial dysfunction [34].

Other Factors

Studies looking for association of HIV disease (or ART use) with surrogate markers for CVD – carotid intimal medial thickness (cIMT) and coronary calcium score (CCS) – have produced conflicting results as detailed by Hsue et al. [3].

Dyslipidemia and HIV Infection

Patients with HIV, either as a result of the disease or its therapies, show alterations in lipid and insulin/glucose metabolism and body composition that are proatherogenic [7]. The prevalence of dyslipidemia in the HIV-infected patients varies widely from 20 to 70% depending on the definition of dyslipidemia and the population studied [35]. In the DAD cohort of 23,437 patients, the prevalence of dysplipidemia at study entry was 42% [10]. In HIV-infected patients, there are increased levels of small, dense LDL which can get incorporated into the vessel wall and easily undergo oxidation, leading to atherosclerosis [36–38]. There is also an increase in recruitment of macrophages into the vessel wall, making them more susceptible to foam cell formation, causing atherosclerosis [38]. Given this risk of atherosclerosis with dyslipidemia, it is important to understand the changes in lipids with HIV infection and/or ART therapy, the mechanism of these changes, and to elucidate, if possible, the most effective approach to reverse or prevent this process.

Lipid Changes with HIV Infection

The lipid profile in HIV-infected persons varies with disease activity [26, 39]. The initial effects of HIV infection on lipid levels is a decrease in total cholesterol with a decrease in HDL-C levels; followed later by a slight decease in LDL-C levels [26, 40, 41]. Likewise, apolipoprotein A-1 (apoA1) – the major apolipoprotein of HDL-C – and apolipoprotein B-100 (apoB100) – the major apolipoprotein of LDL-C – are decreased [26]. By the time signs and symptoms of AIDS occur, very low-density lipoprotein (VLDL) cholesterol levels and triglycerides increase [26, 40]. Unfortunately, the protective effects of the slight reduction in LDL-C are likely offset by the decrease in HDL-C and increase in VLDL [7].

The hypertriglyceridemia associated with HIV infection results from an increase in VLDL, making non-HDL-C a better predictor of CVD risk than LDL-C [7]. The non-HDL-C (total minus HDL-C) is a an important component of the lipid profile because it is the atherogenic component within all lipoprotein particles [42] and tries to account for atherogenesis especially in patients with hypertriglyceridemia [43]. It is equivalent to VLDL + LDL-C; and when calculated, it includes intermediate-density lipoprotein (IDL) [43].

These lipid changes with HIV infection are likely mediated by inflammatory processes occurring with HIV infection; as prior studies have shown a decrease in clearance of triglycerides with increase in lipogenesis associated with disease activity and cytokine levels (particularly, interferon-α) [26, 44]. Despite these changes, there is limited evidence to support contribution of individual alterations in lipid profile to the atherosclerotic process [7, 45]. A study by Duprez et al. is noteworthy however; and showed that total, large and small HDL particles are significantly and independently associated with CVD and non-fatal coronary disease.

Lipid Changes with ART

The lipid profile is altered significantly after initiation of ART with 10–30% increase in plasma levels of total cholesterol, HDL-C, and LDL-C; and 10–50% increase in plasma triglyceride levels within 2 weeks to 1 month after initiation of ART [46, 47]. In the 5-year follow-up study by Shlay et al., the peak levels of the total cholesterol, HDL-C, and LDL-C were achieved within 4 months; with HDL-C plateau at 4 months and LDL-C decline to baseline by 40 months [46]. The triglyceride levels continued to rise slowly for up to 5 years of follow-up [46].

(a) *Protease inhibitors (PIs)*: This class of drugs is associated with dyslipidemia that is more severe and more common than that seen prior to ART therapy. PIs are associated with hypertriglyceridemia (up to >500 mg/dL) and hypercholesterolemia (up to >240 mg/dL) [48] as seen in HIV patients on PI therapy, as compared to those not being treated with PIs [49]. The elevated triglyceride levels in this population is particularly reflective of VLDL levels [50]. PIs do not influence HDL-C levels, and data on the influence of this class of drugs on LDL-C levels are controversial [5]. The greatest worsening in lipid profile, particularly, triglyceride levels, has been observed with ritonavir [50–53]. Atazanavir, on the other hand, has minimal effects on LDL-C levels [54]; and in fact, raises HDL-C levels [54]. Saqunavir and indinavir also have few negative effects on the lipid profile [50, 55]. Furthermore, PIs – particularly lopinavir and ritonavir – have been associated with increased apoB [56] and apoA1 levels [56, 57].
(b) *Nonnucleoside reverse transcriptase inhibitors (NNRTIs)*: The greatest elevations in HDL-C levels, reflecting some favorable effects of ART on lipid profile, have been observed with NNRTIs [53, 58]. However NNRTIs, like other class of antiretrovirals, also have not so favorable effects on the lipid profile. Efavirenz has been shown to increase triglyceride levels in patients with HIV infection [53], while nevirapine has been shown to increase LDL-C levels [58]. A direct comparison of nevirapine and efavirenz showed nevirapine had better effects on the lipid profile; with smaller increases in triglycerides, total cholesterol, and LDL-C levels, and greater increases in HDL-C levels than efavirenz [59].
(c) *Nucleoside reverse transcriptase inhibitors (NRTIs)*: This is the class of ART least associated with dyslipidemia [10, 60]. From this class, stavudine has shown the most significant increase in total cholesterol, LDL-C, and triglyceride levels when compared with zidovudine [61] and tenofovir [62, 63].

In general, since the general population is at risk of dyslipidemia due to genetic and/or environmental factors, the worsening in lipid profile observed with ART is likely a function of each individual's predisposition [7]. Worth mentioning is that the increase in LDL-C observed with ART occurs as a result of effective HIV treatment which actually reverses the initial small decrease in LDL-C typically detected with HIV infection [7].

HIV Treatment-Associated Lipodystrophy

Increased dorsocervical and abdominal fat, as well as visceral adipose tissue (lipohypertrophy), and loss of subcutaneous fat in the arms, legs, face, and buttocks (lipoatrophy) are associated with elevated oxidized LDL [64], low HDL-C, and elevated triglyceride levels [7]. Together with insulin resistance, all three disease processes constitute what is known as the HIV lipodystrophy syndrome (or fat redistribution syndrome) [65]. The associated increase in non-HDL-C levels could be a mechanism for CVD in this population. Some medications in all classes of ART, particularly, the PIs, have been associated with lipodystrophy [64, 66, 67].

Treatment of lipoatrophy has met with limited success. Options include the thiazolidinediones which have shown mixed results [68–71]; uridine [72], and the statins (particularly pravastatin) [73, 74]; both of which have limited data to support their use for this purpose. For lipohypertrophy, metformin has shown mixed results [75, 76] and can worsen lipoatrophy [76]. Other options for the treatment of lipohypertrophy are growth hormone releasing hormone (GHRH) [77], GHRH analog (tesamorelin) [78], and human GH (hGH) [79, 80], at both physiological and supraphysiological doses. In November 2010, tesamorelin was approved by the by the US Food and Drug Administration for treatment of HIV lipodystrophy. The others are not currently approved for this indication. Treatment with tesamorelin significantly reduced visceral fat, triglycerides, and total to HDL-C ratios in one study [78]. Similarly, treatment with hGH is associated with a dose-dependent lipoatrophy as well as a favorable lipid profile, including reduction in LDL-C and non-HDL-C, and an increase in HDL-C [79–81] but with impaired glucose tolerance [81], and some studies showing a transient benefit in the reduction of lipohypertrophy [74]. hGH did not significantly increase or decrease serum triglyceride levels [80].

Evaluation of Lipids and Cardiovascular Risk in the HIV-Infected Patient

Treatment Goals for Abnormal Cholesterol Levels in the HIV Patient

Currently, the target goals for lipid levels/therapy in HIV-infected patients are the same as that of the general population, since there is no evidence so far to suggest otherwise [5]. Based on the National Cholesterol Education Program (NCEP) Expert Panel on Detection, Evaluation, and Treatment of High Blood Cholesterol in Adults (Adult Treatment Panel III [ATP III]) guidelines [82], the following steps can be taken to risk stratify a patient:

(a) Count the number of risk factors (see Table 11.1) that modify LDL-C goals. (Risk assessment of patients with ≥2 risk factors can be carried out using the Framingham model at http://hp2010.nhlbihin.net/atpiii/calculator.asp to estimate the 10-year risk of MI or cardiac death.)
(b) Use these data to estimate LDL-C goals (see Table 11.2).

From these tables, it is obvious that the goals of treatment are dependent on CHD risk as measured by the presence of risk factors and LDL-C levels. Importantly, while Table 11.2 is adapted from the most recent NCEP ATP III guidelines published in 2004, more recent data emphasizing the influence of lower LDL-C and other lipoprotein particles (apoB and non-HDL-C) on cardiometabolic risk have prompted a new consensus statement from the American Diabetes Association (ADA) and the American College of Cardiology (ACC) Foundation (Table 11.3) [42].

Table 11.1 CHD risk factors that modify LDL-C goals

Risk factor	Definition
Cigarette smoking	–
Hypertension	Blood pressure ≥ 140/90 mmHg or an antihypertensive medication
Low HDL-C	<40 mg/dL
Family history of premature CHD	CHD in male first-degree relative <55 years of age; CHD in female first-degree relative <65 years of age
Age	Men ≥ 45 years; women ≥ 55 years

Adapted from Dube et al. [5]

Table 11.2 NCEP ATP III treatment guidelines based on LDL-C

Risk category	High risk (>20% 10-year risk) (mg/dL)	Moderately high risk (10–20% 10-year risk) (mg/dL)	Moderate risk (<10% 10-year risk) (mg/dL)	Lower risk (0–1 risk factors) (mg/dL)
LDL-C goal	<100 (optional: <70)	<130	<130	<160
Initiate TLC	≥100	≥130	≥130	≥160
Consider drug therapy	≥100	≥130	≥160	≥190

Adapted from Grundy et al. [43]

High risk: CHD [history of MI, unstable angina, stable angina, coronary artery procedures (angioplasty or bypass surgery), or evidence of clinically significant myocardial ischemia]; or CHD risk equivalents [other clinical manifestations of atherosclerosis (peripheral arterial disease, abdominal aortic aneurysm, and carotid artery disease), diabetes, ≥2 risk factors]

Moderate risk or moderately high risk: ≥2 risk factors

Goal triglycerides should be < 150mg/dL, and goal HDL-C should be > 40mg/dL. NCEP-ATP III = National Cholesterol Education Program-Adult Treatment Panel III

Table 11.3 ADA/ACC treatment guidelines based on lipoprotein abnormalities

	Highest risk patients (mg/dL)	High-risk patients (mg/dL)
LDL-C goal	<70	<100
Non HDL C goal	<100	<130
ApoB goal	<80	<90

Adapted from Brunzell et al. [42]

Highest risk: known CHD or diabetes plus ≥ additional major CHD risk factor(s)

High risk: diabetes without other major CHD risk factors; ≥2 additional major CHD risk factors without diabetes or known clinical CHD with diabetes

ADA = American Diabetic Association

ACC = American College of Cardiology

In fact, apoB could be a substitute for LDL-C and non-HDL-C in screening and treatment of CVD. Some studies suggest that it is a stronger predictor of CVD [83, 84] and that apoB to apoA1 ratio is superior in prediction of CVD risk than LDL-C/HDL-C, non-HDL-C/HDL-C, or TC/HDL-C ratios [85].

There is no evidence to suggest that raising HDL-C provides the additional benefit of CV risk reduction [86]; and in fact, a recent study of the drug torcetrapib [a cholesteryl ester transfer protein (CETP) inhibitor] which significantly raised HDL-C was associated with higher risk of death from any cause, major cardiovascular events, hypertension, peripheral vascular disease, and hospitalizations for both heart failure and unstable angina [87, 88]. In addition, the AIM-HIGH trial of niacin plus simvastatin was stopped early due to a failure to show a difference in most CV event rates, with a higher rate of strokes observed in the treatment group compared to placebo.

Treatment Goals for Hypertriglyceridemia in the HIV Patient

A lot of HIV-infected patients have severe hypertriglyceridemia; however, the goal of therapy for the management of hypertriglyceridemia (serum triglyceride levels >200 mg/dL) presents a dilemma. This is because although patients with elevated triglycerides are at increased CVD risk, there is lack of data regarding reduction in CHD risk with therapies targeting reduction in serum triglyceride levels [42]. Non-HDL-C levels which is an independent predictor of CV events [89, 90] can however be used as a measure of cardiometabolic risk in patients with elevated serum triglyceride levels. The normal target non-HDL-C levels for each risk category is 30 mg/dL higher than the corresponding LDL-C target [5] (see also Table 11.3).

Lipid Measurement [5]

Serum lipid evaluation (total cholesterol, HDL-C, and triglyceride levels) should be determined prior to initiation of ART and should be performed after an 8–12 h fast. Based on this evaluation, the LDL-C and non-HDL-C levels can be calculated. After the initiation of ART, the lipid profile should be re-evaluated within 3–6 months, then yearly until abnormalities are detected; or lipid-lowering therapy initiated. Patients with elevated triglyceride levels at baseline might require a repeat measurement sooner (1–2 months) after ART initiation.

Goals for Other Risk Factors

The metabolic syndrome (abdominal obesity, atherogenic dyslipidemia including low HDL-C, small LDL-C particles, and elevated triglycerides, elevated blood pressure, insulin resistance ± glucose intolerance, prothrombotic state, and proinflammatory state) which is linked to HIV treatment-associated lipodystrophy is identified by NCEP ATP III as secondary target for intervention [82]. The patients should be encouraged to lose weight, make dietary modifications, and increase physical activity; bearing in mind that excessive weight loss could potentially exacerbate lipoatrophy [5]. Routine interventions should be offered for these modifiable risk factors including smoking, hypertension, physical inactivity, obesity, and DM. Physicians should be on the lookout for exacerbating conditions including excessive alcohol use, hypothyroidism, drug abuse, renal disease, hypogonadism, and/or liver disease. Effects of individual drugs being used by the patients on lipid profile should also be taken into account [5]. Interestingly, there is a debate as to whether the prevalence of metabolic syndrome is increased in HIV patients [91].

Therapy for Dyslipidemia in the HIV Patient

Therapeutic Lifestyle Changes

In order to avoid adverse effects of drug therapy and drug–drug interactions, initial management of dyslipidemia in the HIV-infected patient should consist of nondrug therapies, unless the patient is in the high-risk category or has severely elevated LDL-C (>220 mg/dL) [5]. Lipid management in the HIV patient could be complicated in that a patient might need to increase muscle mass and decrease lipid levels at the same time. Diet and exercise can be effective interventions and resulted in 11% decrease in cholesterol levels in one study [92] and 18% decrease in total cholesterol levels as well as 25% decrease in triglyceride levels in another study [93]. Smoking cessation, aggressive management of DM, reduction in carbohydrate and alcohol intake, and replacement of saturated fat with monounsaturated fat or omega-3 polyunsaturated fats are all measures that could be undertaken to reduce serum triglyceride levels [5]. Smoking cessation should be emphasized since the DAD study found a decrease in relative rate of MI in current vs. former HIV-infected smokers from 2.9 to 1.6 [10]. For patients with severe hypertriglyceridemia and hyperchylomicronemia, very low-fat diets, avoidance of simple sugars, and elimination of alcohol intake are required [5]. A diet of 2 g/day of plant stanols/sterols and 10–25 g/day of viscous (soluble) fiber and reduced intake of saturated fat and cholesterol, in addition to increased physical activity and weight loss, can be used to attempt initial cholesterol control [43]. In order to achieve maximal control of dyslipidemia in the HIV-infected patient while avoiding or maintaining low-dose lipid-lowering agents (thereby avoiding/minimizing drug interactions), employment of the services of a dietician should be considered. It is ultimately important to note that interventions for advanced immunosuppression, opportunistic infections, malignancies, and HIV-associated wasting should take precedence over treatment of dyslipidemia in the HIV-infected patient [5].

Lipid-Lowering Drug Therapy

(a) *HMG Co-A reductase inhibitors*: Also known as statins, this class of drugs is the recommended first-line therapy for hypercholesterolemia [5]. Statins lower non-HDL-C and LDL-C levels to the same degree [43] and demonstrate good evidence for reduction of CHD and CHD event risks [94]. Statins are also the recommended first choice for elevated non-HDL-C and LDL-C when triglyceride levels are between 200 and 500 mg/dL [5], but are not recommended as first-line therapy for isolated hypertriglyceridemia >500 mg/dL [5]. Statins can achieve a 7–30% reduction in triglyceride levels [82]. With triglyceride levels between 200 and 500 mg/dL, statins exhibit equal efficacy in lowering LDL-C as in lowering triglyceride levels [82]. However, with triglycerides >500 mg/dL, statins significantly lose their ability to lower LDL-C [82]. In this situation, a decrement in triglycerides with fibrates is more imperative to avoid pancreatitis (occurs at triglyceride levels >1,000 mg/dL), and statins may be used in combination with fibrates for LDL-C and triglyceride lowering; or used alone for non-HDL-C lowering after triglyceride levels are reasonably controlled (<500 mg/dL) [82]. The Infectious Disease Society of America recommends pravastatin and atorvastatin for treatment of HIV patients [5].

(b) *Fibric acid derivates*: Also known as fibrates, this class of drugs only modestly reduce LDL-C (5–20%) [5]. Some studies have shown that they reduce risk of CHD events in patients with high triglycerides and low HDL-C [82, 95]. This reduction in risk is mostly observed with gemfibrozil [96, 97], rather than fenofibrate [98]. In fact more recently, the ACCORD trial of diabetic participants, showed that the combination of fenofibrate and simvastatin increased HDL-C and decreased triglyceride levels, but failed to show a difference in cardiovascular event rates (during a mean follow-up period of 8 years) compared to placebo. The fibrates have been shown to reduce serum triglyceride levels by 12–40% [57, 99–101] and although controversial [100], can increase HDL-C levels by 10–14% [57, 99]. Significant results can be achieved when fibrates are used in combination with statins; however, there is concern for the development of myopathy with this combination [43]. This concern is less when fenofibrate is used with moderate dose of statins [102–104]. Also, the combination of atorvastatin and gemfibrozil was safe in very small study of <30 patients taking both atorvastatin and gemfibrozil [92]. Pravastatin and fluvastatin are the preferred statin drugs when used in combination with fibrates [5].

(c) *Other drugs*: Niacin is a favored drug for raising HDL-C and is very efficacious when used in combination with the statins for raising HDL-C and lowering LDL-C [105, 106]. It also lowers CHD risk [107, 108], but produces frequent cutaneous flushing, hepatotoxicity (rare), and insulin resistance. If the use of niacin cannot be avoided however, it is recommended that patients taking niacin should have regular evaluation of fasting glucose levels [5]. In this case, consideration should be given to conducting a standard 75 g, 2 h oral glucose tolerance test; especially in the presence of lipodystrophy and/or risk factors for type-2 DM [47, 109]. Niacin was well tolerated in HIV-infected patients with low HDL-C levels [110].

Bile acid sequestering resins (cholestyramine, colestipol, and colesevalam) are not recommended in HIV-infected patients since they are associated with hypertriglyceridemia and their effects on absorption of antiviral drugs have not been studied [5].

Ezetimibe is a cholesterol absorption inhibitor which has been shown to lower LDL-C by 17–21% [111, 112]; and is especially efficacious when used in combination with statins [113, 114]. Some studies have evaluated the safety and efficacy of ezetimibe in HIV-infected patients, and have shown the drug to be well-tolerated with good LDL-C and non-HDL-C (but not triglycerides) lowering ability. Note that despite lowering LDL-C, niacin has not yet been proven to lower the risk of CV events.

Fish oils (omega-3-fatty acid supplements) have been associated with a 15–25% reduction in plasma triglyceride levels [101, 115]. They have been shown to improve hypertriglyceridemia in patients with AIDS wasting [116], but have not been tested in patients receiving PIs.

L-Carnithine at a dosage of 3 g/day reduced serum triglyceride levels by 28% in one open-arm study [117].

An important point to make is that ART-associated dyslipidemia is typically refractory to standard lipid-lowering therapies [104, 118]. This might be related to drug interactions, noncompliance secondary to high pill burden, or the disease process itself [119]. Referral to an expert in treating lipid disorders is generally recommended in HIV-infected patients with refractory lipid disorders [5]. For these refractory cases, consideration should also be given to replacing an ART causing dyslipidemia with another less likely to induce lipid abnormalities [35]. In one study, an old PI was switched to a newer PI (atazanavir) with 33% reduction in triglyceride levels vs. 3% reduction when previous regimen was maintained [120, 121]. Switching to raltegravir-based regimen also demonstrated an increase in HDL-C with a 42% reduction in triglyceride levels, but was associated with a significant increase in viral load compared to a lopinavir-ritonavir based regimen. ART therapy changes should therefore only be made in extreme cases of treatment of refractory dyslipidemia where the benefits of controlling the lipid abnormalities are obvious and outweigh the risks of switching ART therapy.

Interactions Between Lipid-Lowering Drugs and ART in the HIV-Infected Patient

The risk of myopathy is increased in HIV-infected patients on statin therapy for multiple reasons, including the use of other myotoxic medications, e.g., zidovudine [122], the use of agents that inhibit metabolism of statins, e.g., PIs and itraconazole [123], or the HIV disease itself [124].

With the exception of pravastatin and fluvastatin, statin drugs are metabolized by oxidation via the CYP3A4 system [5]. Pravastatin is eliminated via multiple other metabolic pathways, especially glucuronidation [125], while fluvastatin inhibits and is metabolized by CYP2C9 [126] along with rosuvastatin [127, 128]. Likewise, the antiretroviral drug classes – PIs and NNRTIs – are metabolized by or affect the function of the CYP system [129, 130].

(a) *Statins and PIs*: The PIs (particularly ritonavir) potently inhibit CYP3A4 [131]. Statins do not significantly increase plasma levels of PIs [132–135], but PIs increase plasma levels of the statins metabolized via the CYP3A4 including lovastatin, simvastatin, and to a lesser extent, atorvastatin [5, 35]. In fact, rhabdomyolysis has been reported in HIV-infected patients on simvastatin and PI therapy [136, 137]. The use of lopinavir/ritonavir was associated with attenuated efficacy of rosuvastatin, but for reasons not understood, caused a 2.1- to 4.7-fold increase in the area under the plasma concentration time curve (AUC) for rosuvastatin [132]. In a small study with short follow-up period [101], rosuvastatin exhibited a relatively safe profile even when used with PIs. Also, in another small study, atorvastatin was used safely in combination with PIs, in a short follow-up period of about 5–7 months [92, 138]. More recently, an open-label randomized study showed that rosuvastatin was well tolerated and more efficacious that pravastatin in lowering triglycerides and LDL-C in HIV-1 patients treated with ritonavir-boosted ART regimen.

(b) *Statins and NNRTIs*: The NNRTIs – delavirdine and nevirapine – are substrates and inhibitors of CYP3A4 [139, 140]. Conversely, the NNRTI – efavirenz – is more of a potent inducer of CYP3A4, with little inhibitory activity [140]. Statins do not significantly increase plasma levels of efavirenz [141], but because of its inhibitory effect on the CYP3A4, delavirdine increases the concentrations of certain statins particularly lovastatin and simvastatin [5, 35]. More data are required, but it is likely that efavirenz and nevirapine can safely be used with any statin drug [5, 141]. In fact, given its inductive CYP3A4 capabilities, efavirenz may decrease the efficacy of some statins [35]. Unfortunately, there is limited data on drug–drug interactions with NNRTIs and statins [5], including rosuvastatin [119]. It should be noted, however, that the only interaction predicted between rosuvastatin and NNRTIs is a potential reduction in potency of rosuvastatin due to inductive capabilities of the NNRTIs [119].

(c) *Statins and NRTIs*: The NRTIs are metabolized via glucuronidation and phosphorylation and not via the CYP system, and as a result, have no effect on the metabolism of statins.

As a result of the nature of these interactions between statins and ART, the consensus guidelines recommend that pravastatin and fluvastatin be considered first-line agents for the control of hypercholesterolemia in HIV-infected patients [5]. Simvastatin and lovastatin should be avoided in patients taking PIs or delavirdine, while atorvastatin and rosuvastatin should be used with caution in reduced dosages to avoid rhabdomyolysis [5, 35]. Unfortunately, pravastatin and fluvastatin are low potency statins for secondary prevention of CV events, while atorvastatin and rosuvastatin are proven to be superior [119].

Because of other routes of metabolism employed, drug–drug interactions are less likely with other class of ART and other lipid-lowering agents [5]. Note that ritonavir and nelfivavir induce glucuronidation and might potentially diminish the efficacy of the fibrates which undergo conjugation by glucuronidation prior to being renally excreted [142]. Currently, data to support the use of niacin with ART are limited [119], and until more evidence is available, it is recommended that niacin be avoided as first-line therapy in HIV-infected patients who have lipodystrophy or those on PI therapy [5].

Back to the Case

Based on the patient's lipid profile (low HDL-C and high triglycerides), history of diabetes, elevated blood pressure, and abdominal obesity, he has the metabolic syndrome. For his increased abdominal obesity and borderline elevated blood pressure, strategies for weight loss and diet modification are discussed. These include brisk walking for 45 min to 1 h at least 6 days a week, increase intake of fruits and vegetables in the diet, reduce salt intake to less than 2 g/day, reduce daily caloric intake, and avoid white starchy foods. He is also referred to a dietary specialist. In the meantime, he continues glyburide and home blood sugar monitoring

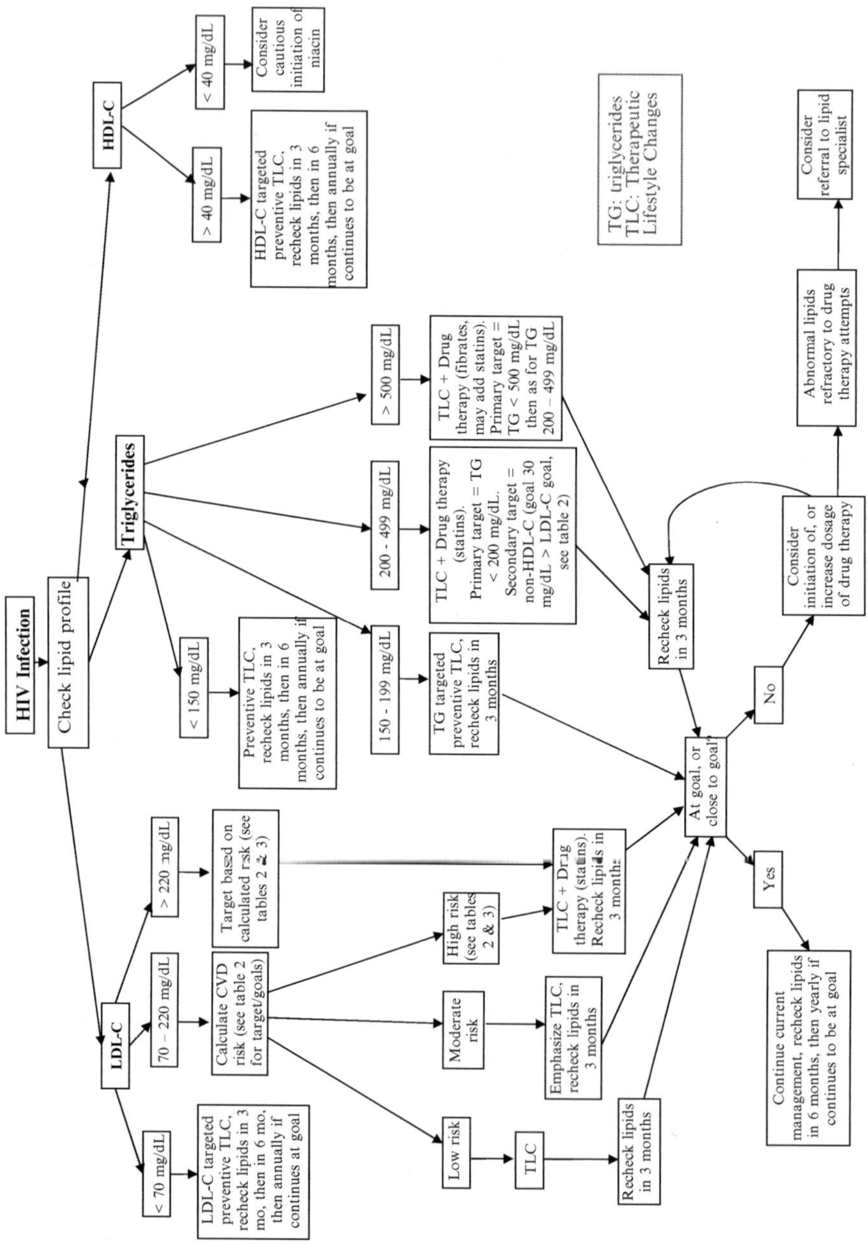
HIV Infection
Check lipid profile
HDL-C
< 40 mg/dL
Consider cautious initiation of niacin
> 40 mg/dL
HDL-C targeted preventive TLC, recheck lipids in 3 months, then in 6 months, then annually if continues to be at goal
Triglycerides
< 150 mg/dL
Preventive TLC, recheck lipids in 3 months, then in 6 months, then annually if continues to be at goal
150 - 199 mg/dL
TG targeted preventive TLC, recheck lipids in 3 months
200 - 499 mg/dL
TLC + Drug therapy (statins). Primary target = TG < 200 mg/dL. Secondary target = non-HDL-C (goal 30 mg/dL > LDL-C goal, see table 2)
> 500 mg/dL
TLC + Drug therapy (fibrates, may add statins). Primary target = TG < 500 mg/dL then as for TG 200 – 499 mg/dL
LDL-C
< 70 mg/dL
LDL-C targeted preventive TLC, recheck lipids in 3 mo, then in 6 mo, then annually if continues at goal
70 – 220 mg/dL
Calculate CVD risk (see table 2 for target/goals)
> 220 mg/dL
Target based on calculated risk (see tables 2 & 3)
High risk (see tables 2 & 3)
TLC + Drug therapy (statins). Recheck lipids in 3 months
Moderate risk
Emphasize TLC, recheck lipids in 3 months
Low risk
TLC
Recheck lipids in 3 months
Recheck lipids in 3 months
At goal, or close to goal?
No
Consider initiation of, or increase dosage of drug therapy
Abnormal lipids refractory to drug therapy attempts
Consider referral to lipid specialist
Yes
Continue current management, recheck lipids in 6 months, then yearly if continues to be at goal
TG: triglycerides
TLC: Therapeutic Lifestyle Changes

Fig. 11.1 Proposed algorithm for lipid management in HIV-infected patients. *Recommended statins:* (a) Pravastatin: starting dose: 20 mg/day; may increase to 40 mg/day. Maximum with caution: 80 mg/db. (b) Fluvastatin: starting dose: 20 mg/day; may increase to 40 mg/day. Maximum with caution: 80 mg/dc. (c) Rosuvastatin (with caution): starting dose: 5–10 mg/day; >10 mg/day not advised. (d) Atorvastatin (with caution): starting dose: 10 mg/day; may increase to 20 mg/day; >20 mg/day not advised. *Fibrates:* (a) Gemfibrozil 600 mg BID. (b) Fenofibrate, up to 200 mg daily. If LDL-C continues to be elevated, and unable to increase statin further, consider adding ezetimibe for further LDL-C reduction [35]. If triglycerides continue to be elevated despite fibrate therapy, consider adding a statin and/or fishoil [35]. Patients with elevated triglyceride levels at baseline might require a repeat measurement sooner (1–2 months) after ART initiation [5]. *Therapeutic lifestyle changes (TLC) for cholesterol lowering*: Includes reduced intakes of saturated fats and cholesterol, therapeutic dietary options to enhance LDL lowering (2 g/day of plant stanols/sterols and 10–25 g/day of viscous (soluble) fiber), weight control, and increased physical activity [82]. *TLC for triglycerides lowering (TG 200–499 mg/dL)* Smoking cessation, aggressive management of DM, reduction in carbohydrate and alcohol intake, and replacement of saturated fat with monounsaturated fat or omega-3 polyunsaturated fats [82]. *TLC for severe hypertriglyceridemia (TG > 500 mg/dL)*: Very low-fat diets, avoidance of simple sugars, and elimination of alcohol intake are required [82]

for his diabetes and is instructed to monitor and record his blood pressure measurements daily.

Based on his LDL-C, his 10-year Framingham risk for CV event is calculated to be 23%, putting him in the high-risk category requiring aggressive lipid management (see Tables 11.2 and 11.3; see also Fig. 11.1). We do not know his LDL-C, but it is likely high given elevated total cholesterol and low HDL-C. Based on the recent ADA/ACC treatment guidelines (Table 11.3), his LDL-C goal should be <100 mg/dL, since he has no known CAD, and is asymptomatic. Similarly, his non-HDL-C goal should be <130 mg/dL (currently calculated to be 264 mg/dL). However, his triglyceride level of 680 mg/dL should be the main focus of therapy at this time to prevent pancreatitis. Also, in order to avoid the risk of myopathy and since statin therapy would not be very effective for LDL-C and non-HDL-C lowering due to severely elevated serum triglyceride levels, statin therapy was not initiated at this time. He was therefore started on gemfibrozil 600 mg twice daily without statin therapy. The initial plan is for conservative management of HDL-C with exercise therapy, so niacin is not initially initiated for HDL-C lowering.

Repeat fasting laboratory data 3 months later revealed total cholesterol of 280 mg/dL, triglycerides 398 mg/dL, and HDL-C 29 mg/dL. His calculated LDL-C is now 171 mg/dL. He had been exercising and had lost 7 lbs since the last visit. His blood pressure is now 135/75 mg/dL (about the same at home). His calculated 10-year Framingham risk for CV events is now 20%, which still places him in the high-risk category. The gemfibrozil has worked somewhat to reduce his triglyceride levels which are still moderately elevated. Since pravastatin is the least likely to interact with his HIV medications (Table 11.4), pravastatin 20 mg daily for LDL-C and non-HDL-C lowering is now initiated; in addition to continued gemfibrozil therapy for continued triglyceride lowering (Fig. 11.1). As a precautionary measure against drug–drug interactions between fibrates and statins (Table 11.4), his CK levels and symptoms suggestive of myopathy are watched closely for every 3–6 months. Also, given that he already has diabetes making risk of glucose intolerance less of a concern in this situation; niacin is initiated at 500 mg daily to increase HDL-C. Laboratory data are again repeated in 3 months and now reveal HDL-C of 41 mg/dL (goal 40 mg/dL), but the rest of his lipid profile is essentially unchanged. Pravastatin is then increased to 40 mg daily lipid profile is again obtained in 3 months. Unfortunately, total cholesterol remains elevated at 273 mg/dL, triglycerides 392 mg/dL, and HDL-C 38 mg/dL, and calculated LDL-C 157 mg/dL.

The patient is now considered to have refractory dyslipidemia with hypercholesterolemia and hypertriglyceridemia likely related to lopinavir/ritonavir therapy. In addition, he continues to maintain a significantly elevated (moderate to severe) Framingham risk for cardiovascular events. A consultation is therefore initiated with lipid and infectious disease specialists and his ART regimen is consequently changed to tenofovir/emtricitabine and efavirenz. Lipid profile is again obtained 3 months later; and this time, total cholesterol is 171 mg/dL, HDL-C 42 mg/dL, triglycerides 163 mg/dL, and LDL-C 97 mg/dL. A follow-up lipid profile will be measured in 6 months, and if this continues to be at goal, annually thereafter.

Table 11.4 Drug–drug interactions with lipid lowering in the HIV-infected patient

Drug	Metabolism	Interaction/effect with ART	Use with ART	Comments
Statins				
Rosuvastatin	CYP2C9	Likely ↓ effect with PIs, but ↑ AUC	Caution with PIs	Interactions with ART mostly unknown
Fluvastatin	CYP2C9	Likely ↓ effect with PIs[a], likely ↑ AUC with delavirdine	Likely safe	
Pravastatin[b]	Mostly glucuronidation	↓ AUC, and likely ↓ effect with PIs[a]	Safe	
Atorvastatin[b]	CYP3A4	↑ AUC with PIs and delavirdine	Caution with PIs/delavirdine	
Simvastatin[b]	CYP3A4	↑↑ AUC with PIs and delavirdine	Contraindicated with PIs/ delavirdine	
Lovastatin	CYP3A4	↑↑ AUC with PIs and delavirdine	Contraindicated with PIs/ delavirdine	
Fibrates	Conjugated by glucuronidation	Likely ↑ AUC with ritonavir/nelfivavir, likely no effect with other ARTs	Relatively safe	Possible myopathy when used with statins[c]
Niacin	Conjugation	Unknown, limited data	Caution	May cause insulin resistance/ hepatotoxicity
Bile acid sequestrants	Binds with bile acids, fecally excreted	Unknown, limited data	Not recommended	May cause hypertriglceridemia
Ezetimibe	Conjugated by glucuronidation	Limited data	Likely safe based on newer data	-
Fish oils	–	Not tested in patients receiving PIs	No data, but likely safe	Improves ↑ triglycerides in AIDS wasting

AUC area under the concentration–time curve, *PI* protease inhibitor, *CYP* cytochrome P-450

[a] Likely reduced effect with ritonavir and nelfinavir, likely no interactions with other PIs

[b] 40–58% decrease in AUC when used concomitantly with efavirenz [141]

[c] Pravastatin, fluvastain, and likely rosuvastatin; are preferred statin drugs to be used with fibrates. Atorvastatin may be cautiously combined with fibrates

Conclusion

CVD is the predominant cause of mortality in the USA and most of the industrialized world, where HIV is also prevalent. In addition, it is fast becoming a major cause of mortality in developing nations where HIV is even more prevalent, and a major cause of morbidity and death. With the advent of ART, HIV-infected persons live longer, unmasking CVD and CHD as a major cause of morbidity and mortality in this population. Atherosclerosis leads to endothelial dysfunction and sets up the milieu for plaque rupture leading to CVD and CHD events. Dyslipidemia with elevated HDL-C, non-HDL-C, apoB, and triglyceride levels provides an atherogenic environment setting up the initial sequence of events that lead to cardiovascular deaths. In the HIV-infected person, dyslipidemia is caused by HIV-related factors; including the HIV disease process, HIV drug therapy, as well as the usual modifiable culprits including diet and physical inactivity. In other words, the HIV patient, by virtue of the HIV disease and its drug therapy, has an added risk of dyslipidemia and atherosclerosis when compared with the general population. This fact becomes more important as the HIV patient lives longer, making it imperative that efforts be made to control as many of the atherosclerotic factors, including dyslipidemia, as possible.

To this end, lipid profile should be obtained prior to initiation of drug therapy. Lifestyle modifications should be instituted regardless of lipid profile status. Lipid-lowering drug therapy should be initiated with caution, being mindful of the anticipated and proven drug–drug interactions between available lipid-lowering agents and ART. The patients should be monitored closely during treatment; and as a last resort (as in the case described in this chapter), a switch to a different ART regimen can be considered after consultation with the infectious disease specialist. Early involvement of a lipid expert is advised in the complicated HIV patient with refractory dyslipidemia.

As new drug therapies are instituted for HIV treatment and lipid management, it is likely that safer options will be available in the near future. Until then, caution is advised in the institution and maintenance of lipid-lowering therapy in the HIV-infected patient, while taking into account the increased risk of cardiovascular events and death in this population. Ultimately, other co-morbidities associated with high mortality in the HIV population, such as opportunistic infections, malignancies, and HIV-associated wasting, constitute a higher priority than treatment of dyslipidemia in the HIV-infected patient.

References

1. Rosamond W et al. Heart disease and stroke statistics–2007 update: a report from the American Heart Association Statistics Committee and Stroke Statistics Subcommittee. Circulation. 2007;115(5):e69–171.
2. Currier JS et al. Epidemiological evidence for cardiovascular disease in HIV-infected patients and relationship to highly active antiretroviral therapy. Circulation. 2008;118(2):e29–35.
3. Hsue PY et al. Screening and assessment of coronary heart disease in HIV-infected patients. Circulation. 2008;118(2):e41–7.

4. Friis-Moller N et al. Class of antiretroviral drugs and the risk of myocardial infarction. N Engl J Med. 2007;356(17):1723–35.
5. Dube MP et al. Guidelines for the evaluation and management of dyslipidemia in human immunodeficiency virus (HIV)-infected adults receiving antiretroviral therapy: recommendations of the HIV Medical Association of the Infectious Disease Society of America and the Adult AIDS Clinical Trials Group. Clin Infect Dis. 2003;37(5):613–27.
6. Sackoff JE et al. Causes of death among persons with AIDS in the era of highly active antiretroviral therapy: New York City. Ann Intern Med. 2006;145(6):397–406.
7. Grunfeld C et al. Contribution of metabolic and anthropometric abnormalities to cardiovascular disease risk factors. Circulation. 2008;118(2):e20–8.
8. Stein JH. Cardiovascular risks of antiretroviral therapy. N Engl J Med. 2007;356(17):1773–5.
9. Schambelan M et al. Development of appropriate coronary heart disease risk prediction models in HIV-infected patients. Circulation. 2008;118(2):e48–53.
10. Friis-Moller N et al. Cardiovascular disease risk factors in HIV patients – association with antiretroviral therapy. Results from the DAD study. AIDS. 2003;17(8):1179–93.
11. Saves M et al. Risk factors for coronary heart disease in patients treated for human immunodeficiency virus infection compared with the general population. Clin Infect Dis. 2003;37(2):292–8.
12. Klein D et al. Do protease inhibitors increase the risk for coronary heart disease in patients with HIV-1 infection? J Acquir Immune Defic Syndr. 2002;30(5):471–7.
13. Currier JS et al. Coronary heart disease in HIV-infected individuals. J Acquir Immune Defic Syndr. 2003;33(4):506–12.
14. Triant VA et al. Increased acute myocardial infarction rates and cardiovascular risk factors among patients with human immunodeficiency virus disease. J Clin Endocrinol Metab. 2007;92(7):2506–12.
15. Obel N et al. Ischemic heart disease in HIV-infected and HIV-uninfected individuals: a population-based cohort study. Clin Infect Dis. 2007;44(12):1625–31.
16. Law MG et al. The use of the Framingham equation to predict myocardial infarctions in HIV-infected patients: comparison with observed events in the D:A:D Study. HIV Med. 2006;7(4):218–30.
17. Kaplan RC et al. Ten-year predicted coronary heart disease risk in HIV-infected men and women. Clin Infect Dis. 2007;45(8):1074–81.
18. Riddler SA et al. Impact of HIV infection and HAART on serum lipids in men. JAMA. 2003;289(22):2978–82.
19. Joy T et al. Dietary fat intake and relationship to serum lipid levels in HIV-infected patients with metabolic abnormalities in the HAART era. AIDS. 2007;21(12):1591–600.
20. Orenstein JM. Replication of HIV-1 in vivo and in vitro. Ultrastruct Pathol. 2007;31(2):151–67.
21. Wolf K et al. Antiretroviral therapy reduces markers of endothelial and coagulation activation in patients infected with human immunodeficiency virus type 1. J Infect Dis. 2002;185(4):456–62.
22. Celermajer DS. Endothelial dysfunction: does it matter? Is it reversible? J Am Coll Cardiol. 1997;30(2):325–33.
23. Grinspoon SK. Metabolic syndrome and cardiovascular disease in patients with human immunodeficiency virus. Am J Med. 2005;118 Suppl 2:23S–8S.
24. Conaldi PG et al. Productive HIV-1 infection of human vascular endothelial cells requires cell proliferation and is stimulated by combined treatment with interleukin-1 beta plus tumor necrosis factor-alpha. J Med Virol. 1995;47(4):355–63.
25. Ren Z, Yao Q, Chen C. HIV-1 envelope glycoprotein 120 increases intercellular adhesion molecule-1 expression by human endothelial cells. Lab Invest. 2002;82(3):245–55.
26. Grunfeld C et al. Lipids, lipoproteins, triglyceride clearance, and cytokines in human immunodeficiency virus infection and the acquired immunodeficiency syndrome. J Clin Endocrinol Metab. 1992;74(5):1045–52.
27. Gupta SK et al. Improvement in HIV-related endothelial dysfunction using the anti-inflammatory agent salsalate: a pilot study. AIDS. 2008;22(5):653–5.

28. Friis-Moller N et al. Combination antiretroviral therapy and the risk of myocardial infarction. N Engl J Med. 2003;349(21):1993–2003.
29. El-Sadr WM et al. CD4+ count-guided interruption of antiretroviral treatment. N Engl J Med. 2006;355(22):2283–96.
30. Rickerts V et al. Incidence of myocardial infarctions in HIV-infected patients between 1983 and 1998: the Frankfurt HIV-cohort study. Eur J Med Res. 2000;5(8):329–33.
31. Holmberg SD et al. Protease inhibitors and cardiovascular outcomes in patients with HIV-1. Lancet. 2002;360(9347):1747–8.
32. Bozzette SA et al. Cardiovascular and cerebrovascular events in patients treated for human immunodeficiency virus infection. N Engl J Med. 2003;348(8):702–10.
33. David MH, Hornung R, Fichtenbaum CJ. Ischemic cardiovascular disease in persons with human immunodeficiency virus infection. Clin Infect Dis. 2002;34(1):98–102.
34. Stein JH et al. Use of human immunodeficiency virus-1 protease inhibitors is associated with atherogenic lipoprotein changes and endothelial dysfunction. Circulation. 2001;104(3): 257–62.
35. Mikhail NE. LIPID abnormalities in patients infected with human immunodeficiency virus. Endocr Pract. 2008;14(4):492–500.
36. Feingold KR et al. The hypertriglyceridemia of acquired immunodeficiency syndrome is associated with an increased prevalence of low density lipoprotein subclass pattern B. J Clin Endocrinol Metab. 1993;76(6):1423–7.
37. Chait A et al. Susceptibility of small, dense, low-density lipoproteins to oxidative modification in subjects with the atherogenic lipoprotein phenotype, pattern B. Am J Med. 1993;94(4):350–6.
38. Steinberg D et al. Beyond cholesterol. Modifications of low-density lipoprotein that increase its atherogenicity. N Engl J Med. 1989;320(14):915–24.
39. Grunfeld C et al. Circulating interferon-alpha levels and hypertriglyceridemia in the acquired immunodeficiency syndrome. Am J Med. 1991;90(2):154–62.
40. Constans J et al. Plasma lipids in HIV-infected patients: a prospective study in 95 patients. Eur J Clin Invest. 1994;24(6):416–20.
41. Shor-Posner G et al. Hypocholesterolemia is associated with immune dysfunction in early human immunodeficiency virus-1 infection. Am J Med. 1993;94(5):515–9.
42. Brunzell JD et al. Lipoprotein management in patients with cardiometabolic risk: consensus statement from the American Diabetes Association and the American College of Cardiology Foundation. Diabetes Care. 2008;31(4):811–22.
43. Grundy SM et al. Implications of recent clinical trials for the National Cholesterol Education Program Adult Treatment Panel III guidelines. Circulation. 2004;110(2):227–39.
44. Hellerstein MK et al. Increased de novo hepatic lipogenesis in human immunodeficiency virus infection. J Clin Endocrinol Metab. 1993;76(3):559–65.
45. Duprez DA, et al. Lipoprotein particle subclasses, cardiovascular disease and HIV infection. Atherosclerosis 2009;207:524–529.
46. Shlay JC et al. Long-term body composition and metabolic changes in antiretroviral naive persons randomized to protease inhibitor-, nonnucleoside reverse transcriptase inhibitor-, or protease inhibitor plus nonnucleoside reverse transcriptase inhibitor-based strategy. J Acquir Immune Defic Syndr. 2007;44(5):506–17.
47. Schambelan M et al. Management of metabolic complications associated with antiretroviral therapy for HIV-1 infection: recommendations of an International AIDS Society-USA panel. J Acquir Immune Defic Syndr. 2002;31(3):257–75.
48. Tsiodras S et al. Effects of protease inhibitors on hyperglycemia, hyperlipidemia, and lipodystrophy: a 5-year cohort study. Arch Intern Med. 2000;160(13):2050–6.
49. Fellay J et al. Prevalence of adverse events associated with potent antiretroviral treatment: Swiss HIV Cohort Study. Lancet. 2001;358(9290):1322–7.
50. Periard D et al. Atherogenic dyslipidemia in HIV-infected individuals treated with protease inhibitors. The Swiss HIV Cohort Study. Circulation. 1999;100(7):700–5.
51. Sadler BM et al. Pharmacokinetics and safety of amprenavir and ritonavir following multiple-dose, co-administration to healthy volunteers. AIDS. 2001;15(8):1009–18.

52. Sullivan AK, Nelson MR. Marked hyperlipidaemia on ritonavir therapy. AIDS. 1997;11(7): 938–9.
53. Fontas E et al. Lipid profiles in HIV-infected patients receiving combination antiretroviral therapy: are different antiretroviral drugs associated with different lipid profiles? J Infect Dis. 2004;189(6):1056–74.
54. Murphy RL et al. Dose-ranging, randomized, clinical trial of atazanavir with lamivudine and stavudine in antiretroviral-naive subjects: 48-week results. AIDS. 2003;17(18):2603–14.
55. Moyle GJ, Baldwin C. Lipid abnormalities during saquinavir soft-gel-based highly active antiretroviral therapy. J Acquir Immune Defic Syndr. 1999;21(5):423–4.
56. Petit JM et al. Increased VLDL-apoB and IDL-apoB production rates in nonlipodystrophic HIV-infected patients on a protease inhibitor-containing regimen: a stable isotope kinetic study. J Lipid Res. 2003;44(9):1692–7.
57. Badiou S et al. Decrease in LDL size in HIV-positive adults before and after lopinavir/ritonavir-containing regimen: an index of atherogenicity? Atherosclerosis. 2003;168(1):107–13.
58. van der Valk M et al. Nevirapine-containing antiretroviral therapy in HIV-1 infected patients results in an anti-atherogenic lipid profile. AIDS. 2001;15(18):2407–14.
59. van Leth F, Phanuphak P, Gazzard B, Cahn P, Wood R, Bloch M, et al. Lipid changes in a randomized comparative trial of first-line antiretroviral therapy with regimens containing either nevirapine alone, efavirenz alone or both drugs combined, together with stavudine and lamivudine (2NN Study). 10th Conference on Retroviruses and Opportunistic Infections, Boston, MA, 2003;10:abstract no. 752.
60. Shikuma CM et al. Metabolic effects of protease inhibitor-sparing antiretroviral regimens given as initial treatment of HIV-1 Infection (AIDS Clinical Trials Group Study A5095). J Acquir Immune Defic Syndr. 2007;44(5):540–50.
61. Kumar P, Rodriguez-French A, Thompson M, Tashima K, Williams V, Wannamaker P, et al. Prospective study of hyperlipidemia in ART-naive subjects taking combivir/abacavir (COM/ABC), COM/nelfinavir (NFV), or stavudine (d4T)/lamivudine (3TC)/NFV (ESS40002). 9th Conference on Retroviruses and Opportunistic Infections, Seattle, WA, 2002;9:abstract no. 33.
62. Eron Jr JJ et al. A comparison of stavudine, didanosine and indinavir with zidovudine, lamivudine and indinavir for the initial treatment of HIV-1 infected individuals: selection of thymidine analog regimen therapy (START II). AIDS. 2000;14(11):1601–10.
63. Gallant JE et al. Efficacy and safety of tenofovir DF vs stavudine in combination therapy in antiretroviral-naive patients: a 3-year randomized trial. JAMA. 2004;292(2):191–201.
64. Duong M et al. Concentration of circulating oxidized LDL in HIV-infected patients treated with antiretroviral agents: relation to HIV-related lipodystrophy. HIV Clin Trials. 2006;7(2): 41–7.
65. Grinspoon S, Carr A. Cardiovascular risk and body-fat abnormalities in HIV-infected adults. N Engl J Med. 2005;352(1):48–62.
66. Carr A et al. A syndrome of lipoatrophy, lactic acidaemia and liver dysfunction associated with HIV nucleoside analogue therapy: contribution to protease inhibitor-related lipodystrophy syndrome. AIDS. 2000;14(3):F25–32.
67. Carr A et al. A syndrome of peripheral lipodystrophy, hyperlipidaemia and insulin resistance in patients receiving HIV protease inhibitors. AIDS. 1998;12(7):F51–8.
68. Carr A et al. No effect of rosiglitazone for treatment of HIV-1 lipoatrophy: randomised, double-blind, placebo-controlled trial. Lancet. 2004;363(9407):429–38.
69. Sutinen J et al. Rosiglitazone in the treatment of HAART-associated lipodystrophy – a randomized double-blind placebo-controlled study. Antivir Ther. 2003;8(3):199–207.
70. Hadigan C et al. Metabolic effects of rosiglitazone in HIV lipodystrophy: a randomized, controlled trial. Ann Intern Med. 2004;140(10):786–94.
71. Slama L et al. Effect of pioglitazone on HIV-1-related lipodystrophy: a randomized double-blind placebo-controlled trial (ANRS 113). Antivir Ther. 2008;13(1):67–76.
72. Sutinen J et al. Uridine supplementation for the treatment of antiretroviral therapy-associated lipoatrophy: a randomized, double-blind, placebo-controlled trial. Antivir Ther. 2007;12(1): 97–105.

73. Mallon PW et al. Effect of pravastatin on body composition and markers of cardiovascular disease in HIV-infected men – a randomized, placebo-controlled study. AIDS. 2006;20(7): 1003–10.
74. Macallan DC et al. Treatment of altered body composition in HIV-associated lipodystrophy: comparison of rosiglitazone, pravastatin, and recombinant human growth hormone. HIV Clin Trials. 2008;9(4):254–68.
75. Hadigan C, Rabe J, Grinspoon S. Sustained benefits of metformin therapy on markers of cardiovascular risk in human immunodeficiency virus-infected patients with fat redistribution and insulin resistance. J Clin Endocrinol Metab. 2002;87(10):4611–5.
76. Kohli R et al. A randomized placebo-controlled trial of metformin for the treatment of HIV lipodystrophy. HIV Med. 2007;8(7):420–6.
77. Koutkia P et al. Growth hormone-releasing hormone in HIV-infected men with lipodystrophy: a randomized controlled trial. JAMA. 2004;292(2):210–8.
78. Falutz J et al. Metabolic effects of a growth hormone-releasing factor in patients with HIV. N Engl J Med. 2007;357(23):2359–70.
79. Grunfeld C et al. Recombinant human growth hormone to treat HIV-associated adipose redistribution syndrome: 12 week induction and 24-week maintenance therapy. J Acquir Immune Defic Syndr. 2007;45(3):286–97.
80. Engelson ES et al. Effect of recombinant human growth hormone in the treatment of visceral fat accumulation in HIV infection. J Acquir Immune Defic Syndr. 2002;30(4):379–91.
81. Lo JC et al. The effects of recombinant human growth hormone on body composition and glucose metabolism in HIV-infected patients with fat accumulation. J Clin Endocrinol Metab. 2001;86(8):3480–7.
82. Executive Summary of the Third Report of the National Cholesterol Education Program (NCEP) Expert Panel on Detection, Evaluation, and Treatment of High Blood Cholesterol in Adults (Adult Treatment Panel III). JAMA 2001;285(19):2486–97.
83. Pischon T et al. Non-high-density lipoprotein cholesterol and apolipoprotein B in the prediction of coronary heart disease in men. Circulation. 2005;112(22):3375–83.
84. Sniderman AD. Apolipoprotein B versus non-high-density lipoprotein cholesterol: and the winner is. Circulation. 2005;112(22):3366–7.
85. Walldius G et al. The apoB/apoA-I ratio is better than the cholesterol ratios to estimate the balance between plasma proatherogenic and antiatherogenic lipoproteins and to predict coronary risk. Clin Chem Lab Med. 2004;42(12):1355–63.
86. Dean BB et al. Can change in high-density lipoprotein cholesterol levels reduce cardiovascular risk? Am Heart J. 2004;147(6):966–76.
87. Barter PJ et al. Effects of torcetrapib in patients at high risk for coronary events. N Engl J Med. 2007;357(21):2109–22.
88. U.S. Department of Health and Human Services: NIH News; Released Thursday, May 26, 2011.
89. Frost PH et al. Serum lipids and incidence of coronary heart disease. Findings from the Systolic Hypertension in the Elderly Program (SHEP). Circulation. 1996;94(10):2381–8.
90. Cui Y et al. Non-high-density lipoprotein cholesterol level as a predictor of cardiovascular disease mortality. Arch Intern Med. 2001;161(11):1413–9.
91. Pao V, Lee GA, Grunfeld C. HIV therapy, metabolic syndrome, and cardiovascular risk. Curr Atheroscler Rep. 2008;10(1):61–70.
92. Henry K et al. Atorvastatin and gemfibrozil for protease-inhibitor-related lipid abnormalities. Lancet. 1998;352(9133):1031–2.
93. Jones SP et al. Short-term exercise training improves body composition and hyperlipidaemia in HIV-positive individuals with lipodystrophy. AIDS. 2001;15(15):2049–51.
94. Gould AL et al. Cholesterol reduction yields clinical benefit: impact of statin trials. Circulation. 1998;97(10):946–52.
95. Rubins HB. Triglycerides and coronary heart disease: implications of recent clinical trials. J Cardiovasc Risk. 2000;7(5):339–45.
96. Rubins HB et al. Gemfibrozil for the secondary prevention of coronary heart disease in men with low levels of high-density lipoprotein cholesterol. Veterans Affairs High-Density

Lipoprotein Cholesterol Intervention Trial Study Group. N Engl J Med. 1999;341(6): 410–8.
97. Manninen V et al. Joint effects of serum triglyceride and LDL cholesterol and HDL cholesterol concentrations on coronary heart disease risk in the Helsinki Heart Study. Implications for treatment. Circulation. 1992;85(1):37–45.
98. The ACCORD investigators. Effects of combination lipid therapy in type 2 diabetes mellitus. N Engl J Med 2010;362(17):1563–74.
99. Martinez E et al. Effects of metformin or gemfibrozil on the lipodystrophy of HIV-infected patients receiving protease inhibitors. Antivir Ther. 2003;8(5):403–10.
100. Neumann T et al. Atherosclerosis in HIV-positive patients. Z Kardiol. 2002;91(11):879–88.
101. Calza L et al. Rosuvastatin for the treatment of hyperlipidaemia in HIV-infected patients receiving protease inhibitors: a pilot study. AIDS. 2005;19(10):1103–5.
102. Pan WJ et al. Lack of a clinically significant pharmacokinetic interaction between fenofibrate and pravastatin in healthy volunteers. J Clin Pharmacol. 2000;40(3):316–23.
103. Prueksaritanont T et al. Effects of fibrates on metabolism of statins in human hepatocytes. Drug Metab Dispos. 2002;30(11):1280–7.
104. Aberg J, Zackin R, Evans S, Yang Y, Alston B, Henry K, et al. A prospective, multicenter, randomized trial comparing the efficacy and safety of fenofibrate versus pravastatin in HIV-infected subjects with lipid abnormalities: ACTG 5087. Int Conf AIDS 2002;14:abstract no. LbPeB901.
105. Brown BG et al. Simvastatin and niacin, antioxidant vitamins, or the combination for the prevention of coronary disease. N Engl J Med. 2001;345(22):1583–92.
106. Bays HE et al. Comparison of once-daily, niacin extended-release/lovastatin with standard doses of atorvastatin and simvastatin (the ADvicor Versus Other Cholesterol-Modulating Agents Trial Evaluation [ADVOCATE]). Am J Cardiol. 2003;91(6):667–72.
107. Clofibrate and niacin in coronary heart disease. JAMA 1975;231(4):360–81.
108. Canner PL et al. Fifteen year mortality in Coronary Drug Project patients: long-term benefit with niacin. J Am Coll Cardiol. 1986;8(6):1245–55.
109. Dube MP. Disorders of glucose metabolism in patients infected with human immunodeficiency virus. Clin Infect Dis. 2000;31(6):1467–75.
110. Fessel WJ, Follansbee SE, Rego J. High-density lipoprotein cholesterol is low in HIV-infected patients with lipodystrophic fat expansions: implications for pathogenesis of fat redistribution. AIDS. 2002;16(13):1785–9.
111. Dujovne CA et al. Efficacy and safety of a potent new selective cholesterol absorption inhibitor, ezetimibe, in patients with primary hypercholesterolemia. Am J Cardiol. 2002;90(10): 1092–7.
112. Gagne C et al. Efficacy and safety of ezetimibe added to ongoing statin therapy for treatment of patients with primary hypercholesterolemia. Am J Cardiol. 2002;90(10):1084–91.
113. Wohl DA, et al. Ezetimibe alone reduces low-density lipoprotein cholesterol in HIV-infected patients receiving combination antiretroviral therapy. Clin Infect Dis. 2008;47(8):1105.
114. Chow D, et al. Short-term ezetimibe is well tolerated and effective in combination with statin therapy to treat elevated LDL cholesterol in HIV-infected patients. AIDS. 2009;23 (16):2133.
115. Wohl DA et al. Randomized study of the safety and efficacy of fish oil (omega-3 fatty acid) supplementation with dietary and exercise counseling for the treatment of antiretroviral therapy-associated hypertriglyceridemia. Clin Infect Dis. 2005;41(10):1498–504.
116. Hellerstein MK et al. Effects of dietary n-3 fatty acid supplementation in men with weight loss associated with the acquired immune deficiency syndrome: relation to indices of cytokine production. J Acquir Immune Defic Syndr Hum Retrovirol. 1996;11(3):258–70.
117. Loignon M, Toma E. L-Carnitine for the treatment of highly active antiretroviral therapy-related hypertriglyceridemia in HIV-infected adults. AIDS. 2001;15(9):1194–5.
118. Johns KW, Bennett MT, Bondy GP. Are HIV positive patients resistant to statin therapy? Lipids Health Dis. 2007;6:27.
119. Bain AM et al. A multimodal, evidence-based approach to achieve lipid targets in the treatment of antiretroviral-associated dyslipidemia: case report and review of the literature. Pharmacotherapy. 2008;28(7):932–8.

120. Martinez E et al. Risk of metabolic abnormalities in patients infected with HIV receiving antiretroviral therapy that contains lopinavir-ritonavir. Clin Infect Dis. 2004;38(7):1017–23.
121. Eron JJ et al. Switch to a raltegravir-based regimen versus continuation of a lopinavirritonavir-based regimen in stable HIV-infected patients with suppressed viraemia (SWITCHMRK 1 and 2): two multicentre, double-blind, randomised controlled trials. Lancet. 2010; 375(9712):396.
122. Dalakas MC et al. Mitochondrial myopathy caused by long-term zidovudine therapy. N Engl J Med. 1990;322(16):1098–105.
123. Neuvonen PJ, Jalava KM. Itraconazole drastically increases plasma concentrations of lovastatin and lovastatin acid. Clin Pharmacol Ther. 1996;60(1):54–61.
124. Dalakas MC. Retroviruses and inflammatory myopathies in humans and primates. Baillières Clin Neurol. 1993;2(3):659–91.
125. Everett DW et al. Biotransformation of pravastatin sodium in humans. Drug Metab Dispos. 1991;19(4):740–8.
126. Transon C et al. In vivo inhibition profile of cytochrome P450TB (CYP2C9) by (+/−)-fluvastatin. Clin Pharmacol Ther. 1995;58(4):412–7.
127. Pasha MK et al. Analysis of five HMG-CoA reductase inhibitors – atorvastatin, lovastatin, pravastatin, rosuvastatin and simvastatin: pharmacological, pharmacokinetic and analytical overview and development of a new method for use in pharmaceutical formulations analysis and in vitro metabolism studies. Biomed Chromatogr. 2006;20(3):282–93.
128. Fujino H et al. Metabolic properties of the acid and lactone forms of HMG-CoA reductase inhibitors. Xenobiotica. 2004;34(11–12):961–71.
129. Smith PF, DiCenzo R, Morse GD. Clinical pharmacokinetics of non-nucleoside reverse transcriptase inhibitors. Clin Pharmacokinet. 2001;40(12):893–905.
130. Flexner C. HIV-protease inhibitors. N Engl J Med. 1998;338(18):1281–92.
131. Hsu A, Granneman GR, Bertz RJ. Ritonavir. Clinical pharmacokinetics and interactions with other anti-HIV agents. Clin Pharmacokinet. 1998;35(4):275–91.
132. Kiser JJ et al. Drug/Drug interaction between lopinavir/ritonavir and rosuvastatin in healthy volunteers. J Acquir Immune Defic Syndr. 2008;47(5):570–8.
133. Fichtenbaum CJ et al. Pharmacokinetic interactions between protease inhibitors and statins in HIV seronegative volunteers: ACTG Study A5047. AIDS. 2002;16(4):569–77.
134. Hsyu PH et al. Pharmacokinetic interactions between nelfinavir and 3-hydroxy-3-methylglutaryl coenzyme A reductase inhibitors atorvastatin and simvastatin. Antimicrob Agents Chemother. 2001;45(12):3445–50.
135. Aberg JA et al. Pharmacokinetic interaction between nelfinavir and pravastatin in HIV-seronegative volunteers: ACTG Study A5108. AIDS. 2006;20(5):725–9
136. Neuvonen PJ, Kantola T, Kivisto KT. Simvastatin but not pravastatin is very susceptible to interaction with the CYP3A4 inhibitor itraconazole. Clin Pharmacol Ther. 1998;63(3):332–41.
137. Aboulafia DM, Johnston R. Simvastatin-induced rhabdomyolysis in an HIV-infected patient with coronary artery disease. AIDS Patient Care STDs. 2000;14(1):13–8.
138. Aslangul E et al. Rosuvastatin versus pravastatin in dyslipidemic HIV-1 infected patients receiving protease inhibitors: a randomized trial. AIDS. 2010;24:77–83.
139. Erickson DA et al. Characterization of the in vitro biotransformation of the HIV-1 reverse transcriptase inhibitor nevirapine by human hepatic cytochromes P-450. Drug Metab Dispos. 1999;27(12):1488–95.
140. von Moltke LL et al. Inhibition of human cytochrome P450 isoforms by nonnucleoside reverse transcriptase inhibitors. J Clin Pharmacol. 2001;41(1):85–91.
141. Gerber JG et al. Effect of efavirenz on the pharmacokinetics of simvastatin, atorvastatin, and pravastatin: results of AIDS Clinical Trials Group 5108 Study. J Acquir Immune Defic Syndr. 2005;39(3):307–12.
142. Adkins JC, Faulds D. Micronised fenofibrate: a review of its pharmacodynamic properties and clinical efficacy in the management of dyslipidaemia. Drugs. 1997;54(4):615–33.

Chapter 12
Treatment of Dyslipidemia in Patients with Renal Insufficiency and End-Stage Renal Disease

Matthew J. Sorrentino

Keywords Chronic kidney disease • Microalbuminuria • Proteinuria • Nephrotic syndrome • Statins

Case Report

A 54-year-old African American male patient comes to the office for a preoperative assessment prior to the placement of an A-V fistula for hemodialysis. He was recently diagnosed with end-stage renal disease and started on hemodialysis through a temporary catheter. He has a long standing history of hypertension which has been poorly controlled due in part to lack of compliance with medications because of side effects. In the office, he has no complaints except for fatigue and pain in his legs when he walks. He has no chest pain. There is no history of prior cardiac disease or diabetes.

His physical exam is notable for a blood pressure of 150/100 mmHg, pulse 64 bpm, and weight 140 pounds. He has no xanthelasmas. He has a dynamic precordium with a prominent fourth heart sound. On neck exam, he has a left carotid bruit. His pedal pulses are diminished bilaterally. He has no edema.

His laboratories are notable for a total cholesterol of 170 mg/dL, high-density lipoprotein cholesterol (HDL-C) 28 mg/dL, triglycerides of 340 mg/dL, and a calculated low-density lipoprotein cholesterol (LDL-C) of 74 mg/dL. His liver enzymes are normal.

What is the role of lipid-lowering therapy in this patient with end-stage renal disease?

M.J. Sorrentino (✉)
Department of Medicine, Section of Cardiology,
University of Chicago Pritzker School of Medicine, Chicago, IL 60637, USA
e-mail: msorrent@medicine.bsd.uchicago.edu

M.J. Sorrentino (ed.), *Hyperlipidemia in Primary Care: A Practical Guide to Risk Reduction*, Current Clinical Practice, DOI 10.1007/978-1-60327-502-6_12,

Introduction

Twenty million Americans have chronic kidney disease (CKD) representing over 10% of the total adult population, and nearly 500,000 people have end-stage renal disease requiring dialysis [1]. Patients with CKD are at high risk of developing heart disease. Most CKD patients will die from a cardiovascular event long before they will require dialysis. An elevated serum creatinine is a potent independent risk factor for all-cause mortality and cardiovascular disease (CVD) [2]. The presence of proteinuria, including microalbuminuria, is a recognized risk factor for cardiovascular events. The National Kidney Foundation Task Force on Cardiovascular Disease in Chronic Renal Disease recommended that patients with CKD be placed into the high-risk category for CVD [3]. CKD patients would therefore be considered as having coronary heart disease risk equivalent disease by the National Cholesterol Education Program (NCEP) criteria. The 10-year risk of a cardiovascular event in patients with CKD would be similar to individuals who already have documented heart disease or have had a previous myocardial infarction.

Cardiovascular Risk Factors in CKD

CKD patients have a high prevalence of cardiovascular risk factors. Many of these factors, such as hypertension and diabetes, have deleterious effects on the kidney as well as increasing the risk for the development of CVD. In addition, CKD patients tend to accumulate a large number of nontraditional risk factors that may increase the CVD risk conferred by the traditional risk factors (Table 12.1).

Table 12.1 Traditional and nontraditional cardiovascular risk factors associated with chronic kidney disease (modified from [5])

Traditional risk factors
Older age and male sex
Hypertension
Diabetes mellitus
Increased LDL-C and low HDL-C
Tobacco smoking
Sedentary lifestyle
Family history of cardiovascular disease
Left ventricular hypertrophy
Nontraditional risk factors
Abnormal lipoproteins, small dense LDL-C, increased lipoprotein(a)
Increased inflammation (C-reactive protein)
Hyperhomocysteinemia
Albuminuria
Anemia
Increased oxidative stress
Abnormal calcium/phosphate metabolism

Older age, hypertension, diabetes mellitus, and a low HDL-C are traditional CVD risk factors that tend to cluster in patients with CKD. An increased total and LDL-C also correlate with mortality in CKD patients. Paradoxically, a low total cholesterol is strongly associated with mortality in patients with end-stage renal disease [4]. This finding may possibly be due to the increased prevalence of malnutrition in this cohort of patients.

The cardiovascular risk attributed to traditional risk factors in CKD patients is similar to the relationship described in the general population [5]. When using the risk factor algorithm based on the Framingham risk equation to calculate CVD risk, the projected risk of CVD events for individuals with CKD is similar to or at most marginally higher than when compared with reference populations from the Framingham cohort [6]. It is possible that the Framingham risk score may be insufficient to capture the full extent of CVD risk in CKD patients because nontraditional risk factors such as increased inflammation and oxidative stress are not represented by the risk score. In addition, CKD patients may have a longer and more severe exposure to risk factors such as hypertension and diabetes making these factors more potent when compared with a general population cohort. Therefore, most investigators would consider the Framingham score as a minimal risk prediction and would consider risk to be higher based on the presence of renal dysfunction, proteinuria, and the clustering of other nontraditional risk factors.

The nontraditional risk factors that are related to CVD in CKD patients may not necessarily be strong independent predictors of risk when put into a multivariate analysis. Observational studies may show an association between a risk factor and CVD but have not yet been proven to be beneficial treatment targets in randomized studies. These factors may be used to better predict long-term cardiovascular risk in a patient and can be used to consider more aggressive treatment strategies targeted at known risk factors to help lower future risk. Trials targeting treatment on novel risk factors will need to be completed before guidelines can be generated with treatment goals relating to these factors.

Risk factors can be divided into those factors known to be associated with CVD in the general population and those factors that appear to be unique to CKD patients. CKD patients have a higher prevalence of lipid abnormalities such as an increased lipoprotein(a), small dense LDL-C, and abnormal apolipoproteins. Increased markers for inflammation and oxidative stress are commonly found in CKD patients. Patients with CKD may have an increased risk for thrombosis possibly due to hyperhomocysteinemia. In addition to these general risk factors, CKD patients have an increased prevalence of renal-specific factors that have been associated with increased CVD risk including proteinuria, anemia, and abnormal calcium/phosphate metabolism.

Dyslipidemia of CKD and End-Stage Renal Disease

It is common for patients with CKD to have multiple lipoprotein abnormalities. Lipid profile patterns in CKD patients are summarized in Table 12.2. The prevalence

Table 12.2 Common lipid profiles in CKD patient with or without nephrotic proteinuria (adapted from [11])

Lipid parameter	Nephrotic range proteinuria	Minimal proteinuria
Total cholesterol	↑	↔ or ↓
LDL-C	↑	↔, ↓ or ↑
Small, dense LDL	↑	↑
HDL-C	↓	↓
Triglycerides	↑	↑
IDL-C	↑	↑
ApoA-I, ApoA-II	↓	↓

LDL low-density lipoprotein, *HDL* high-density lipoprotein, *IDL* intermediate-density lipoprotein, *ApoA* apolipoprotein A

of dyslipidemia in CKD varies with the degree of renal insufficiency [7]. HDL-C decreases and triglycerides increase as glomerular filtration rate (GFR) declines. In addition, proteinuria may have a significant impact on the lipid profile. Increased levels of total and LDL-C, increased triglycerides, and a decreased HDL-C are associated with nephrotic range proteinuria. Increased lipoprotein synthesis in the liver in response to urinary loss of proteins as well as the reduced oncotic pressure from hypoalbuminemia are thought to contribute to the hyperlipidemia of the nephrotic syndrome.

Diabetic patients have a high prevalence of lipid abnormalities and have a similar pattern to CKD patients with elevated triglycerides and low HDL-C. Elevated triglyceride levels are associated with small, dense LDL particles [8]. Small LDL particles are more easily oxidized, bind poorly to the LDL receptor, and have delayed clearance from the plasma. These properties make small, dense LDL particles more atherogenic than larger particles [9]. Therefore, patients with predominantly smaller denser LDL particles may have increased CVD risk even if the total LDL-C level is measured in the desirable range.

CKD patients frequently have elevated plasma triglycerides due to increased plasma concentrations and impaired clearance of very low-density lipoproteins (VLDLs). Low serum albumin, a common finding in nephrotic syndrome, is associated with reduced endothelial-bound lipoprotein lipase (LPL), the enzyme responsible for catabolism of triglycerides from lipoproteins [10]. Low LPL levels are associated with higher VLDL levels and higher triglycerides. In addition, in the nephrotic syndrome, there is reduced binding of VLDL to LPL as a result of dysfunctional HDL particles. High triglyceride levels, therefore, are due to low catabolism from reduced LPL levels and reduced lipoprotein binding to LPL leading to the accumulation of atherogenic VLDL remnants [11]. Insulin resistance, which is frequently associated with renal insufficiency, helps to promote increased production of VLDL particles by the liver. The clearance of chylomicrons is also impaired contributing to the increased triglycerides.

Apolipoprotein abnormalities have been described in CKD patients. Changes in apolipoproteins may precede changes in lipid levels in CKD patients. Apolipoprotein (Apo)A-I and ApoA-II are the major lipoproteins associated with HDL. CKD patients tend to have reduced ApoA levels. The lower apolipoprotein levels may be due to downregulation of hepatic apolipoprotein gene expression [12] or secondary to chronic inflammation leading to lower albumin and HDL-C levels [13].

Once patients have begun dialysis, total and LDL-C levels may be normal or even below normal. HDL-C typically remains low and triglycerides remain elevated. In addition, hemodialysis patients have increased levels of lipoprotein(a) and oxidized LDL [14]. This suggests that even though the LDL-C level is low, the smaller denser particles may have a higher atherogenic potential. The prevalence of dyslipidemia in peritoneal dialysis patients is somewhat different from hemodialysis. Total and LDL-C tend to be higher and lipoprotein(a) levels are markedly higher in peritoneal dialysis subjects than in the hemodialysis population.

Proteinuria as an Additional CKD Risk Factor

Microalbuminuria is defined as an albumin excretion of 30–300 mg/day and overt proteinuria is albuminuria above 300 mg/day. The albumin:creatinine ratio (ACR) assessed in a spot urine specimens is an easy and quick method to screen for microalbuminuria. The definitions of proteinuria are listed in Table 12.3. Proteinuria is common in CKD patients and population studies have shown that 29% of diabetics and 16% of hypertensive patients have microalbuminuria [15].

Proteinuria is a recognized risk factor for cardiovascular outcomes. The presence of proteinuria was associated with adverse outcomes in the Framingham cohort [16]. In diabetic patients, microalbuminuria is an independent risk factor for CVD events [5]. Proteinuria is a risk factor for CVD events in nondiabetics as well. An increased mortality was associated with microalbuminuria in a population study in Norway of healthy hypertensive individuals but no diabetes with an increased risk of mortality of 7.0% in men and 6.3% in women [17]. In the Losartan Intervention

Table 12.3 Definitions of proteinuria [5]

Urine collection method	Normal	Microalbuminuria	Albuminuria or clinical proteinuria
Total protein			
24-h Excretion	<300 mg/day	NA	≥300 mg/day
Spot urine dipstick	<30 mg/dL	NA	≥30 mg/dL
Spot urine protein-to-creatinine ratio	<200 mg/g	NA	≥200 mg/g
Albumin			
24-h Excretion	<30 mg/day	30–300 mg/day	>300 mg/day
Spot urine-specific dipstick	<3 mg/dL	>3 mg/dL	NA
Spot urine albumin-to creatinine ratio	<17 mg/g (men); <25 mg/g (women)	17–250 mg/g (men); 24–355 mg/g (women)	>250 mg/g (men); >355 mg/g (women)

NA not applicable

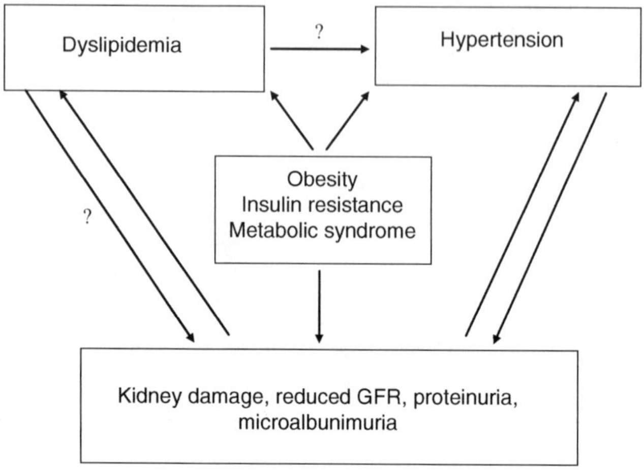

Fig. 12.1 Relationship among dyslipidemia, hypertension, metabolic syndrome, and kidney disease (adapted from [25])

for End-point Reduction (LIFE) study, albuminuria was independently related to LVH [18] and increased CVD morbidity and mortality [19]. Healthy cohort studies have shown a relationship between increasing urinary albumin concentration and mortality after adjustment for other CVD risk factors [20]. Patients with known CVD have also been shown to have increased CVD risk with the presence of albuminuria. The Heart Outcomes Prevention Evaluation (HOPE) study showed that any degree of albuminuria was a risk factor for CVD events in individuals with or without diabetes [21].

There are a number of explanations why proteinuria may be linked with an increased CVD risk. Albuminuria may indicate progressive kidney disease leading to worsening hypertension and dyslipidemia increasing the impact of these risk factors on the cardiovascular system (Fig. 12.1). In addition, proteinuria may be a marker for the severity and duration of risk factors indicating a higher-risk population. Proteinuria may be a surrogate marker for endothelial dysfunction in the kidney and systemic circulation. Proteinuria has been associated with endothelial dysfunction in clinically healthy subjects by impaired flow-mediated dilatation of the brachial artery [22]. Finally, albuminuria may indicate the presence of chronic inflammation.

How to Use Proteinuria as a Risk Marker

Proteinuria, both microalbuminuria and overt albuminuria, can be used with other nontraditional risk factors to help modify the risk assessment for an individual patient. The presence of one or more nontraditional risk factors may indicate a risk level that is higher than predicted by traditional risk factor assessment such as from the Framingham risk algorithm. Although estimates of risk from traditional risk factors have been shown to predict the majority of the risk, additional factors may raise an individual higher in their risk category or into a higher category, e.g., from intermediate to high 10-year risk. The presence of these factors may help to decide treatment goals such as more aggressive treatment targets for LDL-C and blood pressure.

Progression of Renal Disease

The risk factors associated with CKD not only increase the risk for cardiovascular events but also lead to the progression of renal disease. In the Physician's Health study, a low HDL-C and an increased non-HDL-C was associated with reduced kidney function [23]. CVD risk factors cause both vascular injury and direct damage to the kidney glomeruli and tubules. The presence of microalbuminuria represents some degree of glomerular vascular injury. Microalbuminuria is commonly associated with the metabolic syndrome suggesting that the clustering of factors seen in the metabolic syndrome may have deleterious effects on the kidney. As kidney function declines, there is a reduced clearance in a variety of proteins and nitrogenous byproducts that can cause injury to the vascular system [24]. Ongoing kidney dysfunction can raise blood pressure and promote the development of insulin resistance and dyslipidemia leading to further vascular injury (Fig. 12.1) [25]. In this way, cardiovascular risk factors cause kidney dysfunction which leads to new and worsening vascular injury.

The dyslipidemia of CKD may cause direct kidney damage both at the glomerular and tubular level. Lipoproteins have been shown to accumulate in the glomerular mesangium. Mesangial cells can take up LDL via the scavenger receptor and form foam cells [26]. Glomerular foam cells are associated with focal segmental glomerulosclerosis [25]. Tubular epithelial cells reabsorb fatty acids, phospholipids, and cholesterol contained in the filtered proteins causing increased tubulointerstitial inflammation and foam cell formation leading to kidney tissue injury [11].

There is evidence to support the fact that high cholesterol levels are associated with a decline in renal function even in healthy individuals [23]. In addition, animal studies suggest that dyslipidemia can directly cause kidney tissue injury. Lipid-lowering medications are able to blunt renal injury in an animal model of progressive renal disease supporting the contention that lipids contribute to the renal dysfunction [27]. In another study, treatment with atorvastatin prevented glomerular changes in hypercholesterolemic rabbits [28]. Finally, treatment to raise HDL levels slowed the progression of renal disease in a rat model [29]

Dyslipidemia and the progression of renal disease have also been assessed in a number of clinical studies. An association among obesity, proteinuria, and the development of glomerulosclerosis has been noted [30]. The Helsinki Heart study, a primary prevention trial of middle-aged dyslipidemic men, showed that individuals with a higher LDL:HDL ratio had a 20% faster decline in renal function compared with individuals having a lower ratio suggesting that blood lipids and especially a low HDL may effect kidney function [31]. An increased serum total cholesterol level is an independent risk factor for the development of microalbuminuria in noninsulin-dependent diabetics [32]. Elevated triglycerides were found to be a risk factor for microalbuminuria in a study of newly diagnosed type 2 diabetic patients [33]. The Atherosclerosis

Risk in Communities (ARIC) study, a prospective observational cohort study of over 15,000 white and African American participants, also showed that elevated triglycerides were an independent risk factor for the development of end-stage renal disease over a median 16-year follow-up [34].

Some trials have suggested that lipid-lowering therapy may have a beneficial effect on kidney function. Statin therapy may reduce albuminuria [35]. Analysis of the Cholesterol and Recurrent Events (CARE) study, a secondary prevention trial of postmyocardial infarction patients comparing pravastatin vs. placebo, showed that the pravastatin group had a significantly reduced rate of decline in kidney function in individuals with more advanced kidney dysfunction (GFR < 40 mL/min) at baseline. Patients with proteinuria were more likely to benefit from statin therapy [36]. A meta-analysis of 50 trials representing over 30,000 patients, however, failed to show an improvement in GFR with statin therapy although a significant reduction in proteinuria was noted [37]. From these data, it is unclear if the reduction in proteinuria observed with statin therapy translates into a substantial benefit in the preservation of kidney function.

Lipid-Lowering Therapy in Patients with CKD

Few trials have been done evaluating patients with CKD and no known CVD. The Prevention of Renal and Vascular End Stage Disease Intervention Trial (PREVENT IT) of 864 patients with microalbuminuria randomized to pravastatin 40 mg daily or placebo is the only completed prospective randomized clinical trial evaluating statin therapy in primary prevention patients with early CKD [38]. A nonsignificant 13% reduction in the primary end point of cardiovascular mortality and morbidity was seen in the pravastatin arm although the trial was statistically underpowered to prove a benefit due to the small number of observed events. A subgroup analysis of the primary prevention Air Force/Texas Coronary Atherosclerosis Prevention Study (AFCAPS/TexCAPS) comparing lovastatin to placebo in 304 individuals with and without CKD and lower than average HDL showed that the incidence of fatal and nonfatal CVD events was lower in CKD patients receiving lovastatin compared with placebo.

Meta-analyses and subgroup analyses of lipid-lowering studies in predialysis patients with CVD, however, suggest that active therapy achieves a similar benefit in CKD patients as in patients with preserved renal function. A meta-analysis of 50 trials performed to analyze the potential benefits of statins in patients with CKD found a significant reduction in all-cause mortality, cardiovascular mortality, and cardiovascular events in predialysis patients with CKD [37]. Subgroup analysis of over 1,300 patients with renal dysfunction in the Heart Protection Study, a comparison of simvastatin 40 mg vs. placebo in patients with coronary heart disease or coronary heart risk equivalent disease, showed that simvastatin was as effective at reducing the primary end point in renal impaired patients as in patients with normal renal function [39]. Analysis of the Aggressive Lipid-Lowering Initiation Abates New Cardiac Events (ALLIANCE) study, investigating atorvastatin therapy vs. usual care on CVD outcomes in patients with coronary heart disease with and without

CKD, found that atorvastatin therapy decreased CVD events with no significant difference observed between patients with and without CKD [40]. A subgroup of the Treat to New Targets (TNT) trial investigated the effect of intense lipid lowering with high-dose atorvastatin compared with low-dose atrovastatin in patients with coronary heart disease, diabetes, and mild-to-moderate CKD and showed a marked reduction in CVD events with intensive lipid lowering that was significantly greater than those treated with low-dose therapy [41]. These trials all support the treatment of lipids with LDL-directed therapy in patients with known CVD and CKD.

Data from trials done in end-stage renal disease patients have generated further questions about the role of lipid-lowering and statin therapy in particular in this cohort of high-risk patients. A study using 20 mg of atorvastatin among 1,255 patients with type 2 diabetes mellitus who were receiving hemodialysis showed a lack of benefit of the statin therapy despite a high rate of CVD events [42]. Likewise, the Rosuvastatin and Cardiovascular Events in Patients Undergoing Hemodialysis (AURORA) study investigating rosuvastatin 10 mg in 2,776 patients undergoing hemodialysis had no significant effect of the end points of death from cardiovascular causes, nonfatal myocardial infarction, or nonfatal stroke despite a significant lowering of LDL-C [43]. Sample sizes may have compromised the results of the hemodialysis trials and both trials were plagued by a large number of patients who discontinued treatment. In addition, the cause of death of patients on hemodialysis may differ from the general population and therefore these patients may not receive the same risk reduction benefit from statin therapy. About 75% of deaths due to CVD in patients undergoing hemodialysis are due to sudden death or arrhythmia: causes that may not be modified by statin therapy [44].

The National Kidney Foundation Task Force on Cardiovascular Disease in Chronic Renal Disease recommended that CKD patients should be considered high risk for the development of CVD [3]. The National Cholesterol Education Program Adult Treatment Panel III recommends that LDL-C should be the primary target of therapy for at-risk patients. Non-HDL-C (total cholesterol minus HDL-C) is a secondary lipid target for patients with fasting triglyceride levels greater than 200 mg/dL. Table 12.4 shows the LDL and non-HDL-C targets according to risk categories. CKD patients without documented CVD would have an LDL-C goal

Table 12.4 LDL-C and non-HDL-C goals according to risk categories

Risk category	LDL-C goal (mg/dL)	Non-HDL-C goal (triglycerides ≥ 200 mg/dL) (mg/dL)
Very high risk	<100 (<70 optional goal)	<130 (<100 optional goal)
High risk (CHD or CHD risk equivalent, 10-year risk >20%)	<100	<130
Moderate high risk (≥2 risk factors, 10–20% 10-year risk)	<130 (<100 optional goal)	<160 (<130 optional goal)
Moderate risk (≥2 risk factors, <10% 10-year risk)	<130	<160
Low risk (0 or 1 risk factor)	<160	<190

Adapted from NCEP ATPIII guidelines [51] and the National Heart, Lung, and Blood Institute update [52]

<100 mg/dL and non-HDL-C goal <130 mg/dL. Patients with CKD and documented CVD would be placed in the very high-risk category with an optional LDL-C goal of <70 mg/dL and non-HDL-C goal of <100 mg/dL.

Treatment

A therapeutic lifestyle program is the cornerstone of any treatment plan for the reduction of CVD events. Lifestyle changes that have been shown effective in modifying cardiovascular risk factors and reducing CVD events include reducing the intake of saturated fat and cholesterol, increasing physical activity, and weight loss if overweight or obese.

Statins are the drug of first choice to reduce LDL-C. Patients with mild-to-moderate renal insufficiency require no dose adjustments of the statin. Caution is needed with some of the statins for severe renal insufficiency (creatinine clearance <30 mL/min) [45]. Atorvastatin and pravastatin require no dose adjustment. If rosuvastatin is used, it is recommended to start with 5 mg/day and not to exceed 10 mg/day. The starting dose for simvastatin is 5 mg/day and lovastatin doses above 20 mg need to be used cautiously in patients with severe renal impairment. Fluvastatin doses above 40 mg/day have not been studied in severe renal insufficiency.

Combination therapy will need to be considered in patients when statin monotherapy cannot achieve the LDL-C goal. Intestinal agents such as bile acid resins or ezetimibe can be safely added to statin therapy for additional LDL lowering. The bile acid resin colesevelam has been shown to improve glycemic control in patients with type 2 diabetes mellitus with a mean reduction in hemoglobin A_{1c} between 0.5 and 1% compared with placebo [46]. There are no completed outcome studies showing that combination therapy with a statin and an intestinal agent can lead to further CVD risk reduction in CKD patients. When considering combination therapy, the potential benefit of further LDL lowering needs to be balanced with the potential for side effects from the medications. The patients in the very high-risk category would be the group most likely to have the greatest absolute benefit justifying combination therapy until further studies better define the groups most likely to benefit from this approach.

After the LDL-C is at goal, non-HDL-C is the secondary target of therapy. Since CKD patients typically have elevated triglycerides with a low HDL-C, the non-HDL-C will be commonly above the desired range and a target for therapy. This may require combination therapy to achieve the non-HDL-C goal. Unfortunately, few combination therapy studies have been completed, so caution will need to be used when combining medications. Three general strategies for lowering non-HDL-C can be considered: more aggressive LDL-C lowering, reducing triglyceride levels, or raising HDL-C. It has not been determined if one strategy is superior to another in reducing CVD events. The strongest data are seen with more aggressive LDL-C lowering.

More aggressive LDL-C lowering has been shown to lead to greater CVD risk reductions. The Treating to New Targets (TNT) trial evaluating low-dose atorvastatin 10 mg vs. high-dose atorvastatin 80 mg in chronic coronary heart disease patients achieved a further 22% relative risk reduction (2.2% absolute risk reduction) in cardiovascular events in the high-dose group compared with the low-dose cohort [47]. The mean LDL-C achieved in the high-dose group was 77 mg/dL. This outcome was similar in the subgroup of CKD patients. More aggressive LDL lowering may be a reasonable strategy for very high-risk patients who cannot achieve their non-HDL-C goal.

Reducing triglycerides can also lower non-HDL-C. Small, dense LDL particles may shift to larger more buoyant particles as triglycerides are reduced. A combination of lifestyle modification and pharmacological therapy is required to significantly reduce triglycerides. Dietary therapy concentrates on reducing complex carbohydrates and improving glycemic control in diabetics. A reduction or elimination of alcohol is recommended. Triglycerides can be reduced by about 35% with 3–4 g/day of a combination of the marine fish oils eicosapentaenoic acid (EPA) and docosahexaenoic acid (DHA) [48]. Gemfibrozil and fenofibrate are two available fibrates that are effective triglyceride-lowering agents. Note that fibrates may increase creatinine levels although this usually returns to baseline when the fibrate is discontinued [49]. The National Lipid Association (NLA) Safety Task Force recommends that gemfibrozil be reduced to 600 mg/day and fenofibrate reduced to 48 mg/day for individuals with a GFR from 15 to 59 mL/min/1.73 m^2. Both drugs should be avoided if the GFR is <15 mL/min/1.73 m^2.

There is one completed study using the combination of statins and fibrates that showed no additional outcome advantage to the combination of simvastatin and fenofibrate in type 2 diabetes mellitus when compared with a statin alone (Action to Control Cardiovascular Risk in Diabetes – ACCORD study) [50]. Subgroup analysis of ACCORD, however, suggested that patients with high triglyceride levels (≥204 mg/dL) and low HDL-C levels (≤34 mg/dL) may achieve a benefit although this subgroup did not reach statistical significance for benefit. In addition, there is a safety concern with a statin–fibrate combination because of the possible increase risk for muscle toxicity and rhabdomyolysis. This may be a greater concern when gemfibrozil is added to a statin. Fenofibrate is the preferred fibrate to combine with a statin because fenofibrate is metabolized by a different hepatic enzyme that does not interfere with the metabolism of statins [49]. If a fibrate is to be used with a statin, it is advised not to use the maximal statin dose to avoid toxicity.

Increasing HDL-C can also reduce non-HDL-C levels. Currently, the best drug available to raise HDL-C is niacin. There have been few outcome studies, however, that document cardiovascular risk reduction with niacin in combination with statins and limited data in CKD patients. Tolerability may limit its use for many patients. Long-term combination of statin and niacin trials are ongoing.

Should Hemodialysis Patients Receive Statins?

The two negative studies using statin therapy in patients on hemodialysis raise the question about efficacy of this treatment strategy in this patient population. Also, muscle side effect concerns are important in this group especially with some of the statins that may have increased serum levels in advanced renal insufficiency. Patients with end-stage renal disease are at significantly increased risk for a cardiovascular event. Many of these events, such as sudden cardiac death, may not be reduced by statin therapy. In hemodialysis patients with documented atherosclerotic disease, however, it is reasonable to consider lipid-lowering therapy until larger and longer-term studies indicate that this strategy would not be useful.

Back to the Case

How should the patient in the case report be treated? He has evidence for the presence of CVD with the history of claudication, decreased peripheral pulses, and a carotid bruit. He would be in the high-risk group based on the presence of peripheral vascular disease. His LDL-C is 74 mg/dL, very near the optional goal of LDL<70 mg/dL. His non-HDL-C value is 142 mg/dL. His optional goal would be a non-HDL-C of <100 mg/dL. Since he is at high risk and his non-HDL-C is not at goal, it is reasonable to consider lipid-lowering treatment. A statin would be a reasonable treatment to begin with even though the two end-stage renal failure studies failed to show a benefit in dialysis patients. Since the triglycerides are significantly elevated, a strategy to lower triglycerides is also reasonable using both dietary change and fish oils and possibly adding a fibrate.

References

1. K/DOQI clinical practice guidelines for chronic kidney disease: evaluation, classification, and stratification. Am J Kidney Dis 2002;39(2 Suppl 1):S1–266.
2. Shulman NB, Ford CE, Hall WD, et al. Prognostic value of serum creatinine and effect of treatment of hypertension on renal function. Results from the hypertension detection and follow-up program. The Hypertension Detection and Follow-up Program Cooperative Group. Hypertension. 1989;13(5 Suppl):I80–93.
3. Levey AS, Beto JA, Coronado BE, et al. Controlling the epidemic of cardiovascular disease in chronic renal disease: what do we know? What do we need to learn? Where do we go from here? National Kidney Foundation Task Force on Cardiovascular Disease. Am J Kidney Dis. 1998;32(5):853–906.
4. Iseki K, Yamazato M, Tozawa M, Takishita S. Hypocholesterolemia is a significant predictor of death in a cohort of chronic hemodialysis patients. Kidney Int. 2002;61(5):1887–93.
5. Sarnak MJ, Levey AS, Schoolwerth AC, et al. Kidney disease as a risk factor for development of cardiovascular disease: a statement from the American Heart Association Councils on Kidney in Cardiovascular Disease, High Blood Pressure Research, Clinical Cardiology, and Epidemiology and Prevention. Hypertension. 2003;42(5):1050–65.
6. Uhlig K, Levey AS, Sarnak MJ. Traditional cardiac risk factors in individuals with chronic kidney disease. Semin Dial. 2003;16(2):118–27.
7. Kasiske BL. Hyperlipidemia in patients with chronic renal disease. Am J Kidney Dis. 1998;32 (5 Suppl 3):S142–56.
8. Austin MA. Triglyceride, small, dense low-density lipoprotein, and the atherogenic lipoprotein phenotype. Curr Atheroscler Rep. 2000;2(3):200–7.
9. Roheim PS, Asztalos BF. Clinical significance of lipoprotein size and risk for coronary atherosclerosis. Clin Chem. 1995;41(1):147–52.

10. Shearer GC, Stevenson FT, Atkinson DN, Jones H, Staprans I, Kaysen GA. Hypoalbuminemia and proteinuria contribute separately to reduced lipoprotein catabolism in the nephrotic syndrome. Kidney Int. 2001;59(1):179–89.
11. Vaziri ND. Dyslipidemia of chronic renal failure: the nature, mechanisms, and potential consequences. Am J Physiol Renal Physiol. 2006;290(2):F262–72.
12. Vaziri ND, Deng G, Liang K. Hepatic HDL receptor, SR-B1 and Apo A-I expression in chronic renal failure. Nephrol Dial Transplant. 1999;14(6):1462–6.
13. Vaziri ND, Moradi H. Mechanisms of dyslipidemia of chronic renal failure. Hemodial Int. 2006;10(1):1–7.
14. Holdaas H. Preventing cardiovascular outcome in patients with renal impairment: is there a role for lipid-lowering therapy? Am J Cardiovasc Drugs. 2005;5(4):255–69.
15. Jones CA, Francis ME, Eberhardt MS, et al. Microalbuminuria in the US population: third National Health and Nutrition Examination Survey. Am J Kidney Dis. 2002;39(3):445–59.
16. Kannel WB, Stampfer MJ, Castelli WP, Verter J. The prognostic significance of proteinuria: the Framingham study. Am Heart J. 1984;108(5):1347–52.
17. Romundstad S, Holmen J, Kvenild K, Hallan H, Ellekjaer H. Microalbuminuria and all-cause mortality in 2,089 apparently healthy individuals: a 4.4-year follow-up study. The Nord-Trondelag Health Study (HUNT), Norway. Am J Kidney Dis. 2003;42(3):466–73.
18. Wachtell K, Olsen MH, Dahlof B, et al. Microalbuminuria in hypertensive patients with electrocardiographic left ventricular hypertrophy: the LIFE study. J Hypertens. 2002;20(3):405–12.
19. Wachtell K, Ibsen H, Olsen MH, et al. Albuminuria and cardiovascular risk in hypertensive patients with left ventricular hypertrophy: the LIFE study. Ann Intern Med. 2003;139(11):901–6.
20. Hillege HL, Fidler V, Diercks GF, et al. Urinary albumin excretion predicts cardiovascular and noncardiovascular mortality in general population. Circulation. 2002;106(14):1777–82.
21. Gerstein HC, Mann JF, Yi Q, et al. Albuminuria and risk of cardiovascular events, death, and heart failure in diabetic and nondiabetic individuals. JAMA. 2001;286(4):421–6.
22. Clausen P, Jensen JS, Jensen G, Borch-Johnsen K, Feldt-Rasmussen B. Elevated urinary albumin excretion is associated with impaired arterial dilatory capacity in clinically healthy subjects. Circulation. 2001;103(14):1869–74.
23. Schaeffner ES, Kurth T, Curhan GC, et al. Cholesterol and the risk of renal dysfunction in apparently healthy men. J Am Soc Nephrol. 2003;14(8):2084–91.
24. Yerkey MW, Kernis SJ, Franklin BA, Sandberg KR, McCullough PA. Renal dysfunction and acceleration of coronary disease. Heart. 2004;90(8):961–6.
25. Sahadevan M, Kasiske BL. Hyperlipidemia in kidney disease: causes and consequences. Curr Opin Nephrol Hypertens. 2002;11(3):323–9.
26. Ruan XZ, Varghese Z, Powis SH, Moorhead JF. Dysregulation of LDL receptor under the influence of inflammatory cytokines: a new pathway for foam cell formation. Kidney Int. 2001;60(5):1716–25.
27. Kasiske BL, O'Donnell MP, Cleary MP, Keane WF. Treatment of hyperlipidemia reduces glomerular injury in obese Zucker rats. Kidney Int. 1988;33(3):667–72.
28. Vazquez-Perez S, Aragoncillo P, de Las HN, et al. Atorvastatin prevents glomerulosclerosis and renal endothelial dysfunction in hypercholesterolaemic rabbits. Nephrol Dial Transplant. 2001;16 Suppl 1:40–4.
29. Vaziri ND, Liang K. ACAT inhibition reverses LCAT deficiency and improves plasma HDL in chronic renal failure. Am J Physiol Renal Physiol. 2004;287(5):F1038–43.
30. Kasiske BL, Crosson JT. Renal disease in patients with massive obesity. Arch Intern Med. 1986;146(6):1105–9.
31. Manttari M, Tiula E, Alikoski T, Manninen V. Effects of hypertension and dyslipidemia on the decline in renal function. Hypertension. 1995;26(4):670–5.
32. Gall MA, Hougaard P, Borch-Johnsen K, Parving HH. Risk factors for development of incipient and overt diabetic nephropathy in patients with non-insulin dependent diabetes mellitus: prospective, observational study. BMJ. 1997;314(7083):783–8.

33. Kohler KA, McClellan WM, Ziemer DC, Kleinbaum DG, Boring JR. Risk factors for microalbuminuria in black Americans with newly diagnosed type 2 diabetes. Am J Kidney Dis. 2000;36(5):903–13.
34. Bash LD, Astor BC, Coresh J. Risk of incident ESRD: a comprehensive look at cardiovascular risk factors and 17 years of follow-up in the Atherosclerosis Risk in Communities (ARIC) Study. Am J Kidney Dis. 2010;55(1):31–41.
35. Douglas K, O'Malley PG, Jackson JL. Meta-analysis: the effect of statins on albuminuria. Ann Intern Med. 2006;145(2):117–24.
36. Tonelli M, Moye L, Sacks FM, Cole T, Curhan GC. Effect of pravastatin on loss of renal function in people with moderate chronic renal insufficiency and cardiovascular disease. J Am Soc Nephrol. 2003;14(6):1605–13.
37. Strippoli GF, Navaneethan SD, Johnson DW, et al. Effects of statins in patients with chronic kidney disease: meta-analysis and meta-regression of randomised controlled trials. BMJ. 2008;336(7645):645–51.
38. Asselbergs FW, Diercks GF, Hillege HL, et al. Effects of fosinopril and pravastatin on cardiovascular events in subjects with microalbuminuria. Circulation. 2004;110(18):2809–16.
39. Heart Protection Study Collaborative Group. MRC/BHF Heart Protection Study of cholesterol lowering with simvastatin in 20,536 high-risk individuals: a randomised placebo-controlled trial. Lancet. 2002;360(9326):7–22.
40. Koren MJ, Davidson MH, Wilson DJ, Fayyad RS, Zuckerman A, Reed DP. Focused atorvastatin therapy in managed-care patients with coronary heart disease and CKD. Am J Kidney Dis. 2009;53(5):741–50.
41. Shepherd J, Kastelein JP, Bittner VA, et al. Intensive lipid lowering with atorvastatin in patients with coronary artery disease, diabetes, and chronic kidney disease. Mayo Clin Proc. 2008;83(8):870–9.
42. Wanner C, Krane V, Marz W, et al. Atorvastatin in patients with type 2 diabetes mellitus undergoing hemodialysis. N Engl J Med. 2005;353(3):238–48.
43. Fellstrom BC, Jardine AG, Schmieder RE, et al. Rosuvastatin and cardiovascular events in patients undergoing hemodialysis. N Engl J Med. 2009;360(14):1395–407.
44. Baigent C, Burbury K, Wheeler D. Premature cardiovascular disease in chronic renal failure. Lancet. 2000;356(9224):147–52.
45. Harper CR, Jacobson TA. Managing dyslipidemia in chronic kidney disease. J Am Coll Cardiol. 2008;51(25):2375–84.
46. Bays HE, Goldberg RB, Truitt KE, Jones MR. Colesevelam hydrochloride therapy in patients with type 2 diabetes mellitus treated with metformin: glucose and lipid effects. Arch Intern Med. 2008;168(18):1975–83.
47. LaRosa JC, Grundy SM, Waters DD, et al. Intensive lipid lowering with atorvastatin in patients with stable coronary disease. N Engl J Med. 2005;352(14):1425–35.
48. Harris WS. n-3 fatty acids and serum lipoproteins: human studies. Am J Clin Nutr. 1997;65 (5 Suppl):1645S–54.
49. Davidson MH, Armani A, McKenney JM, Jacobson TA. Safety considerations with fibrate therapy. Am J Cardiol. 2007;99(6A):3C–18.
50. ACCORD Study Group, Ginsberg HN, Elam MB, Lovato LC, Crouse 3rd JR, Leiter LA, et al. Effects of combination lipid therapy in type 2 diabetes mellitus. N Engl J Med. 2010;362(17):1563–74.
51. Third Report of the National Cholesterol Education Program (NCEP) Expert Panel on Detection, Evaluation, and Treatment of High Blood Cholesterol in Adults (Adult Treatment Panel III) final report. Circulation 2002;106(25):3143–21.
52. Grundy SM, Cleeman JI, Merz CN, et al. Implications of recent clinical trials for the National Cholesterol Education Program Adult Treatment Panel III guidelines. Circulation. 2004;110(2):227–39.

Index

M.J. Sorrentino (ed.), *Hyperlipidemia in Primary Care: A Practical Guide to Risk Reduction*, Current Clinical Practice, DOI 10.1007/978-1-60327-502-6,

N

O

P

Made in the USA
Monee, IL
13 September 2026

62976960R10133